Smart 4 Your Heart

four simple ways to
easily manage your cholesterol

Margaret Pfeiffer, MS, RD, CLS

KING
Publishing

Library of Congress Control Number: 2008904108

Includes bibliographical references and index.

ISBN 13:   978-0-9799626-2-2
ISBN 10:   0-9799626-2-5

Printed in the United States of America

To Rex and Joe

Note to Readers

This book is written to provide information to help you make informed decisions. It is not intended to replace the medical advice of your doctor. If you think you have a medical problem seek help for your particular health concerns from your personal qualified medical health professional before following any of the suggestions in this book.

Every effort has been made to make this book as accurate as possible. However content is only up to date as of the printing date and there may be unintentional mistakes as new research occurs. The author and publisher cannot be held responsible for any liability, loss or damage personal or otherwise from the use or application of the information contained in this book.

Acknowledgments

I am indebted to all of the people who made this book possible. Through the years, there have been many who have in some way contributed to the ideas in this book. Even though everyone is not listed personally, I am grateful to each of them for their insight, suggestions and encouragement. *Special thanks to the following:*

To Phyllis Haak of Computer Communiqué for book design and typography. I relied on Phyllis' expertise, attention to detail, and incredible patience with numerous changes – all while she fought a personal battle with cancer until she was no longer able to continue with the project.

To complete the design and production of the book, Tyra Baumler of Tessera Design graciously stepped in to complete the job Phyllis started.

To Kris Sobczak of Sobczak Communications for expert editing which helped to make the copy in the book more reader friendly.

To Tara Dall, M.D., who shared her passion about lipids and tirelessly mentored me in their study, along with reviewing many chapters, especially the one on advanced testing.

To Majed Abujahir, M.D., who reviewed the vitamin K and warfarin (*Coumadin*) chapter and with whom I shared many hours exploring and discussing foods and cooking. Our talks helped me with the development of the recipes.

To Sandra Plach, Ph.D., R.N., an amazing registered nurse whose friendship and expertise has guided me over the years. Thank you for finding time to read chapters and provide valuable feedback.

To Jennifer A. Ehrhardt, R.C.E.P., A.C.S.M., registered clinical exercise physiologist, for her review of the chapter on physical activity.

To Ana Weerts, M.L.I.S., R.D., for technical editing and whose many questions helped to reveal areas that needed further clarification. I always enjoy our sessions in search of the facts.

To Laurel Dauer, R.D., of Dauer Dietary Consulting, for content review of all chapters of the first draft. Early in the writing process, she convinced me that I should continue the project and provided helpful comments.

To Susan Barnhardt for tireless hours spent typing the recipes with speed and accuracy.

To Sergio Casarino, for his positive attitude and belief in this project. His optimism kept me writing.

Thank you to my family and friends who willingly and enthusiastically taste tested recipes as they were being developed, often offering helpful suggestions. To my family, Rex, Joe, Leah and Jake; Amy, Keith, Amanda, Ben and Audrey; Jay and Virginia. To my mom, Theresa for her love and support who cheerfully washed many dishes following recipe experiments. To Monika and Joe Pfeiffer who have loved and encouraged me like their own daughter.

Finally, to the many people who attended my nutrition lectures, classes, grocery store tours and cooking programs. Special thanks to those who provided ideas, asked questions, gave suggestions, read some or all of the chapters, and provided ideas and encouragement that inspired this book. While there are too many of you to name, I will be forever grateful to you. Because you kept asking if all of the class information was available in a book, I was motivated to see this project through so that you can reference it as many times as you need.

To those who have helped along the way and those who seek answers and encouragement within the pages of this book, I wish you all a happy, healthy life.

Foreword

Heart disease, unlike many other causes of death, is highly preventable. All we need to do is modify what puts us at risk as early in life as possible. It may be high blood pressure; high cholesterol; diabetes; obesity; or certain lifestyle choices, such as smoking, poor diet or lack of activity. It's important that we take responsibility for the risk factors that we can control.

Most of us live busy lives. We devote time and energy to our jobs and our families, but find it difficult to take the time to do the things that improve our health. What have you done recently to care for and nourish your body? The fact that you are reading this book suggests you are interested in doing something to care for your health. You are interested in learning more about how you can modify your diet to help reduce your chances of having a heart attack or stroke. Maybe you have a heart problem already and want to make the best choices possible to prevent another one. I commend you for taking this important step toward leading a healthier life.

Unfortunately, many of us don't care about heart disease until it affects us or someone we love. Statistics show that 25 percent of people who die from heart disease never knew they had it. Their first cardiac event was their last.

We have become a culture of convenience. We buy ready-made meals and processed food from superstores that are supplied by bulk manufacturers and suppliers who often choose the cheapest way to deliver the goods. We eat what is convenient. Unfortunately, convenient food is often unhealthy.

We exercise – if we have time – but it's not always a priority. We may have bad genes, which is something we can suspect if people in our family have suffered a heart attack or stroke at an early age (men younger than age 55 or women younger than 65). We may think there is nothing we can do. However, once risk factors have been identified, we can "trump" genetics. For some, that means taking medication for blood pressure or high cholesterol, in addition to improving their lifestyle by quitting smoking, exercising more and eating healthier.

The information in this book will be invaluable in your journey toward better health. The author, Margaret Pfeiffer, has unique expertise. A superb educator, she has taught nutrition for many years, offering high-power classes that have benefited many patients and professionals. She is one of only a small handful of dietitians in the United States who are board certified as clinical lipid specialists. Margaret obtained this certification in 2007, the first year such certification became available to nonphysicians. Her certification was earned after accumulating 3,000 clinical hours caring for heart disease patients and obtaining more than 200 hours of continuing education credits in the field of lipidology. She has successfully passed a rigorous board examination.

As an expert in the science of food, she also has an advanced understanding of the genetic disorders of cholesterol metabolism – and how to diagnose and treat these disorders. She understands the role dietary changes play, but also knows the role of medication in treating cholesterol abnormalities when diet and exercise alone fail to prevent disease. This is a unique perspective. You will find this book to be a resource not just for understanding the role of food in our health, but also the role of genetics and medication. You will find information on the latest blood tests available to better identify the genetic factors of heart disease. Some of these simple, inexpensive blood tests will be invaluable to understanding your heart disease risk.

Smart 4 Your Heart is comprehensive and sophisticated, yet easily understood by the average reader. Ultimately, you will be empowered to reduce your risk of having a heart attack or stroke.

Congratulations for taking this journey. Your life may be forever changed as a result.

Tara Dall, M.D.
Diplomate, American Board of Clinical Lipidology
Advanced Lipidology, S.C., Early Detection Center for Heart Disease & Diabetes
524 Milwaukee Street, Suite 180, Delafield, WI 53018

CONTENTS

Chapter 1   Introduction..1
Chapter 2   Four Simple Ways To Manage Your Cholesterol..................3
Chapter 3   How "Smart 4 Your Heart" Is Your Lifestyle? 7
Chapter 4   Eight Steps To Determine Your Nutritional Needs 13
Chapter 5   Cholesterol Terminology 21
Chapter 6   Lipid Profile Blood Test - Know Your Heart Numbers 25
Chapter 7   Beyond A Lipid Profile - Advanced Testing 31
Chapter 8   Picture The Risk. Heart Scan, Calcium Scores
             and Angiogram 39
Chapter 9   Metabolic Syndrome 41
Chapter 10   How To Lower Triglycerides.......................................45
Chapter 11   How To Increase HDL 47
Chapter 12   A Heart Healthy Plate..49
Chapter 13   Fat 57
Chapter 14   Saturated Fat 67
Chapter 15   Meat 69
Chapter 16   Organic Vs. Grass Fed 75
Chapter 17   Poultry..79
Chapter 18   Harmful Fat - Trans Fat 83
Chapter 19   Cholesterol In Foods 89
Chapter 20   Fish - Omega-3 (EPA and DHA) 93
Chapter 21   Fish Oil Supplements...103
Chapter 22   Flaxseed - Omega-3 (ALA).......................................113
Chapter 23   Nuts..119
Chapter 24   Soluble Fiber (Viscous) 127
Chapter 25   Psyllium, Oats and Barley 137
Chapter 26   Whole Grain 143
Chapter 27   Beans and Legumes 151
Chapter 28   Soy Foods 157
Chapter 29   Carbohydrates - Making Better Choices 163
Chapter 30   Type 2 Diabetes 177
Chapter 31   Sodium 181
Chapter 32   Blood Pressure...189
Chapter 33   Beverages (Water, Coffee, Tea, Cocoa and Alcohol) 197
Chapter 34   Vitamin K and Warfarin 203
Chapter 35   Multivitamin/Mineral Supplement 211
Chapter 36   Other Supplements 227
Chapter 37   Niacin 235
Chapter 38   Healthy Dining Out 241
Chapter 39   Physical Activity..251
Chapter 40   A Healthy Weight..263

Quiz Answers 279

THE RECIPES

Recipe Ingredients...283
Preparing A Recipe With Ease 289
Safe Cooking Temperatures..291
Vegetable Preparation 291
Menu Planning 293
7-day Menu Plan (no wheat or refined grains) 294
7-day Menu Plan (with whole grains) 296
Quick Breakfast Ideas 298
Quick Meals 299

Breakfast 303
Breads/Muffins...319
Cooking Whole Grains 325
Soup/Sandwich/Pizza 337
Vegetables 351
Salads 369
Meatless Main Dishes 383
Main Dishes 399
Fish 409
Great Snack Ideas 423
Desserts...433

Recipe Index 447
Book Index 452
Further reading and resources..456
Appendix A: Web Sites 462
Appendix B: List Of Tables 463
Appendix C: Tips and Assessments......................................464

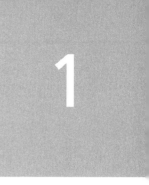

Introduction

Heart disease is the number one killer of Americans. Most major risk factors for heart disease can be controlled with lifestyle changes and/or medications.

You may already be aware of the obvious lifestyle changes that prevent heart disease: avoid smoking, be physically active, lose weight if you are overweight, and eat a healthy diet. The first three factors are self-explanatory. But the last, eating a healthy diet, is often confusing.

Do you think "fat free" or "low fat" when you hear the words, heart healthy eating? If you do, then it is time to deprogram yourself from the "FAT IS BAD" thinking. There are good fats that are important for heart health. We will explore that topic later in this book.

You may think avoiding all carbohydrates is healthy. Did you also know that carbohydrates are not all the same? There are both bad carbohydrates and good carbohydrates. You will also learn more about carbohydrate choices later in this book. Eating healthy carbohydrates and less of the bad fats and unhealthy carbohydrates is good for your heart.

Keeping your heart healthy involves more than looking at your cholesterol numbers. When you eat heart protective foods, you decrease your risk of having a heart attack even if there is very little change in cholesterol numbers. Healthy foods such as vegetables and fruits add potassium and magnesium that protect the heart. If your diet is rich in omega-3 fats from fish, you reduce inflammation and protect yourself from heart disease. Even if you need medications, a healthy diet may lower inflammation and help you maintain a healthy weight, which allows your medications to work better. Lowering your cholesterol does not guarantee you will live a longer, healthier life, but changing your diet and lifestyle will lower your risk for many other diseases related to diet and lifestyle. Did you know that more than 90 percent of the cases of Type 2 diabetes and 70 percent of the cases of colon cancer could also be prevented by eating a heart healthy diet?

Start by taking the self-assessment on Page 7 titled "How *Smart 4 Your Heart* is Your Lifestyle?" to identify your individual challenges. For more in-depth information refer to the pages listed.

Each person is different in how much they are willing to change their habits and how they respond to those changes. For some all it takes is healthy eating and lifestyle changes. For others, adding cholesterol-lowering drugs may be necessary.

I want this book to be a resource for you on your journey to a healthier heart. In the beginning of that journey, there may be chapters you skip because you are not ready for them. They may appear too complex and contain more information than you desire. That's okay. When you are ready for the next change or for more information, it will be here waiting for you.

Questions You May Have

How soon can I expect diet and lifestyle to work?

It has been my experience that you may see a change in a month, with additional changes seen two to three months later. Raising your HDL may take as long as a year. These are only general guidelines of what you can expect. Your experience may be more or less than the average response.

If diet and lifestyle can help, why is my doctor skeptical?

You may find your doctor less than enthusiastic about using diet and lifestyle to change your cholesterol.

Even though your doctor will admit that these modifications can affect your cholesterol, with all the powerful medications doctors have at their disposal it's easy to overlook the power of diet. They may not understand all the diet tools required to get the 35 percent reduction in LDL that lifestyle changes may make. For example, the American Heart Association's low-fat diet, which gives you a 7 percent drop in cholesterol, is not enough. They wonder if you will change your diet and exercise patterns enough to make a difference and how long you will stick to the changes.

If you have not had a heart event that puts you at high risk, ask your doctor to give you three to six months to try lifestyle modification. Use the self-assessment on Page 7 to determine what changes you can make. After a month, check your progress with a cholesterol blood test. Keep making changes and testing. Frequent testing will motivate you. You will see that these changes are making a difference.

If I'm on cholesterol medications, when can I stop taking them?

Your cholesterol must continue to be managed to stay at the desired goal. Talk to your physician before making any changes with your medications. Ask your doctor to work with you to see if the drugs can be reduced or modified. If you are at very high risk, have a strong family history of heart disease, or have already had a procedure such as a stent or heart bypass, your doctor will probably not want you to stop.

If you have a history of heart disease, stroke or peripheral vascular disease, the anti-inflammatory benefits of statins will be lost if the dose is reduced or stopped.

Four Simple Ways To Manage Your Cholesterol

There are four simple ways that will allow you to naturally manage your cholesterol and keep your heart healthy. Each will be discussed in greater detail throughout the book.

Number 1: Eat A Heathy Diet

Eat **whole, real, unprocessed foods** in their simplest form, with the least amount of processing to make them edible. Select foods that most closely resemble how you would find them in their natural state. Often these foods don't have labels, and if they do, the ingredient list is a short list of words you recognize as foods. Forget highly processed packaged foods listing artificial sugar substitutes, partially hydrogenated fats and high fructose corn syrup in the ingredients. If choosing foods from animals, select those fed diets they were designed to eat such as grass-fed beef, antibiotic-free chickens and wild salmon.

Eat **whole, intact grains** such as brown rice, barley, wild rice, quinoa and steel-cut oats more often than foods made from grains ground into flour.

Include **healthy fat**. A low-fat diet may lower cholesterol but may also lower the good HDL (cholesterol), raise blood fats (triglycerides), increase the number of small dense LDL cholesterol particles, and decrease insulin sensitivity. Include nuts and seeds. Eat fatty fish, low in mercury and rich in omega-3 fats, such as wild salmon, sablefish, herring, sardines and troll-caught tuna.

Eat **more plants**. You don't have to become a vegetarian, unless you choose to, but you want to eat more like one. A diet rich in whole plant foods has twice the power to lower cholesterol than simply eating low fat.

Fill half your plate with vegetables and salads. Eating vegetables lowers the risk of heart disease. Choose more dark green, leafy vegetables. Aim for a wide variety of deeply colored vegetables. The colors indicate they are rich in antioxidants which fight inflammation.

Have **fruit for dessert.** Naturally sweet, nutrient-packed fruits are the perfect way to end a meal.

Prepare your food at home. Health starts in the kitchen. Learn a few simple ways to prepare whole foods. You do not have to be a gourmet chef or spend hours in the kitchen. Fresh ingredients prepared simply are best. Involve your spouse or other family members so everyone is eating healthy foods they enjoy with less effort.

Number 2: Exercise Daily

We are meant to be active and move our bodies. Aim to be more physically active or exercise most if not all days of the week. Blood fats called triglycerides are lowered and the good cholesterol is increased with activity. Exercise seems to change the type of cholesterol the body produces from the type that builds plaque to a form that is less harmful. Blood sugars are more easily cleared from the blood when you are active. Exercise also helps to maintain a healthy weight and keeps off weight you lose.

Number 3: Maintain A Healthy Lifestyle

Eliminate causes of **inflammation**. The high-sensitivity C-reactive protein blood test (hs-CRP) measures inflammation. See Page 35 for more on this test.

Finding ways to **manage stress** is important to a healthy heart. Find what works for you. It could be listening to relaxing music or doing relaxation exercises such a yoga or tai chi. Learn how to breath deeply, meditate or use prayer to find what is effective. Each day it is important to spend some time doing something that allows escape from the usual stress we all experience.

Get **adequate sleep**. The average amount is eight hours although you may need more or less. Adjust the amount of time you sleep so that you feel refreshed and not sleepy during the day.

Drink **water** as your primary beverage. Develop a lifetime plan to achieve a healthy weight without "diets." Control blood sugar and blood pressure.

If you smoke, quit. Avoid secondhand smoke. Smoking is particularly bad for heart health. Smoking lowers your healthy HDL cholesterol. Individuals who smoke are much more likely to have a heart attack than those who do not. Smoking doubles your risk of having a stroke. Secondhand smoke also puts you at risk, even if you are a nonsmoker. If you smoke, make it your top priority to quit. Avoid situations that expose you to secondhand smoke.

NUTRITION NOTE

Exercise benefits can't be stored while you take a break. Get some most days of the week.

NUTRITION NOTE

Smoking is equivalent to adding 25 years of risk to males.

Supplement Wisely. Work with an expert in nutrition to sort out what your individual nutrient requirements are and what supplements you may need. Fish oil, soluble fiber and vitamin D are needed for most people.

Number 4: Undergo Testing To Assess Your Overall Risk Of Heart Disease

Know your cholesterol numbers and how cholesterol is carried. A simple lipid panel test may not be enough. To more clearly evaluate and differentiate your risk, consider advanced blood testing of lipoproteins that carry cholesterol. Have lipoprotein particles assessed. Check for the presence of plaque in your arteries with a heart scan. Seek the help of a lipidologist who uses a variety of testing to more accurately identify your cardiovascular risk. Have your vitamin D levels tested. Measure your waist, and check your blood pressure. Evaluate your lifestyle with the self-assessment on Page 7.

If you have a genetic disorder of lipid metabolism or already have heart disease, medications are often required along with diet, exercise, supplements and lifestyle changes to achieve desirable lipid numbers.

Testing

- Fasting Lipid Profile – to determine total cholesterol, HDL, LDL, and triglycerides (Page 25)
- Blood pressure, fasting blood sugar and waist circumference
- NMR *LipoProfile* – to assess particle size of LDL (Page 32) or Apo B (page 34). Higher levels Apo B indicates more LDL particles.
- Homocysteine – higher levels increase risk of heart attack (Page 34)
- Lp(a) – inherited risk factor. When high, increases chance for heart attack and stroke. (Page 34)
- High sensitivity C-reactive protein (hs-CRP) – to measure inflammation (Page 35)
- Calcium score heart scan – to determine amount of plaque in arteries (Page 39). Individuals with two or more risk factors (obesity, smoking, metabolic syndrome, etc.) plus a family history of heart disease would be good candidates for having a scan.
- Vitamin D – a 25(OH)D test to determine blood levels (Page 217)

Some individuals may require

- GTT glucose tolerance testing, 2-hour measurement of blood glucose
- APO E genetic testing (Page 36)
- Other tests based on your individual risks as determined by your physician, cardiologist or lipidologist.

Smart 4 Your Heart

How "Smart 4 Your Heart" Is Your Lifestyle?
(Self-Assessment)

Answer the following questions to find out how many heart healthy habits you have and which ones you need to work on.

Some questions refer you to the appropriate page to get more information if you need it.

Take this assessment again after you have worked on changing your diet to see how you have improved.

	Page	Date ___/___/___		Date ___/___/___	
1. I know how many grams of saturated fat I can have each day and stay within those guidelines 90% of the time.	P. 16	Yes ❏	No ❏	Yes ❏	No ❏
2. I choose olive, high-oleic safflower or canola oil for cooking.	P. 62	Yes ❏	No ❏	Yes ❏	No ❏
3. I eat at least 2 servings of low-mercury fatty fish (salmon, etc.) per week (but not deep-fried fish).	P. 96	Yes ❏	No ❏	Yes ❏	No ❏
4. I eat 1-2 oz. of raw or dry roasted, unsalted nuts or seeds daily.	P. 119	Yes ❏	No ❏	Yes ❏	No ❏
5. I include milled or ground flax daily.	P. 113	Yes ❏	No ❏	Yes ❏	No ❏
6. I do not use margarine that lists partially hydrogenated in the list of ingredients (choose non-hydrogenated). If butter is used, I limit my intake to stay within my allowed grams of saturated fat.	P. 85	Yes ❏	No ❏	Yes ❏	No ❏
7. I avoid foods with partially hydrogenated fats in the ingredient list.	----	Yes ❏	No ❏	Yes ❏	No ❏
8. I do not eat breaded or deep fried foods in restaurants. (trans fats)	----	Yes ❏	No ❏	Yes ❏	No ❏

			Yes	No	Yes	No
9.	I choose plant protein (veggie burger, legumes), fish and poultry more often than red meat such as beef, pork or lamb.	----	Yes ❏	No ❏	Yes ❏	No ❏
10.	If I eat meat, I use lean cuts of meat such as round and loin (ideally 100% grass-fed).	P. 75	Yes ❏	No ❏	Yes ❏	No ❏
11.	I avoid high-fat, processed deli meats, cold cuts, sausage, bacon and hot dogs and limit products even if low fat to less than once a week.	----	Yes ❏	No ❏	Yes ❏	No ❏
12.	If I eat poultry, I remove the skin.	P. 79	Yes ❏	No ❏	Yes ❏	No ❏
13.	Each week, at two or more of my main meals (dinner or supper), I have a meatless or vegetarian meal.	----	Yes ❏	No ❏	Yes ❏	No ❏
14.	I eat 2 Tbsp. or more of cooked dry beans (legumes) per day.	P. 151	Yes ❏	No ❏	Yes ❏	No ❏
15.	If I eat dairy products (milk, yogurt, ice cream), I choose nonfat, or limit amounts to stay within saturated fat allowance or choose those made from soy.	----	Yes ❏	No ❏	Yes ❏	No ❏
16.	I limit cheese to stay within my saturated fat allowance.	----	Yes ❏	No ❏	Yes ❏	No ❏
17.	My plate is 1/4 protein; 1/4 whole, intact grains; and 1/2 vegetables and salads.	P. 49	Yes ❏	No ❏	Yes ❏	No ❏
18.	I have eliminated most refined high-glycemic carbohydrates from my diet.	P. 165	Yes ❏	No ❏	Yes ❏	No ❏
19.	I eat more whole, intact grains than I do foods made from whole grains ground into flour.	P. 146	Yes ❏	No ❏	Yes ❏	No ❏
20.	If I eat cereal for breakfast, it is high fiber, low glycemic, low sugars, such as steel-cut oats.	P. 168	Yes ❏	No ❏	Yes ❏	No ❏
21.	I limit desserts and sweets to twice a week or less even if they are healthier versions. I usually eat fruit instead.	----	Yes ❏	No ❏	Yes ❏	No ❏
22.	I rarely drink soda, pop, fruit drinks, lemonades, sweetened teas, punch or other sweetened and artificially sweetened beverages.	P. 197	Yes ❏	No ❏	Yes ❏	No ❏

		Yes	No	Yes	No
23. I eat at least 2 cups of fruits and 2-1/2 cups of cooked (5 cups raw) vegetables each day (9 servings).	P. 272	❏	❏	❏	❏
24. I eat 2 servings of vegetable for each 1 serving of fruit.	----	❏	❏	❏	❏
25. I eat a good source of vitamin C daily (citrus, kiwi, strawberries, broccoli, tomato, cabbage).	P. 215	❏	❏	❏	❏
26. I eat a purple, red/blue fruit or vegetable daily. (See side bar.)	----	❏	❏	❏	❏
27. I eat dark green vegetables, especially dark, leafy greens daily (iceberg doesn't count).	----	❏	❏	❏	❏
28. I eat a deep orange or yellow fruit or vegetable daily. (see side bar)	----	❏	❏	❏	❏
29. I eat at least 4 different colors of fruits and vegetables each day.	----	❏	❏	❏	❏
30. I get 10 grams *soluble* fiber each day.	P. 132	❏	❏	❏	❏
31. I participate in physical activity for 30 minutes (to maintain weight) to 60 minutes (to lose weight) on most days of the week.	P. 251	❏	❏	❏	❏
32. I find ways to incorporate physical activity into my regular routine.	----	❏	❏	❏	❏
33. I get at least 10,000 steps daily. A pedometer is a way to keep track.	P. 253	❏	❏	❏	❏
34. I read ingredient lists and avoid foods with high fructose corn syrup.	P. 168	❏	❏	❏	❏
35. I limit foods with added sugars, natural or artificial, to a few times a week.	----	❏	❏	❏	❏
36. I limit processed and restaurant foods to keep sodium moderate. (2,300 mg sodium a day or less)	P. 249	❏	❏	❏	❏
37. I drink 6 (8-oz.) glasses of water daily.	P. 197	❏	❏	❏	❏
38. I take fish oil supplements (EPA & DHA) if not eating enough omega-3 from fish.	P. 103	❏	❏	❏	❏

NUTRITION NOTE
A serving of vegetables is:
1/2 cup cooked
    or
1 cup raw
    or
2 cups green, leafy

NUTRITION NOTE
Anthocyanins in purple, red/blue fruits and vegetables act as powerful antioxidants to help protect cells from damage and disease.

Purple, Red/ Blue Fruits:
Berries
    Blackberries
    Black currants
    Blueberries
    Elderberries
Plums
Prunes
Purple figs
Purple grapes
Raisins

Purple, Red/ Blue Vegetables:
Eggplant
Potatoes
    (Purple fleshed)
Purple asparagus
Purple (red)
    cabbage
Purple carrots
Purple (red) onion
Purple peppers
Purple heirloom
    tomatoes

Deep Orange/Yellow:
Carrots
Butternut squash
Sweet potato
Cantaloupe
Apricot
Mango

		Yes	No	Yes	No
39. I include at least 3 cups of tea daily. (5 cups preferred)	P. 200	❏	❏	❏	❏
40. If I drink alcohol, I limit my intake to one serving per day for women or two per day for men.	P. 201	❏	❏	❏	❏
41. If I eat out I make requests to increase vegetables and limit unhealthy fats and limit portions.	P. 241	❏	❏	❏	❏
42. I have had my LDL particles and vitamin D levels evaluated.	P. 31 P. 217	❏	❏	❏	❏

How did you do?

Add up the number of yes answers. If your yes answers total:

- 1-20: There are many ways you can eat heart healthier.
- 21-34: There is still room for improvement.
- 35-41: You are making many heart healthy choices.
- 42: No one is expected to have a perfect score.

Look over the self-assessment and pay close attention to the questions to which you answered "no." Do not be discouraged if there are many negative responses.

Next, select three you think you can begin to change right now. Try to make the changes you selected on most days. You do not have to do them perfectly every day. Making one or two small changes in your diet that you can consistently maintain is better than attempting to change too many things at once. Overdoing it may result in your giving up and going back to where you started. You can succeed by making small changes.

When a change seems automatic on most days, add another change to your list. Some may be easier but remember it takes at least a month before a change becomes a habit.

Track your changes by writing in the three changes you are willing to make on Page 11, then place an X in each day that you are able to make the change.

Example of 3 changes	Day 1	Day 2	Day 3	Day 4	Day 5	. . . . .	Day 30
I will not eat deep-fried foods.		X				. . . . .	x
I will wear a pedometer and try to get 5,000 steps a day.	1,000	1,100	980	1500	forgot to wear	. . . . .	5,000
I will eat a dark green or deep orange vegetable daily.	X			X	X	. . . . .	X

MY CHANGES

LIST CHANGES		DAY																													
	1	2	3	4	5	6	7	8	9	10	11	12	13	14	15	16	17	18	19	20	21	22	23	24	25	26	27	28	29	30	31
1.																															
2.																															
3.																															
4.																															
5.																															
6.																															
7.																															
8.																															
9.																															
10.																															
11.																															
12.																															
13.																															
14.																															

TABLE 3.1

The Effect Diet and Lifestyle Can Have
On LDL, HDL and Triglycerides

NUTRITION NOTE

For every 2 grams
of soluble fiber,
LDL decreased 1%.

Diet and Lifestyle Modification	Amount of Change	Effect on LDL *BAD*	Effect on HDL *Good*	Effect on Triglycerides
Saturated fat	Less than 7% of total calories	↓ 8-10%		
Soy protein	25 grams daily	↓ 3%	No effect	
Soluble fiber (viscous)	10 grams daily	↓ 5%	No effect	
Psyllium	10 gram	↓ 6-7%		
Oat bran	7 Tbsp. dry	↓ 16%	↑ 15%	
Barley	3-6 grams beta glucan (see Page 137)	↓ 6-17% LDL particle size decrese and VLDL	No change	No effect
Plant stanols	2 grams daily	↓ 6-15% LDL	No effect	No effect
Weight loss	Lose 10 pounds	↓ 5-8%	↑ HDL	
Almonds	20% of calories or (2-1/2 ounces)	↓ 7%		
Nuts	1/2-1 cup	↓ 12-13% as long as weight is not gained	No effect	No change or slight decrease
Trans fats	Any amount	↑ LDL	↓ HDL	
Carbohydrates	More than 60% of calories		↓ HDL	
Exercise	1,000-1,200 calories of exercise per week		↑ HDL	↓ for 24-48 hours after
Omega-3 fish oil	3-4 grams EPA + DHA	No change or small increase	Variable may ↑ HDL 9%	↓ 45%
Portfolio of foods (soy protein, almond, soluble fiber, phytosterols)	(See Page 56) lowered c-reactive protein 28%	↓ 35%		↓ 30%
Mediterranean diet rich in whole foods	more vegetables, fish, olive oil, grains, nuts, fruit, vegetables	↓ 11%		

Eight Steps To Determine Your Nutritional Needs

AUTHOR'S ALERT

Use this chapter if you enjoy details and want to know "how much" you can have of each nutrient.

This chapter is for those who enjoy details and want to know "how much" they can have of each nutrient. If you prefer, you may use the plate method (Page 49) instead. Use 10 grams saturated fat if you are female and 15 grams saturated fat if you are male for your daily allowance.

STEP 1: Determine your level of physical activity

We all like to think we are more active than we are. No one will see this other than you, so be honest.

Sedentary

Sedentary individuals walk less than 5,000 steps a day if using a pedometer. They have no regular physical activity other than the average, typical day-to-day activities such as routine office work; light housework such as preparing dinner, cleaning the kitchen, taking out the trash and watering plants; walking leisurely at a two-mile per hour or slower rate. You might have an occasional evening or weekend activity such as golfing, biking, swimming, ballroom dancing, or horseback riding. You are in this category if you are just starting to add physical activity but have not reached 30 minutes a day.

Moderately active

You are in this category if you walk more than 5,000 but less than 10,000 steps each day if using a pedometer. In addition to day-to-day living, you do a regular activity on most days of the week at a moderate level for at least 30 to 60 minutes. For example, walking at about three to four miles an hour is a moderate activity. You would walk one and a half to two miles in 30 minutes. Moderate activities include housework requiring more effort, such as mopping and vacuuming, gardening, mowing the lawn with a power mower that is not self-propelled, raking leaves, and shoveling snow. (See Page 255 for a list of activities.)

Active

Active people walk more than 10,000 steps each day if using a pedometer. In addition to the average day-to-day living, you do a regular activity on most days of the week that is longer (60 minutes or more) or at a greater intensity than the moderately active level. Walking at the active level means that you walk more than an hour a day at a pace greater than three to four miles per hour. It could also mean you do physical activity that is at a more intense level for less time; for example jogging 20 to 30 minutes for four to seven days of the week. Vigorous activities include jogging, walking a mile in 10 minutes or less, rope skipping, tennis, moderate cycling, aerobic dancing, surfing or chopping wood.

STEP 2: Find your daily calorie estimation needed to *maintain* your current weight (Table 4.1) or *lose* weight (Table 4.2).

Based on your gender, age, whether you want to maintain or lose weight, and your activity level from Step 1, circle the calorie level in the appropriate table. Remember, this is only an estimate of calories needed for ideal body weight.

TABLE 4.1
Average Calories To Maintain Ideal Weight

Gender	Age (Years)	Sedentary	Moderately Active	Active
Female (maintain weight)	19-25	2,000	2,200	2,400
	26-30	2,000	2,000	2,400
	31-50	1,800	2,000	2,200
	51-60	1,600	1,800	2,200
	61 +	1,600	1,800	2,000
Male (maintain weight)	19-20	2,600	2,800	3,000
	21-25	2,400	2,800	3,000
	26-30	2,400	2,600	3,000
	31-35	2,400	2,600	3,000
	36-40	2,400	2,600	2,800
	41-45	2,200	2,600	2,800
	46-50	2,200	2,400	2,800
	51-55	2,200	2,400	2,800
	56-65	2,200	2,400	2,600
	61-65	2,000	2,400	2,600
	66-70	2,000	2,200	2,600
	71-75	2,000	2,200	2,600
	76+	2,000	2,200	2,400

Smart 4 Your Heart

Table 4.2
Calories If Weight Loss Desired

Gender	Age (Years)	Sedentary	Moderately Active	Active
Female (lose weight)	19-25	1,500	1,700	1,900
	26-30	1,500	1,500	1,900
	31-50	1,300	1,500	1,700
	51-60	1,200	1,300	1,700
	61 +	1,200	1,300	1,500
Male (lose weight)	19-20	2,100	2,300	2,500
	21-25	1,900	2,300	2,500
	26-30	1,900	2,100	2,500
	31-35	1,900	2,100	2,500
	36-40	1,900	2,100	2,300
	41-45	1,700	2,100	2,300
	46-50	1,700	1,900	2,300
	51-55	1,700	1,900	2,300
	56-65	1,700	1,900	2,100
	61-65	1,500	1,900	2,100
	66-70	1,500	1,700	2,100
	71-75	1,500	1,700	2,100
	76+	1,500	1,700	1,900

SOURCE: Dietary Guidelines for Americans 2005, Department of Health and Human Services USDA Center for Nutrition Policy and Promotion. For weight loss, 500 calorie reduction but not less than 1,200 calories daily.

My Goal Is _____ Total Calories Per Day.
see page 266 to calculate more specifically for weight loss

STEP 3: Circle your saturated fat allowance

In the table below, use the calories from Step 2. Next, locate in the column below the calories, your grams of total fat, saturated fat and trans-fat.

TABLE 4.3
Saturated Fat Allowance (Grams Per Day)

Calories from Step 2	1,200	1,300	1,500	1,600	1,700	1,800	1,900	2,000	2,100	2,200
Total fat (grams) *	27-47	29-50	33-58	35-62	38-66	40-70	42-74	44-78	47-81	49-85
Saturated Fat (grams) **	9 or less	10 or less	12 or less	12 or less	13 or less	14 or less	15 or less	15 or less	16 or less	17 or less
Trans fat ***	0	0	0	0	0	0	0	0	0	0

Calories from Step 2	2,300	2,400	2,500	2,600	2,700	2,800	2,900	3,000
Total fat (grams) *	51-89	53-93	55-97	58-101	60-105	62-109	64-113	66-117
Saturated Fat (grams) **	18 or less	19 or less	19 or less	20 or less	21 or less	22 or less	22 or less	23 or less
Trans fat ***	0	0	0	0	0	0	0	0

* Total fat
20 to 35 percent of your calories from fat stated in grams.

** Saturated fat
Goal is not more than 7 percent of calories from saturated fat if you have elevated cholesterol,[2] are at risk, or being treated for heart disease.

*** Trans fats
Your desired goal is zero grams. Note that if an item contains up to a half gram (0.5) of trans fats per serving, it can state "0 grams" trans fats. Check the ingredient list for partially hydrogenated oils and eliminate those foods from your diet.

> My Goal For Total Fat _____ Grams Per Day.
> My Goal For Saturated Fat _____ Grams Per Day.
> My Goal For Trans Fats __zero__ Grams Per Day.
> **Note: Try to meet these goals at least 90 percent of the time.**

Smart 4 Your Heart

Step 4: Determine Fiber

Total Dietary Fiber

The total dietary fiber found on food labels includes both soluble fiber and insoluble fiber. As your calorie intake increases, so does your fiber recommendation. As you get older, you need fewer calories so your fiber requirements decrease.

TABLE 4.4

Adequate Intake For Fiber

MALE ADEQUATE INTAKE FOR FIBER: (30-38 GRAMS)
9-13 years old . . . . 31 grams daily
14-50 years old . . . . 38 grams daily
50 years and older . . . . 30 grams daily

FEMALE ADEQUATE INTAKE FOR FIBER: (21-26 GRAMS)
9-13 years old . . . . 26 grams daily
14-50 years old . . . . 25 grams daily
50 years and older . . . . 21 grams daily

My Total Dietary Fiber Goal Is _____ Grams Per Day.

Soluble Fiber

The government regulated food labels are not required to list soluble fiber, although some labels will choose to list it. See the table on Page 132 for the amount found in various foods. It is important to note that no animal foods have fiber. Soluble fiber, which is part of the total fiber, is the type that lowers cholesterol levels.

YOUR SOLUBLE FIBER GOAL
10 to 25 grams of soluble fiber daily to lower LDL cholesterol. If you are currently eating a low-fiber diet, start with a goal of 5 grams. See Page 129 for a plan to increase soluble fiber.
My Soluble Fiber Goal Is _____ Grams Per Day.

AUTHOR'S ALERT

Fiber guidelines are different for children than for adults. After the age of 2, the fiber guidelines are the child's age plus five. For example, a 6 year old would require 11 grams of total fiber, (6 years + 5 = 11 grams).

Step 5: Determine the Amount Of Protein

About 10 percent to 35 percent of total calories in your diet should come from protein. See the table on Page 162 for a list of foods and protein content.

TABLE 4.5
PROTEIN — HOW MUCH YOU NEED

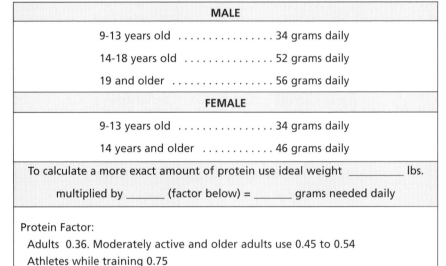

MALE		
9-13 years old . . . . 34 grams daily		
14-18 years old . . . . 52 grams daily		
19 and older . . . . 56 grams daily		
FEMALE		
9-13 years old . . . . 34 grams daily		
14 years and older . . . . 46 grams daily		
To calculate a more exact amount of protein use ideal weight _____ lbs. multiplied by _____ (factor below) = _____ grams needed daily		

Protein Factor:
  Adults 0.36. Moderately active and older adults use 0.45 to 0.54
  Athletes while training 0.75		

My Goal For Protein Is_____ Grams Per Day.

Step 6: Cholesterol From Foods

Individuals with heart disease or diabetes or those who wish to lower blood cholesterol levels, should strive for 200 mg or less per day. For healthy individuals or those who have achieved their blood cholesterol goal, 300 mg or less of cholesterol is recommended per day.

Most of your blood cholesterol comes from what your body makes – not the foods you eat – so this is less important than saturated or trans fats.

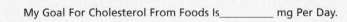

My Goal For Cholesterol From Foods Is_____ mg Per Day.

Smart 4 Your Heart

Step 7: Sodium Allowance

The daily allowance is 2,300 mg of sodium. If your blood pressure is still elevated at this level, the sodium levels may need to be lowered to 1,600 mg to 1,800 mg per day.

> My Sodium Goal Is _____ mg Per Day.

Step 8: Carbohydrates

Total Carbohydrate

Between 35 and 50 percent of your calories should come from carbohydrates. You want most of them from whole, intact grains; fruits; vegetables and legumes. Eat fewer carbohydrates from refined foods and added sugars. You will not need to count grams of carbohydrate unless you have diabetes and have been instructed to follow a carbohydrate counting plan.

Sugars

Since sugars on a food label include both added and natural sugars, it is often difficult to tell if the sugars are in the food naturally or have been added. The "added" sugars should be no more than 10 percent of total caloric intake. If you have diabetes, check total carbohydrates, not only "sugars."

OPTIONAL MY CARBOHYDRATE GOAL:
Calories from Step 2 _____ X 0.35 = _____ ÷ 4 = _____ grams/day
Or
Calories from Step 2 _____ X 0.50 = _____ ÷ 4 = _____ grams/day

Choose the lower percent of carbohydrates if you have metabolic syndrome. The more physicaly active you are the higher the percent of calories from carbohydrates can be. Do not exceed 60 percent of calories from carbohydrates.

NUTRITION NOTE

For carbohydrate counting, the amount of food that contains 15 grams of carbohydrate equals one carbohydrate choice.

NUTRITION NOTE

Carbohydrates are in:
- Fruits
- Vegetables
- Legumes
- Whole Grains
- Milk

MY DAILY ALLOWANCE

Nutrient	Recommendation	My Amount
Calories	Balance intake with calories burned to maintain a desirable weight	
Total Fat	20-35% of total calories	_____ grams
Saturated Fat	Less than 7% of calories	_____ grams
Trans Fat	None Check ingredient lists to avoid partially hydrogenated oils	Zero grams
Dietary Fiber (total)	Based on calorie intake	_____ grams
Soluble Fiber	At least 10 grams	_____ grams
Protein	10-35% of calories	_____ grams
Cholesterol	Less than 200 mg a day	_____ mg
Sodium	2,300 mg or less	_____ mg
Carbohydrates	35-50% of total calories	_____ grams

Note: If needed, seek the help of a registered dietitian or other qualified health professional to individualize your diet.

5

Cholesterol Terminology

Before you begin your journey toward a heart healthy diet, it will be helpful to become familiar with cholesterol terms and what causes a heart attack to occur.

Blood Cholesterol

Cholesterol is a soft, waxy, fatty substance called a lipid. Cholesterol is not all bad; too much may cause harm but you do need some for your body to work properly. Your body requires cholesterol to make bile to digest foods; make hormones such as estrogen and testosterone; and along with sunlight, produce vitamin D. Cholesterol is so important that the body makes most of it primarily by your liver, with a small amount coming from foods you eat. High cholesterol could be from what you eat, but more often it becomes high because your body makes more than it needs.

Saturated fat raises blood cholesterol more than eating foods high in cholesterol, which is the reason you want to limit saturated fat. A cholesterol-free food that is high in saturated fat may raise blood cholesterol. Partially hydrogenated fat or trans fats raise bad cholesterol, but unlike saturated fat, they also lower the good cholesterol. This makes trans fats even worse than saturated fat when trying to control your cholesterol.

Cholesterol in food is called dietary cholesterol and can only be found in animal foods, including meat, chicken, fish and dairy products. In a typical American diet, with large portions of meat, cheese and dairy, cholesterol intake is often excessive. Cholesterol is never found in plant foods. Even high-fat plant foods, such as avocado, peanut butter and olives, do not contain cholesterol.

Cholesterol needs to travel from your liver, through your blood, to where it is needed in the body. Since fats and water do not mix, cholesterol must be packaged as a lipoprotein, made up of fat, protein and cholesterol, to be carried in the blood, which is 90 percent water. Once packaged, cholesterol travels through the bloodstream much like beach balls bounce along in a pool of water. The lipoproteins have different names based on their composition and size. Lipoproteins come in the form of HDL, LDL, IDL, chylomicrons and VLDL. Your total cholesterol is the sum of all five of them. Triglycerides are carried predominantly by chylomicrons and VLDL. Cholesterol that is not used by cells is recycled through the intestinal tract where it is reabsorbed and recycled.

NUTRITION NOTE

Cholesterol is only found in animal foods.

HDL Cholesterol

HDL Cholesterol is often called "good" cholesterol. Remember it by thinking "H" for healthy. You want this number to be HIGH. The HDL lipoprotein picks up cholesterol and returns it to your liver where it can be disposed of. If you have a low HDL, you are at greater risk for heart disease. If you have a high HDL, it protects you against heart disease, **in most cases**, but not always.

LDL Cholesterol

LDL Cholesterol is the "bad" cholesterol. Remember it by thinking "L" for lousy. You want this number to be LOW. Reducing LDL cholesterol makes the lipid core of plaque smaller and thickens the fibrous cap making plaque more stable and less likely to rupture and cause a heart attack. The LDL carries cholesterol through the blood to other tissues. LDL has different sizes – large or "Pattern A," and small, dense "Pattern B." Your LDL cholesterol only partially determines your risk. If you have small dense LDL particles, or a high particle number (LDL-P) you will be at risk even if your LDL cholesterol is not high. See Page 32 for more information.

Triglycerides

Calories from food that you don't use immediately are converted to triglycerides and transported to your fat cells where they will be stored. Your body uses triglycerides as a source of energy. A high triglyceride level is a risk factor for heart disease. If you are a woman, a high triglyceride number is a greater indicator of risk than if you are a man. Triglycerides are high when diabetes is poorly controlled, when too little thyroid hormones are being produced, when a person is obese, or when too many calories are being taken in, especially high carbohydrate, high saturated fat or high alcohol foods or drinks. Genetic factors are also involved in some individuals.

Eating a low-fat diet that replaces fat with high glycemic, simple carbohydrates such as sugars and white flour may cause your triglycerides to increase quickly. See Page 165 for more about the glycemic index.

If your triglycerides are very high (over 1,000), you are at an increased risk of pancreatitis. If you have these very high levels, it requires you to eliminate all fat for a short time. Very quickly, usually within a week, the triglycerides will drop. When they decrease, the diet is switched to a moderate, healthy fat diet. This is best done with the help of a registered dietitian along with close monitoring of triglyceride levels by your physician. To lower triglycerides see Page 45.

VLDL

When you eat excess calories, your body makes fat in the liver to store the calories that are not needed. The very low density lipoprotein (VLDL) carries this fat from the liver to the cells for storage. The fat is composed mostly of triglycerides with a little cholesterol, protein and other lipid molecules surrounding the core. When VLDL delivers the triglycerides, what remains is LDL cholesterol.

If your triglycerides are below 100, VLDL is usually not excessive. If you have a high VLDL level, it is treated the same as a high triglyceride level.

When VLDL passes through blood vessels of muscle cells, an enzyme called lipoprotein lipase located in the cell walls allows the muscle to use the fat in the form of triglyceride from the inside for fuel. The more you exercise, the more lipoprotein lipase your muscles have and the more efficiently your muscles can burn fat as a fuel.

What Causes A Heart Attack

Your heart is a muscle that pumps blood to all parts of your body. Your heart has a left and a right side. There are two chambers on each side – the atrium and the ventricle. Blood rich with oxygen comes from the lungs and enters the atrium. When the atrium contracts, blood is forced into the left ventricle and from there is pumped to the body. Blood returns from the body to the right atrium of the heart and is then pumped into the right ventricle. It returns back to the lungs where it will get oxygen and repeat the process.

Three coronary arteries supply the heart with oxygen rich blood: the right coronary artery (RCA), the left anterior descending (LAD) artery, and the circumflex (CFX) artery. Coronary artery disease (CAD) affects this flow. Lipids or fatty substances (cholesterol and triglycerides) build up fatty deposits or streaks within the artery walls affecting the blood supply. This process is called atherosclerosis (ath-row-sklee-rosis). When blockages narrow the opening by 50 percent or more, the amount of oxygen the heart needs during times of stress or exercise may not be enough. This can result in chest pain called angina, along with shortness of breath.

If the plaque has a thin covering (fibrous cap), it may develop a tear or rupture. The majority of heart attacks are caused by a blockage of plaque that ruptures. A clot develops, and along with plaque, may block the artery. When blocked, the blood supply is cut off to the heart and the result is a heart attack.

NUTRITION NOTE

A heart attack occurs when the oxygen rich blood supply to the heart becomes blocked.

HOW TO CONVERT CHOLESTEROL

Blood lipids in the United States are reported as milligrams per deciliter (mg/dl). The International Standard is millimoles per liter (mmol/l)

Converting total cholesterol, HDL or LDL.

To convert mmol/l of HDL or LDL cholesterol to mg/dl, multiply by 39.
To convert mg/dl of HDL or LDL cholesterol to mmol/l, divide by 39.

Converting triglycerides.

To convert mmol/l of triglycerides to mg/dl, multiply by 89.
To convert mg/dl of triglycerides to mmol/l, divide by 89.

6

Lipid Profile Blood Test —
Know Your Heart Numbers

NUTRITION NOTE

LDL in this chapter refers to:
LDL-C (cholesterol)
<u>not</u>
LDL-P (particles)

To screen for risk of heart disease, your blood can be tested. There are a number of blood tests that are used to assess your risk for a heart attack. The most common test is a fasting lipid profile that measures:

- ❖ **Total cholesterol**
- ❖ **LDL**
- ❖ **HDL**
- ❖ **Triglycerides and VLDL**

Preparing For A Lipid Test

It is necessary for you to fast for 12 hours before the lipid test. Blood is taken from your arm or finger. Total cholesterol and HDL are accurate even if you have not been fasting, but triglycerides and LDL are not. If you have not fasted, triglycerides will be higher and calculated LDL will be lower.

Weight fluctuations, diet changes or excessive alcohol consumption may affect lipid profile results. It is best if you are at a stable weight, as well as following your usual diet, for at least two weeks prior to your test.

Total cholesterol
Total cholesterol = HDL + LDL + VLDL
VLDL = triglycerides ÷ 5

TOTAL CHOLESTEROL	
	Desirable . . . . Less than 200 mg/dL
	Borderline High . . . . 200-239 mg/dL
	High . . . . 240 mg/dL

Note: mg/dl (milligrams per deciliter) are the units used to measure blood cholesterol in the United States. See Page 24 to convert to mmol/l.

LDL

In a standard lipid profile, the LDL is calculated using the Freidewald equation as follows:

$$\textbf{LDL} = \text{Total cholesterol} - \text{HDL} - (\text{triglycerides} \div 5)$$

Testing LDL directly is costly and is not done on a standard lipid profile unless specifically requested by your doctor. When LDL is directly measured, it is typically higher than when it is calculated. Directly measured LDL is more accurate for those with high triglycerides, Type 2 diabetes or coronary artery disease.

If triglycerides are greater than 200, it is recommended that you calculate non-HDL. Even better is to obtain a test (see advanced testing on Page 31) to determine particle number and directly measure LDL particle concentration.

NUTRITION NOTE

When triglycerides are greater than 200 mg/dl, calculated LDL cholesterol underestimates small dense LDL particles.

LDL goal for those with heart disease or any of the following:

- ❖ Heart attack
- ❖ Angioplasty
- ❖ Coronary bypass surgery
- ❖ Coronary stent
- ❖ Stroke
- ❖ Peripheral artery disease
- ❖ Abdominal aortic aneurysm
- ❖ Diabetes
- ❖ Chronic kidney disease

LDL GOAL WITH HEART DISEASE OR ANY OF THE ABOVE	Below 100 mg/dL or Very high risk below 70 mg/dL

LDL goal for those who do not have heart disease

If you have not been diagnosed with any of the conditions listed above, your LDL goal will depend upon the number of risk factors you have and your 10-year risk factor. Your doctor takes into consideration other risks such as being overweight and may adjust your LDL goal lower according to your unique risks. If you had advanced lipid testing for particle size and number, your doctor will use those to adjust your LDL goal.

Risk Factors

First, determine how many risk factors you have that affect your LDL goal.

1. Check your risk factors listed below:
   - ❏ Currently smoke
   - ❏ High blood pressure (140/90 or higher, or you are taking a blood pressure medication)
   - ❏ HDL less than 40 mg/dL (If your HDL is 60 or more, you can subtract one risk factor from your total count)
   - ❏ Father or brother with heart disease before age 55 or a mother or sister with heart disease before age 65
   - ❏ Age: Male 45 years or older or Female 55 years or older
2. Add up the boxes checked (from above) _____ = number of risk factors.
3. If you have two or more risk factors and do not take lipid lowering drugs, calculate your 10-year risk of having a heart attack (see Page 37).

(see Page 37)

LDL GOAL WITHOUT HEART DISEASE[2]	Zero or 1 risk factor. Goal is <160 mg/dl ❖ Recommend start drugs if LDL over 190 mg/dl If 1 risk factor but 10-year risk is 10% or more. Men with 2 or more risk factors with 10-year risk score less than 10%, women less than 20%. Goal is <130 mg/dl. ❖ Recommend start drugs if LDL over 160 mg/dl If 2 or more risk factors with 10-year risk score Men 10 to 20%, women 20 to 23%. Goal is <130 mg/dl. ❖ Recommend start drugs if LDL over 130 mg/dl With any number of risk factors, if 10-year risk greater than 20% men, 23% women. Goal is <100 mg/dl. ❖ Recommend start drugs if LDL over 100 mg/dl

Drugs That Raise LDL and/or Triglycerides

Some drugs will raise LDL. Your doctor must decide how much you need the drug compared to what happens to your LDL when taking it.

- ❖ Progestins, oral
- ❖ Anabolic steroids
- ❖ HIV protease inhibitors
- ❖ Glucocorticoids
- ❖ Accutane
- ❖ Beta-blockers
- ❖ Diuretics

Non-HDL = Total Cholesterol – HDL

Your non-HDL cholesterol is your total cholesterol minus HDL, or put another way, the total of all the bad type of cholesterol LDL, VLDL, IDL and Lp(a). This takes into account other types of cholesterol besides LDL that increase risk. It is a stronger predictor of heart attack than LDL cholesterol.

The AHA Guidelines for preventing cardiovascular disease in women indicate expanded risk factors to be considered include:
- weight
- nutrition/diet
- physical activity

Calculating this is second best to actually measuring non-HDL with a test such as the Apo B, or particle number discussed in Chapter 7. If you have diabetes, high triglycerides or a large waist circumference, you are at increased risk for high non-HDL.

IF YOUR LDL GOAL IS	YOUR NON-HDL GOAL SHOULD BE:
Less than 160 mg/dl	Less than 190 mg/dl
Less than 130 mg/dl	Less than 160 mg/dl
Less than 100 mg/dl	Less than 130 mg/dl
Less than 70 mg/dl	Less than 100 mg/dl

HDL Cholesterol

Low levels of HDL put you at increased risk of heart disease. An advanced lipid test can determine subclasses of HDL and better predict risk since the subclass HDL2 is more protective than HDL3.

HDL

high density lipoprotein

HDL CHOLESTEROL	Low: Less than 40 mg/dL in men, less than 50 mg/dL in women
	Desirable: 60 mg/dL or more

HDL is lowered by:
- ❖ Smoking
- ❖ Being overweight
- ❖ Lack of physical activity
- ❖ Type 2 diabetes
- ❖ High triglycerides
- ❖ A diet with more than 60 percent of calories from carbohydrates
- ❖ Beta-blockers — a drug given to patients who have had a heart attack to reduce the risk of angina and sudden death. This drug is also used in those with heart failure.
- ❖ Anabolic steroids used for body building

Ratio

In the past, a cholesterol ratio was used to determine risk, with smaller numbers being better. The ratio is obtained by dividing your total cholesterol number by your HDL number. The higher your HDL cholesterol the lower your ratio will be. You want a ratio less than 5 with an optimum ratio being 3.5 or less. The American Heart Association states that the ratio is less useful for treatment purposes than using your separate HDL and LDL cholesterol numbers, so not all doctors will calculate the ratio.

Triglycerides

See Page 45 for specific information on lowering triglycerides.

TRIGLYCERIDES	Desirable: less than 150
	Borderline high: 150-199
	High: 200 or above
	Very high: 500 and above

NUTRITION NOTE

A high triglyceride level when not fasting, especially in women, may be related to a high risk for heart-related events independent of other cardiovascular risk factors.[5]

VLDL

In a standard lipid profile, VLDL is estimated with a calculation. If triglycerides are greater than 400 mg/dl, a calculated number is not accurate. In some advanced lipoprotein tests, it is measured directly. You can calculate as follows:

$$\text{VLDL} = \text{triglycerides} \div 5$$

VLDL

very low density lipoprotein

IDL

When your LDL is measured with a standard lipid profile, intermediate-density lipoprotein or IDL is included in the LDL number. IDL can be separately measured in advanced testing such as by NMR *LipoProfile* or VAP. It is an inherited risk factor for heart disease. A high number means that after eating, you are slow to clear fat from the blood. The longer these particles are around, the more likely plaque may be formed. Not everyone who has heart disease has an elevated IDL. If you have Type 2 diabetes, you have a greater chance of having a high IDL.

IDL

intermediate density lipoprotein

TABLE 6.1
What Your Numbers Should Be

YOUR NUMBERS	GOAL	
Total Cholesterol *Lower is better*	Less than 200 mg/dL	
HDL *Higher is better*	Goal: 60 mg/dl or more At risk if: Less than 40 mg/dL (men) Less than 50 mg/dl (women)	
LDL *Lower is better*	LDL with existing heart disease or risk equivalent: *Heart attack, angioplasty, coronary bypass surgery, peripheral artery disease, abdominal aortic aneurysm, diabetes or 10-year risk >20%* Less than 100 mg/dL For high risk, less than 70 mg/dl	LDL without heart disease RISK FACTORS (Page 27) • 0-1 risk factors <160 mg/dL • 2 or more risk factors <130 mg/dL *Note: your doctor may set your goal lower based on your additional individual risks.*
Non-HDL *Lower is better*	Add 30 points to LDL goal	
Triglycerides *Lower is better*	Less than 150 Ideal is probably lower, less than 100 has been suggested	
Blood Pressure	• Desirable/Normal: systolic less than 120 & diastolic less than 80 • Pre-hypertension: systolic 120-139 & diastolic 80-89 • Hypertension Stage 1: systolic 140-159 & diastolic 90-99 • Hypertension Stage 2: systolic 160-179 & diastolic 100-109	
Waist Measurement	Greater risk if: • 40" or greater for men • 35" or greater for women	

Beyond A Lipid Profile — Advanced Testing

7

Traditional testing can successfully predict only 50 percent of coronary artery disease. The Framingham Heart Study[9-11] found that after tracking patients who developed heart disease, 80 percent of them had average cholesterol levels very close to the cholesterol numbers of those who did not develop heart disease. This tells us that the standard lipid profile screening is missing many who are at risk.

A standard cholesterol test measures LDL-C which is the main offender in heart disease, but there are other bad particles that are not measured such as VLDL and IDL, that increase the risk.

There are other specialized tests to measure all the particles that can be used to help determine your risks, along with the standard lipid profile. These screening tests may be ordered by your doctor to further establish your threat of heart disease. Some doctors believe that these provide a better determination of your risk.

These tests may be especially helpful when there is a strong family history yet the standard lipid profile test indicates a low risk. Or, if the lipid profile is slightly elevated, further testing may reveal whether there are any areas of concern that should be treated. If there is uncertainty, the more tests you can do, the easier it is to confirm or rule out concerns.

While these tests are not standard, they may be ordered by your doctor if you request them. Discuss these tests with your doctor. Check with your insurance to see if they cover these tests and what the costs are if you don't have coverage.

Who Would Benefit From Advanced Testing?

❖ Individuals with a family history of premature heart disease.
❖ Those with a moderate risk on the 10-year Framingham risk score, but a standard lipid profile that is within normal range. Testing may reveal hidden disease.
❖ Those with a triglyceride level over 400 since the calculated LDL-C on a standard lipid profile is inaccurate when triglycerides are excessive.
❖ Individuals who have heart disease and have reached their LDL-C goals but have another heart event. Advanced testing may reveal hidden risk such as a high LDL particle number that requires additional treatment.
❖ Isolated low HDL.

KEY:

LDL-C
(low density lipoprotein cholesterol)

LDL-P
(low density lipoprotein particles)

NUTRITION NOTE
LDL-P is a strong predictor of heart disease in women.

Testing may also help your doctor in deciding how aggressive your treatment should be based on your risk. If you have high cholesterol, but lipoprotein testing reveals particle numbers and size within safe guidelines, you may not need further treatment to lower cholesterol. Yet those with low cholesterol made up of too many particles have "hidden" disease that require treatment.

To have these tests, find a doctor such as a lipidologist who understands and is familiar with the tests. Insurance plans vary, some may not cover the cost.

Lipidologist

Board certified lipidologists are doctors with advanced training who specialize in lipid disorders and deal with difficult lipids which do not respond to treatment. They become certified by the American Board of Clinical Lipidology after extensive training. They may consult with your doctor on how to best manage your lipids and often use advanced testing to determine treatment.

Advanced Tests Beyond A Lipid Panel

1. The Berkeley Heart Lab, www.bhlinc.com, includes the largest variety of tests and is the most costly. The test directly measures LDL-C, LDL particle sizes, HDL subclasses, Apo A-I, CRP, homocysteine, Lp(a), Apo B-100, Apo E isoforms and others.
2. The NMR *LipoProfile*, www.liposcience.com, uses nuclear magnetic resonance (NMR) or NMR spectroscopy to directly measure the number of lipoprotein particles and LDL particle size, as well as receive a direct measurement of HDL and VLDL subclasses.
3. The Vertical Auto Profile or VAP test, www.thevaptest.com, directly measures LDL, HDL, VLDL, IDL, Lp(a) and LDL pattern size but not particle number.
4. Apo B-100. Levels are directly measured from a blood sample. Helpful when triglycerides are high since LDL-C cannot be accurately calculated. At any given LDL-C, a higher Apo B level indicates higher LDL-P.

Explanation Of The Various Test Results

Each of the above tests will measure a number of things beyond the standard lipid profile test that has already been discussed. Some of the tests you will find are described here. Keep in mind that you may not have all of these as each varies in what is tested.

LDL particle number

An LDL cholesterol level obtained from a standard lipid test does not indicate the number of particles since the amount of cholesterol each particle carries can vary. A large number of particles, whether small or large, increase

LDL PARTICLES

The more particles you have carrying cholesterol the greater the risk of heart disease.

your risk of heart disease. LDL particle number, more than LDL cholesterol, determines the risk for heart disease. When LDL-C is normal but LDL particle numbers are high, as in those with familial hypercholesterolemia, there is very high risk of early death from heart disease. Those individuals often die in their 30s and 40s or even sooner.

Small particle size, LDL pattern B

You may have a normal LDL cholesterol number, yet be at increased risk due to too many particles. If this is the case, your risk would be underestimated with a standard lipid profile. Your LDL-C number is expressed as the number of milligrams per deciliter (volume), but within a given volume, you could have a few large particles or you could have many small particles. If you have Pattern B with too many small, dense particles, you are **three times** as likely to have heart disease. If you have high blood pressure, Type 2 diabetes or metabolic syndrome, it is more likely that you have Pattern B. This pattern is found more often in women than men.[11]

If you carry your weight in your abdomen, have a high LDL-C, or have high triglycerides with a low HDL, you probably have small, dense LDL. If your triglycerides are greater than 150 mg/dl, there is a very high chance you have the small LDL-P trait.

Treating small particles

To treat small particles, you should exercise, lose abdominal fat, and eat a diet of less refined carbohydrates, more fish, fish oil supplements and soluble fiber such as oats, oat bran, barley, legumes, fruits and vegetables.

If you eat a very low fat diet that is high in refined carbohydrates, you do more harm than good as it may increase small, dense particles. A moderate diet of 25 percent of calories from good fat works better.

Large particle size, LDL pattern A

If you have large particles, also called Pattern A, it is the opposite of small particle size. If you are typical Pattern A, you will also have low triglycerides along with large LDL particles. However, if you have a high LDL-C, you are still at risk even with large particles because there are too many particles.

The optimal goal for an LDL particle number as measured by the NMR *LipoProfile* test is less than 1,000 millimoles per litre (mmol/L).

If you have a high number of particles, it is treated the same as small particles (addressed above). Lifestyle changes have a greater impact on LDL particle numbers than on LDL-C. To reduce LDL particles to optimal levels of less than 1,000, combination drug therapy is often required with lifestyle changes.

NUTRITION NOTE

Greater chance of small LDL particles if:

$$\frac{\text{Triglycerides}}{\text{HDL}} > 3.8$$

NUTRITION NOTE

In most cases, statin drugs are also necessary to eliminate small LDL particles

Soluble fiber also lowers LDL particles see Page 139

NUTRITION NOTE

The American
Diabetes
Association and
the American
College of
Cardiology agree
that a more
appropriate way
to evaluate risk is
to measure Apo B
or LDL particle
number instead of
LDL-C.

Apo B (Apolipoprotein B-100)

This is another test that measures the number of particles. Every particle carries a protein called Apo B. This test measures the protein portion of the LDL-C, IDL and VLDL. As the number gets larger, the risk of heart attack increases. About 25 percent of individuals would be treated differently if Apo B was used instead of LDL-C because it finds hidden disease. When triglycerides are greater than 150, as is often the case in those with diabetes, metabolic syndrome and renal disease, LDL-C is less accurate. Canada recommends the use of Apo B in their cholesterol management guidelines and its use is becoming more widely accepted in the U.S. because Apo B is a superior predictor of LDL-P.

Lp(a)

Pronounced "LP little a," this is made up of the bad LDL cholesterol particle with an attached protein called "apoprotein a" or "apo(a)." It is an inherited risk factor for heart disease. Lp(a) teams up with LDL-C and increases by 10 times the chance that it will cause plaque build up. High levels mean there is a greater chance of a clot forming when plaque ruptures; an event that may lead to a heart attack or stroke.

Lp(a) levels are genetically determined; about 50 percent of children whose parent has high Lp(a) will also have an elevated level. Lifestyle, diet and drugs, except for niacin and estrogen for post-menopausal women, have little impact.

Lp(a) is a test recommended for those with a family history of heart disease at a young age. This test is also recommended for women because the Framingham Heart Study found that high levels doubled the risk of heart attack in women.[12]

Treatment for LDL-C may not lower Lp(a). Lipidologists who often use advanced tests to determine Lp(a) typically recommend aggressively lowering LDL-C to 100 mg/dl or less in order to reduce risk if Lp(a) is elevated. They may use *Niaspan*, a prescription form of niacin, at 2 to 4 grams, which may lower Lp(a) levels by 35 to 50 percent. (For additional information on niacin, see Page 235.) The drug fenofibrate has shown some effect on Lp(a). Bile acid sequestrant (resins) and statin drugs have little effect.

The only other drug that lowers Lp(a) is estrogen, but it is not used for this purpose.

Trans-fatty acids may raise Lp(a); therefore, avoiding fried foods when eating out or avoiding all foods with "partially hydrogenated" listed in the ingredients is important.

NUTRITION NOTE

Small effects on
Lp(a) reduction in
some studies
occurred from:
• fish oil
• milled
  flaxseed[13]
• tea[14]
• raw almonds[16]
• L-carnitine[17]
  (2 grams a day)

Lp(a)
is an inflammatory
marker that
promotes blood
clot formation.

Apo E Genotype DNA test

The Berkley Heart Lab can test the most common gene affecting LDL cholesterol levels, Apo E, which has three major variations, E2, E3 and E4.

You inherit one of these genes from each of your parents, so you have two copies. This is genetically fixed; therefore, it is tested only once since it never changes.

The most common form, E3, occurs in approximately 78 percent of the population. Normal is E3/E3 in which genes from both parents are E3. E4 has a frequency of 15 percent; E2 a frequency of 7 percent. E4 presents the highest risk of heart disease and diseases of the other blood vessels outside of the heart and brain.

Genetic test to determine diet and other treatment

If you have genetic testing, it can be used to determine what treatment and diet is best. If you have E2, you will respond best to fibrates and/or niacin and a higher "healthy" fat diet. If you have E3 or E4, you will respond to lifestyle and diet. If it is E4 you will get the best response with a low saturated fat diet.

When to test for Apo E

You would test for Apo E if your total cholesterol is greater than 240 and triglycerides are greater than 150 or when high cholesterol along with high triglycerides does not respond to diet and exercise. In addition, the test should also be given if a family member has the E2/E2 pattern. Early testing is important to tailor treatment as it may prevent early heart disease.

Homocysteine

If you eat a typical American diet which includes a generous amount of animal protein, including the amino acid methionine, and processed foods low in B vitamins, excess homocysteine may be created. In 1969, it was proposed that a high homocysteine level was the cause of atherosclerosis.

Epidemiologic studies show a higher homocysteine level increases the risk of heart attack, but this type of observation only proves it *could* and not that it *actually does* cause atherosclerosis. Taking B vitamins lowers homocysteine levels, but it is uncertain if taking B vitamins helps reduce the risk of heart attack or stroke. Three trials, VISP, NORVIT and HOPE, were designed to determine if the use of B vitamins would decrease cardiovascular events. All three found that taking folic acid, B_{12} and B_6 did indeed lower homocysteine levels; however, taking B vitamins made no difference in the number of heart attacks or sudden death from heart disease. The trials did find the B vitamins reduced the incidence of stroke. More studies need to be conducted to know all the answers about the benefits of using B vitamins.

Since B vitamins are safe when upper limits (UL) are not exceeded and have other benefits, such as improved memory, decreased depression and increased energy, including them in a multivitamin and mineral supplement is reasonable. If you choose a separate vitamin B supplement, choose one such as a B-50 supplement that does not exceed the UL of 100 mg for B_6 which could cause nerve damage to occur in the arms and legs. Some older adults could have delayed diagnosis of a vitamin B_{12} deficiency when high levels of folic acid are taken. (See discussion under B vitamins on Page 214.)

NUTRITION NOTE

High levels of homocysteine are harmful to the cells that line the artery walls (endothelium).

Homocysteine is lowered by
Vitamin B
Exercise

NUTRITION NOTE

CRP is most useful to measure if 10-year risk is 10-20% with an LDL that is less than 130 mg/dl. If a high level hs-CRP is found with low LDL cholesterol, there is increased risk of having a heart attack.

High sensitivity C-reactive protein (hs-CRP)

A high-sensitivity hs-CRP test measures inflammation. A level between 3 mg/L and 10 mg/L is high risk. Your lab results will have a specific reference range based on the test method. A high number means there is a greater chance of plaque rupturing. If you have a high hs-CRP, you have a 1.5 to 4 times higher risk of having a heart attack or stroke than if your hs-CRP is low.

The levels of hs-CRP levels can be raised by an infection anywhere in your body. Having a cold, the flu, arthritis, high blood pressure, smoking, inactivity, coffee, diabetes, Crohn's disease, gum disease, urinary tract infection, a high protein diet, and even lack of sleep may increase CRP levels. Diets that are high in refined carbohydrates, including white bread, potatoes, cookies, etc., may also cause CRP levels to rise. Large amounts of omega 6 fats, such as corn oil, soybean oil, and a lack of omega-3 fats, also promotes inflammation.

The same recommendations that lower your cholesterol also lower CRP levels. If you have an elevated hs-CRP, an anti-inflammatory diet is effective, along with aspirin and fish oil. Salicylic acid is one of the active ingredients in aspirin that provides anti-inflammatory benefits.

Salicylates are produced in plants as a defense against disease. Organic vegetables grown without pesticides produce higher levels of salicylic acid. Food sources are berries, cherries, oranges and peppers. Spices such as curry powder, hot paprika and thyme are also good sources.

To reduce inflammation, reduce your intake of saturated fats; include plenty of fruits and vegetables; add soluble fiber in the form of oats, barley and psyllium; and increase omega-3 fatty acids. Replace cooking oils with extra-virgin olive oil, high-oleic safflower oil or canola oil in a Mediterranean-type diet. Lifestyle changes may also help reduce inflammation. These include not smoking, weight loss if overweight, exercise on a regular basis, blood pressure control, and blood sugar control. If diet and lifestyle changes are not enough to lower hs-CRP, drugs such as statins and fibrates can be used.

TABLE 7.1
Find Your 10-Year Risk With
Framingham Heart Disease Risk Assessment

The Framingham risk score estimates your 10-year chance of having a heart attack or other coronary event. It was developed to evaluate risk if you **do not already have a diagnosis of heart disease.**

It may **not** be a good determinant of a women's risk if there are two or more factors such as obesity, blood clotting disorders, smoking or metabolic syndrome, as well as a family history for heart disease. In those cases, even if you score at low risk you may want to consider additional testing such as Apo B, NMR *LipoProfile,* for particle number or a heart scan to further identify risk. These tests can help to better determine risk levels and needed treatments.

Review the results with your doctor or ask your health care provider for help if you are unsure which numbers to circle.

1. Age: find age and circle the points below   Your points [   ]

Age	20-34 Years	35-39 Years	40-44 Years	45-49 Years	50-54 Years	55-59 Years	60-64 Years	65-69 Years	70-74 Years	73-79 Years
Points Men	-9	-4	0	3	6	8	10	11	12	13
Points Women	-7	-3	0	3	6	8	10	12	14	16

2. Total cholesterol at different ages   Your points [   ]

If Cholesterol is	Below 160	160-190	200-239	240-279	280 or more
20-39 yr. men	0	4	7	9	11
20-39 yr. women	0	3	6	8	10
40-49 yr. men	0	3	5	6	8
40-49 yr. women	0	3	6	8	10
50-59 yr. men	0	2	3	4	5
50-59 yr. women	0	2	4	5	7
60-69 yr. men	0	1	1	2	3
60-69 yr. women	0	1	2	3	4
70-79 yr. men	0	0	0	1	1
70-79 yr. women	0	1	1	2	2

3. HDL level   Your points [   ]

HDL	60 or more	50-59	40-49	Below 40
Men	-1	0	1	2
Women	-1	0	1	2

NOTE

Does not apply to people on lipid drugs. Use this table to determine risk if you are not taking cholesterol-lowering drugs.

THE REYNOLDS RISK SCORE

By adding two more measurements to the 10-year risk it more accurately predicts the risk of having a heart attack.
- -hs-CRP
- -if a parent died of a heart attack before age 60

www.reynoldsriskscore.org

Adapted from the Third Report of the National Cholesterol Education Program (NCEP) Expert Panel on Detection, Evaluation and Treatment of High Blood Cholesterol in Adults (Adult Treatment Panel III). JAMA. 2001 May 16; 285(19): 2486-97

4. Blood pressure (the top number or first number)   Your points [   ]

Systolic	Below 120	120-129	130-139	140-159	160 or more
Men treated	0	1	2	2	3
Women treated	0	3	4	5	6
Men not treated	0	0	1	1	2
Women not treated	0	1	2	3	4

5. Smoking   Your points [   ]

Age	20-39 yr.	40-49 yr.	50-59 yr.	60-69 yr.	70-79 yr.
Nonsmoker men & women	0	0	0	0	0
Smoker men	8	5	3	1	1
Smoker women	9	7	4	2	1

6. Add up your points from items 1-5. In chart below, use points to find your 10-year risk and LDL goal.   Your points (add1-5) [   ]

Men Total Points (add 1-5)	Your Chance of Having Heart Disease in the Next 10 Years	LDL Goal	Women Total Points (add 1-5)	Your Chance of Having Heart Disease in the Next 10 Years
<0	<1%	0-1 risk factor*	<9	<1%
0	1%	LDL Goal	10	1%
2	1%	<160	12	1%
3	1%		13	2%
4	1%		14	2%
5	2%		15	3%
6	2%	2 risk factors*	16	4%
7	3%	LDL Goal	17	5%
8	4%	<130	18	6%
9	5%		19	8%
10	6%			
11	8%			
12	10%	LDL Goal	20	11%
13	12%	<130	21	14%
14	16%		22	17%
15	20%	LDL Goal	23	22%
16	25%	<100, with	24	27%
17 or more	30% or more	<70 option	25 or more	30% or more

* risk factors listed on Page 27

Picture The Risk
Heart Scan, Calcium Scores and Angiogram

I f you are in the intermediate risk category where decision making is more difficult, adding a scan may be helpful in making the correct decision for you. A CT scan may be a simple coronary calcium score or a more complex and involved angiography. Consider getting a heart scan if you have a strong family history of heart conditions or other risk factors for heart disease.

Calcium Score

A calcium score is a measure of the amount of calcium in your coronary arteries. The higher your score, the more calcium you have. In the past, it was only available in centers that had very expensive electron beam CT scanners (EBCT), but with a multidetector (also called multislice), CT technology Coronary Calcium Scoring is more widely available. The calcium score heart scan uses a minimal amount of radiation. For less than $200 in some areas, you can have a heart scan which is fast, painless and noninvasive, that provides your calcium score. Calcium makes up 20 percent of plaque, so measuring calcium deposits is a good measure of total plaque. As we get older, we have more fat and calcium buildup in the arteries, so if you are young, having a high calcium score is more predictive that you are at risk.

The higher the score, the more plaque you have; however, there are also different ways that you may accumulate plaque. You could have thin layers throughout the arteries or several large clumps. There are some experts who believe that having a lot of small calcium deposits may be riskier since each one weakens the artery making it more likely to tear.

If your plaque score is high, the next step, if it has not already been done, is to assess your other risk factors. Do you have high blood pressure? Is there a family history? Do you have high cholesterol, and what are the results of cholesterol particle size from advanced blood testing? (See Page 33.)

You can follow a program of diet, exercise and supplements as described in this book. Lifestyle changes may be enough to lower your score when you check it a year later. If not, then adding drug therapy would be necessary.

For further information on a program designed around your calcium score, visit www.trackyourplaque.com.

NOTE

Calcium develops as plaques grow in your coronary arteries.

A calcium score involves a very small amount of radiation exposure.

Who should be screened with a calcium score scan?

Risk factors and the Framingham score often fail to predict half of the cardiovascular events which occur, and are therefore, not the best criteria to determine who to screen.

❖ Age may be a good guideline since higher risk begins to appear in men over 40 and women past menopause or over 50.

❖ Cholesterol levels that are not within normal guidelines, including advanced testing.

❖ If you have several other risk factors, such as:
  ◆ Obesity
  ◆ Cigarette smoking or regular exposure to secondhand smoke
  ◆ Diabetes
  ◆ High blood pressure
  ◆ Physical inactivity
  ◆ Metabolic syndrome

Coronary computer tomography angiogram (CT or CTA scan)

This is not a test used for simple routine screening. It is performed when you have symptoms that suggest it may be helpful. In some cases, a CT scan may be used instead of a cardiac catherization.

Coronary computed tomography angiogram provides detailed, three-dimensional images of the blood vessels. It is noninvasive but requires an iodine-containing contrast dye to be injected into your arm through an IV. It provides similar information as a heart catheterization. However, the heart catherization is invasive. It requires inserting a long, thin tube called a catheter through the groin into a blood vessel and then guided to the heart where dye is injected and viewed on X-ray images. The radiation required for an angiogram is similar to what you would be exposed to for a heart catheterization. If the CT scan reveals that you need a cardiac catherization for a stent placement you will have been exposed to extra radiation from having both procedures.

Scanners are becoming widely available throughout the U.S. and are rapidly changing, providing more detailed pictures. Technology has decreased the amount of radiation exposure. The new 64-slice CT scanners can take pictures in spite of the heart constantly moving. This technology can also detect soft plaque or fatty material that has not yet hardened into calcium plaque without doing the invasive procedure of catheterization, some doctors are using sophisticated scanning machines to figure out which of their patients may need to take further steps to lower their risk. The radiation exposure of the multidetector scanner is 50 percent less than traditional CT scans but not a screening method people should have done every year. The test costs between $1,800 and $4,000.

NOTE

CT or CTA scans expose you to a higher amount of radiation than a calcium score scan.

9

Metabolic Syndrome

Metabolic Syndrome may be called Insulin Resistance Syndrome, Syndrome X, cardio-metabolic risk or pre-diabetes. It is estimated that more than 60 million Americans have this syndrome. Obesity and a sedentary lifestyle are often the forces that drive metabolic syndrome.

Are You At Risk For Metabolic Syndrome?

The more questions you answer with a "yes," the greater the chances you have insulin resistance and are at risk for developing metabolic syndrome.

AUTHOR NOTE

To measure your waist:
1. Find the top of your hip bone (iliac crest).
2. Place tape measure on bare skin, horizontal to floor at this level.
3. Measure as you breathe out.

SELF-ASSESSMENT FOR METABOLIC SYNDROME		
Date ____ /____ /____		
1. I have a waist that is greater than half my height.	❏ Yes	❏ No
2. I don't do any physical activity other than daily life activities.	❏ Yes	❏ No
3. My triglycerides are over 128.	❏ Yes	❏ No
4. My HDL is less than 50 if I'm female, or less than 40 if I'm male.	❏ Yes	❏ No
5. I am over 40 years old.	❏ Yes	❏ No
6. I have high blood pressure.	❏ Yes	❏ No
7. There is a history of Type 2 diabetes in my immediate family, such as a parent, brother or sister.	❏ Yes	❏ No
8. I have or had polycystic ovarian syndrome or gestational diabetes during a pregnancy.	❏ Yes	❏ No
9. I am African American, Hispanic/Latino, Asian American, Pacific Islander or Native American.	❏ Yes	❏ No

According to the National Cholesterol Education Program Adult Treatment Panel (NCEP ATP III), you have metabolic syndrome if you have three or more of the following:

AUTHOR NOTE

As waist measurement increases so does:
- insulin resistance
- metabolic syndrome
- triglycerides
- risk of heart disease

❖ Waist measurement*
- Men 40 inches or more
- Women 35 inches or more

❖ Blood pressure
- 130 over 85 mmHg or greater
- Taking blood pressure lowering drugs

❖ Triglycerides
- 150 mg/dl or greater

❖ HDL
- Men less than 40
- Women less than 50

❖ Fasting blood sugar
- 100 mg/dl or higher

Note: some studies have found risk for Asians with a waist size of 31.5" or greater for women and 35.5" or greater for men.

Having metabolic syndrome puts you at high risk to become a diabetic within 10 years. You could have metabolic syndrome for a number of years before you develop diabetes, but once you develop it, there is no turning back. You want to do something before that happens. One in four people who have metabolic syndrome will develop Type 2 diabetes.

Insulin Resistance

When you eat food, it eventually is broken down to glucose. Insulin is used to move glucose to your cells where it is used for fuel. Those with metabolic syndrome are insulin resistant. The body is unable to respond to insulin no matter how much insulin is made. The pancreas works overtime to secrete more and more insulin as it tries to move the glucose from the bloodstream into cells. As the resistance worsens, the pancreas continues to make more insulin, but it is less and less effective in handling blood sugar. As your blood insulin levels increase, the liver overproduces cholesterol in the form of VLDL particles and IDL particles, which indicate you are not clearing fat from the blood as quickly as you should.

Lifestyle Changes

Most Americans who have metabolic syndrome have not been diagnosed. This means that many have a hidden risk for developing heart disease that is not being treated. When triglycerides are high and HDL is low, it is a sign that you have insulin resistance. Metabolic syndrome happens when too many calories are eaten along with too little physical activity. Calories from highly refined carbohydrates (white flour) and bad fats are especially harmful. There is little in the way of drugs that help, but there is much that lifestyle can change. A few simple lifestyle changes may prevent serious future health concerns by increasing your sensitivity to insulin and reducing inflammation.

Being more active is one of those lifestyle changes. Those who don't exercise build a type of dangerous fat around internal organs called visceral fat. Even people who appear thin on the outside can have visceral fat around organs. Women who are not active gain visceral fat twice as fast as men. Adding some daily physical activity helps.

What and how much you eat can also reduce your risk. Cutting out high glycemic refined carbohydrates (foods made from white flour such as crackers, cookies, pastries, pretzels and sweetened beverages) is another change that makes a big difference. Read ingredient lists of foods and avoid high fructose corn syrup. Cut down on the starch or grain portion of your plate (see Pages 294-297 for sample menus). Try eating a little less at each meal. Eat more fish but don't eat it fried. Eat leaner meats and poultry. Have fish more often. Look for ways to include more fruits and vegetables in your diet and snacks. Snack on nuts, but keep the portions small if weight loss is a goal.

Getting your vitamin D levels checked is another important step. (See Page 217 for more on this.) If your vitamin D level is low, correcting it with an over-the-counter supplement of vitamin D_3 may help to raise HDL, lower triglycerides, lower small particles LDL, and increase insulin sensitivity.

Lack of sleep can also affect how insulin works. Getting enough sleep is another lifestyle change that helps. Aim for seven to eight hours every night.

Take fish oil supplements to lower triglycerides (see Page 103).

NUTRITION NOTE

Metabolic syndrome is a result of:
- overweight
- being inactive
- diets high in carbohydrates

Insulin resistance is indicated when
- Low HDL
- High Triglycerides

How Metabolic Syndrome Is Treated

❖ Weight reduction. Losing 5 to 7 percent of body weight, which is 9 to 12 pounds for someone who weighs 180 pounds, with modest diet and exercise may change your risk. For some, it may take an ideal BMI of less than 25.

❖ Increased physical activity will significantly reduce insulin sensitivity even without weight loss. Exercise at least 30 minutes a day, but 60 minutes is even better. Any activity is better than none. Ideally do a combination of resistance (weight lifting) and aerobic exercise.[21] If you have been sedentary, start slowly with walking and gradually increase duration and intensity. See Chapter 39 for guidelines.

❖ Mediterranean-type diet, which helps to fight inflammation.

❖ Less carbohydrates and choose those with a low glycemic load.

❖ Fish oil.

❖ Blood pressure treatment if blood pressure is elevated.

❖ Aspirin (if coronary disease is present).

❖ Reduction of triglycerides (Page 45).

❖ Increase HDL levels (Page 47).

❖ Sufficient amounts of vitamin D. Test and correct if low levels.

❖ Adequate sleep. Correction of sleep apnea if it exists.

10

How To Lower Triglycerides

Triglycerides are raised by:

❖ Drugs, such as beta-blockers in high doses; bile acid sequestrants; corticosteroids, such as prednisone; drugs that block natural estrogen called SERMS, such as tamoxifen and raloxifene; estrogen (oral, not patch)
❖ Alcohol
❖ Very low fat diets that are high in carbohydrates (more than 60 percent of your calories from carbohydrates)

Triglycerides that are in the range of 150 to 400 mg/dl are typically, though not always, a result of insulin resistance. Try the following to lower triglycerides:

❖ Lose weight if overweight.
❖ Increase physical activity. Exercise 30 minutes on most, if not all days; 60 minutes to lose weight. Burning off 1,200 to 2,200 calories a week as exercise can lower triglycerides by 5 to 38 mg/dl.
❖ Restrict/avoid intake of alcohol.
❖ Avoid high glycemic, simple sugars from sweets, pastries, jams, jelly, sugar, honey, maple syrup, jelly beans, licorice, angel food cake, fat-free cookies, sherbet, fat-free ice cream and sorbet.
❖ Choose yogurts that do not have added sugars. Limit sugars to no more than 12 grams for 8 ounces of yogurt which is the amount found naturally in the milk. Greek style yogurt has the least amount of sugar.
❖ Limit fruit juice to one 4-ounce serving a day. Choose whole fruit, especially berries. Avoid soda, punch, lemonades, beverages or teas that are sweetened.
❖ Eat more vegetables than fruits. For every serving of fruit you choose, eat two servings of vegetables. (except potato, baked beans and corn)
❖ Check ingredient list of breads, crackers, cereals, pretzels, chips, snack bars, granola bars, cakes, cookies, pancakes, waffles, tortillas, pasta and

NUTRITION NOTE

Triglycerides: the form in which fat is stored in the body.

Causes of high triglycerides:
- Being overweight
- Lack of activity
- Diets high in carbohydrates
- Type 2 diabetes
- Chronic kidney failure
- Genetic factors
- Excessive alcohol use
- Some drugs

rice. You want the first grain listed to be "whole" wheat, "whole" rye, brown rice, oats or stone-ground corn.

AUTHOR NOTE

Your doctor may prescribe:
- Fibrates
- Prescription niacin (*Niaspan*)
- Prescription fish oil (*Lovaza*)

❖ Cut out refined carbohydrates.
- ◆ White bread, French bread, hard rolls, bagels or any other bread product that does not list a "whole" grain first.
- ◆ Don't rely on the package name, such as wheat crackers, bran cereal, oatmeal bread, multigrain, rye. You must check the ingredient list. If wheat, corn, rice or high-gluten wheat flour are listed first, the product is "refined" not "whole."
- ◆ Enriched wheat means part (but not all) of the nutrients have been added back so, it, too, is refined, not whole.
- ◆ Refined carbohydrates are used in most cookies, cakes, donuts, cereal and breakfast bars, etc. Check the ingredients.

❖ Increase intake of high soluble fiber foods such as oat bran and barley.

❖ Choose more whole, intact grains like brown rice, barley, bulgur, millet, oats, quinoa, rye and teff.

❖ Choose cereals with a low Glycemic Index (Page 165) such as steel-cut oats; oat bran; old-fashioned oats; cooked, hulled barley; *Heart Balance* barley cereal and *Nature's Path* Smart Bran cereal (oat bran and psyllium.)

❖ Sprinkle 1/2 teaspoon (1 gram) cinnamon on your cereal or stir cinnamon into plain yogurt, unsweetened applesauce, warm milk or soy milk. Sprinkle cinnamon on apple slices. You can make cinnamon tea by adding 1/2 teaspoon to a cup of boiling water and letting it stand for five minutes before drinking. Cinnamon may reduce blood glucose, triglycerides, LDL cholesterol, and total cholesterol. Cinnamon appears to enhance the efficiency of insulin.

NUTRITION NOTE

Fish oil more effectively lowers triglycerides than any prescription drug.

❖ Use a plant-based, Mediterranean-style diet (Page 51) that includes healthy fats.
- ◆ Use salad dressing made with olive or canola oil instead of fat-free salad dressings, which are higher in added sweeteners or fake sugars. Check ingredients to avoid those with high fructose corn syrup.
- ◆ Limit saturated fat (beef, pork and cheese) and avoid trans fats.
- ◆ Eat more fatty fish such as salmon, troll-caught albacore tuna, sardines, and herring.
- ◆ Use flaxseed (ground or milled)

❖ Eat nuts – raw, dry roasted, unsalted (go easy if you need to lose weight). Walnuts contain omega-3 fats, but all nuts have healthy fats.

❖ Snack on vegetables (dark green, leafy vegetables have omega-3) and a half ounce of nuts instead of foods made from flour such as crackers, granola bars, muffins, bagels, pretzels.

❖ Take fish oil, The American Heart Association has suggested 2,000 to 4,000 mg EPA + DHA from fish oil supplements for lowering triglycerides with consent of your doctor.

11

How To Increase HDL

 healthy diet and lifestyle may increase your good HDL cholesterol by 10 to 13 percent.[22]

Ways To Raise HDL

❖ Include some good fat. About 30 percent of calories from healthy types of fats (Page 16).
❖ Eat less saturated fat (Page 16) and more monounsaturated fat.
❖ Consider a Mediterranean-style diet (Page 51).
❖ Replace some carbohydrates with lean plant protein and healthy fats.
❖ Be more physically active.
❖ Maintain a healthy body weight.
❖ Include a moderate amount of alcohol intake, with health care provider's approval.
❖ Use niacin (Page 235).
❖ Keep vitamin D levels in the healthy range of 50 to 80 ng/ml (Page 217).

What Lowers or Causes Low HDL

❖ Very low-fat, high-carbohydrate diets
❖ Trans fats (partially hydrogenated)
❖ Smoking
❖ Taking anabolic steroids
❖ Obesity
❖ Physical inactivity
❖ High Triglycerides
❖ Metabolic syndrome
❖ Type 2 diabetes
❖ Genetic factors

NUTRITION NOTE

A healthy diet and lifestyle may increase good HDL cholesterol by 10 to 13 percent.

NUTRITION NOTE

For every 10 pounds excess weight lost, you can expect a 2 mg/dl increase in HDL.

NUTRITION NOTE

Do not take
over-the-counter,
no-flush niacin;
it doesn't work.

When total fat is decreased and carbohydrates are increased, HDL will decrease and triglycerides increase. Neither change is desired.

A better way is to replace the saturated and trans fats with good monounsaturated fats such as nuts, canola and olive oil or to replace some of the simple sugar and refined carbohydrates with lean protein. A diet with 30 percent of the calories from healthy fat may raise HDL by 2 percent.

Excess weight, especially if that fat is in the abdominal area, lowers HDL. While you are losing weight, HDL will be lower, but once you stabilize at your new lower weight, HDL will go up. For every 10 pounds lost, you can expect a 2 mg/dl increase in HDL.

Taking steroids for the purpose of bulking up muscles may cause HDL to drop to 20 mg/dl or less.

Alcohol consumption, whether wine, beer or distilled spirits, raises HDL. Your doctor won't prescribe alcohol to raise your HDL because alcohol is not recommended to people who do not already drink, but it seems that those who are moderate drinkers generally have higher HDL.

When daily physical activity is the equivalent of walking for 45 minutes at a pace of four miles per hour (three miles), HDL can increase 2 to 8 mg/dl. This benefit can also be attained at a lower intensity if the time spent on physical activity is longer. Exercise may raise HDL by 5 to 14 percent.

Smokers who quit and do not gain weight may increase their HDL by 4 mg/dl. If quitting causes a weight gain, HDL benefit is offset.

Niacin may raise HDL 25 to 30 percent. At the same dose of niacin, HDL will continue to rise slowly for months. The flushing caused by niacin decreases with time, but if niacin is stopped and restarted, the flushing starts again. See Page 238 for more information on how to take niacin. Do not take over-the-counter, no-flush niacin; it doesn't work.

12

A Heart Healthy Plate

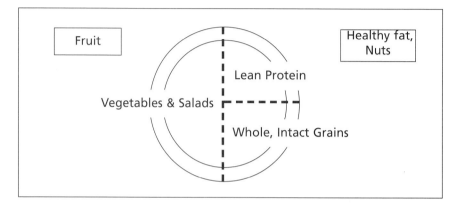

Fruit

Healthy fat, Nuts

Lean Protein

Vegetables & Salads

Whole, Intact Grains

Eating heart healthy involves more than eating chicken, low-fat cheese, skim milk and avoiding eggs. Yes, those are all changes that may help, but the amounts you choose and the other foods eaten with them, make an even bigger difference. If you fill your plate with skinless chicken breast but are skimpy on the vegetable, salad, fruit and whole grains, you are missing out on the benefits that a healthy plant-based diet provides. Hundreds of studies continue to show a strong link between diets that are filled with vegetables and less chronic disease.

If you don't like to count calories or fat grams and prefer general guidelines to a specific diet plan, the method of filling your plate in the right proportions with healthy foods is amazingly close to being on target. I have tried many techniques with my patients: menus with recipes, measuring all their foods, having them keep records of foods eaten. While these work, they are time consuming. In an attempt to simplify things, I often ask people to try to make all their meals and snacks balanced as in the diagram above. With this method, you choose healthy foods and eat them in the correct amounts.

If one of your goals is weight loss, amounts do matter. Use a nine-inch plate instead of platter which encourages huge amounts. Don't pile foods as high as you can. Even healthy foods will provide too many calories when eaten in excess. If you want a second helping or are still hungry, eat more from the vegetables and salads group.

1. On one half of your plate, put vegetables and salads along with some healthy fats such as olive oil dressing, chopped nuts or some avocado.

2. Divide the other half into two equal sections.

3. In one of those quarters goes lean protein. Select fish and legumes more often than poultry. If you enjoy red meat, choose it even less often than poultry.

4. The last quarter is for whole grains such as brown rice, quinoa, wheat kernels, etc. Less often, but also in this spot, would be products made from whole grains that have been ground into flour such as "100%" whole-wheat bread, crackers or whole-wheat pasta. Potatoes go here instead of in the vegetable section.

5. Next to your plate goes a small bowl for fruit, which should be your dessert most of the time. A few times a week, if you enjoy chocolate, include a small piece of dark chocolate with 70 percent or higher cocoa.

6. If you are not lactose intolerant and consume dairy, add a glass of skim or 1% milk. Other options are calcium-fortified beverages, such as soy milk, rice milk, almond milk and oat milk. If none of these are options you enjoy, you may need to take a calcium supplement to meet your calcium requirements, along with consuming other calcium-rich foods (Page 221).

7. Beverages: Choose water most often. Cocoa, tea or red wine are other options. Limit fruit juice to one 4-ounce serving a day. Grapefruit interferes with an enzyme the body uses to breakdown certain statins which means they will stay in your body longer and may increase the risk for developing serious muscle problems. If taking a statin drug such as atorvastatin (*Lipitor*), lovastatin (*Mevacor*) or simvastatin (*Zocor*), avoid grapefruit. However, pravastatin (*Pravachol*) and rosuvastatin (*Crestor*) are metabolized differently, and grapefruit juice won't interact with them. You should check with the pharmacist if you have questions about other drugs you may be taking.

8. Snacks: Choose vegetables and fruits, especially if any of your meals were lacking in those. Snack on an ounce of nuts if you have not used them in another meal.

9. OTHERS: Foods such as desserts, donuts, candy, chips, and highly refined foods such as pretzels and granola bars do not fit into your balanced plate. Limit these if you want optimal health and weight loss. If you do eat them, give up something in the "grain" section of your plate and increase physical activity to compensate for the extra calories.

Healthy Lunch Or Dinner Plate
(Mediterranean-style)

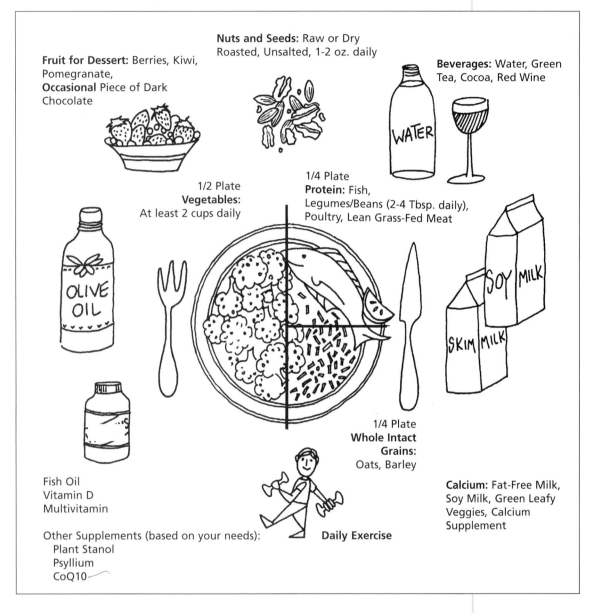

Fruit for Dessert: Berries, Kiwi, Pomegranate, **Occasional** Piece of Dark Chocolate

Nuts and Seeds: Raw or Dry Roasted, Unsalted, 1-2 oz. daily

Beverages: Water, Green Tea, Cocoa, Red Wine

1/2 Plate
Vegetables:
At least 2 cups daily

1/4 Plate
Protein: Fish, Legumes/Beans (2-4 Tbsp. daily), Poultry, Lean Grass-Fed Meat

OLIVE OIL

WATER

SOY MILK

SKIM MILK

1/4 Plate
Whole Intact Grains:
Oats, Barley

Fish Oil
Vitamin D
Multivitamin

Other Supplements (based on your needs):
  Plant Stanol
  Psyllium
  CoQ10

Daily Exercise

Calcium: Fat-Free Milk, Soy Milk, Green Leafy Veggies, Calcium Supplement

Let's give it a try. Imagine that you are dining out and ordering the grilled chicken sandwich:

- ❖ **1/4 protein:** grilled chicken filet
- ❖ **1/4 starch/grain:** bun, ideally whole grain but the best you can do in most restaurants is "wheat" with some whole grains, but this still consists mostly of white flour.
- ❖ **1/2 vegetable and salad:** Yes, that piece of iceberg lettuce, tomato and perhaps a pickle are a start, but don't quite add up to what is healthy. You could order a side salad or a bowl of vegetable lentil soup. Or, pick a snack that fills in the missing part of the plate by having some carrots, tomatoes or an apple. If you chose pretzels or a low-fat granola bar for a snack, they would add to the grains section which further unbalances your plate.

Let's do it again, this time ordering pizza:

- ❖ **1/4 protein:** Cheese is the protein.
- ❖ **1/4 starch/grain:** Crust is the grain.
- ❖ **1/2 vegetable and salad:** If you have a veggie pizza and you measured all those onions, mushrooms and peppers, you might have a couple tablespoons, at best. Have a few less slices of pizza and add a big salad. You get the idea.

Breakfast Plate

Picture your plate as three equal sections and fill them with:
- ❖ **Protein and good fats:** soy milk, skim milk, yogurt, reduced-fat cheese, eggs, egg whites or egg substitute. Fats such as nut butters and chopped nuts or seeds such as flax.
- ❖ **Whole grains:** Oatmeal (steel-cut or old-fashioned not instant or quick), Muesli, cooked grains such as brown rice
- ❖ **Fruit:** Fresh preferred, frozen or canned without sugars are acceptable.

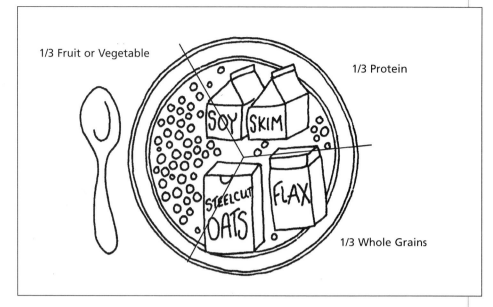

1/3 Fruit or Vegetable

1/3 Protein

1/3 Whole Grains

Tips To Make Your Plate Healthier

❖ Choose healthier fats. Instead of butter, shortening or margarine, use extra-virgin olive oil, high oleic safflower or an expeller-pressed canola oil.

❖ Go easy on red meat. If you do eat it, look for 100% grass-fed meat or wild game. Choose more poultry than beef, lamb, veal or pork.

❖ Choose low mercury, high omega-3 fish such as wild salmon, sablefish, sardines or herring several times a week. Wild fish is preferred over farmed. Skip fish that are battered, breaded or deep fried.

❖ If you eat meat, include a few meatless meals each week. Include plant protein sources from legumes, dry beans and lentils. Lentil soup or hummus sandwiches are easy for lunch.

❖ Fill half your plate with dark green, leafy vegetables such as spinach, kale, broccoli and rapini, along with deep orange vegetables such as butternut squash, sweet potatoes and carrots.

❖ Include a big, green, leafy salad daily with either lunch or dinner. Make the salad with the darkest greens, such as romaine or spinach. Top it with a dressing, preferably one you made with vinegar and olive oil (see recipe Page 371). Add some garbanzo beans, avocado and chopped nuts to the salad. Skip the croutons, bacon bits, cheese and creamy, French or fat-free dressings.

❖ Switch from processed, packaged, manufactured snacks such as pretzels, granola bars and low-fat cookies to foods as close to their natural form as possible Foods such as fresh or dried fruits, vegetables, raw nuts like almonds and walnuts, and pumpkin seeds make great snacks.

- ❖ Explore cooking with whole grains, such as barley, quinoa, brown rice or bulgur for side dishes, salads and soups. Make most of your grain choices whole, intact grains instead of foods made from ground-up grains (flour). Check the recipe sections to get started.
- ❖ When you do choose foods made from flour, such as breads, crackers, granola bars, etc. make sure the first ingredient listed states "whole" before the grain and does not have any **partially hydrogenated** oils or **high fructose corn syrup** listed.
- ❖ Choose whole foods with the least amount of processing possible, such as an apple instead of applesauce or apple juice. Try steel-cut oats or old-fashioned rolled oats or rolled barley instead of instant oats or highly processed oatmeal breakfast bars.
- ❖ Enjoy fruit for dessert rather than the processed, low-fat manufactured treats. Berries are especially good choices. For a splurge, add some dark chocolate that is at least 70 percent cocoa.
- ❖ If you drink alcohol, limit it to no more than one or two servings a day. Drink alcohol with your meal and don't "bank it" for a weekend splurge.
- ❖ Slow down your pace of eating. Take time to savor and enjoy your food. How you eat is as important as what you are eating. Avoid eating in the car, in front of the TV or at your desk. Don't eat food that is disappointing just because it is in front of you. Never feel guilty about eating a food you enjoy. If you eat with others, don't discuss unpleasant topics at dinner; save them for another time.
- ❖ Find ways to be more physically active. Turn off the TV and follow the long-standing tradition of the Italians who enjoy the *passeggiata* ("little walk") a leisurely evening stroll through the streets and plazas before or after dinner.

The Studies That Support Plant-Based Eating

Plant-based diets include the Mediterranean diet, DASH diet and the Portfolio diet. Plant foods seem to be especially good for heart health.

The Dietary Approaches to Stop Hypertension trial **(DASH)** diet[23] found that a diet rich in fruits (four to six servings) and vegetables (four to six servings), was more effective in lowering blood pressure than sodium restriction alone. The DASH diet also lowered LDL cholesterol by 9 percent. (See Page 194)

A **Mediterranean**-style diet was studied by two French scientists in the Lyon Diet Heart Study. Those following the Mediterranean diet had 30 to 73 percent less deaths from heart disease.[24] The diet is associated with lower levels of inflammation and blood-clotting markers.

Portfolio Diet. Several studies found that a diet that included a portfolio of four healthy plant foods was as effective in lowering cholesterol as taking drugs.[25,26] It included almonds, soy, soluble fiber and plant phytosterols. See Page 56 for sample menu plans.

In the **Family Heart Study**,[27] the fruit and vegetable intake of men and women and its affect on LDL was studied. The more fruits and vegetables they ate, the more LDL decreased. This lower LDL blood cholesterol was seen regardless of age, activity level or smoking status.

The **Polymeal Study**[28] included more plant foods, including fish and almost a pound of fruits and vegetables daily, and was able to cut the risk of heart disease by an amazing 76 percent while significantly increasing the life expectancy of people over age 50.

The **INTERHEART Study**[29] found that regular fruit and vegetable intake cut risk for heart attack by 30 percent over those who seldom ate fruits and vegetables.

28% calories from fat, 2.7% calories from saturated fat, 1,386 mg sodium, 54 grams of fiber, 15 grams soluble fiber, 1.5 grams plant phytosterols, 31 grams soy protein

FOOD ITEM	Phytosterol Goal: 1.5 g or 1,500 mg	Soluble Fiber Goal: 13 g	Almonds Goal: 21 g or 3/4 ounce	Soy Protein Goal: 34 g
BREAKFAST				
Cooked steel-cut oats 1/2 cup		1.0 g		
1/2 apple, chopped	5 mg	0.7 g		
Almond, chopped, 2 Tbsp.	20 mg	0.3 g	7.5 g	
Ground flax, 2 Tbsp.		1.3 g		
Plain soy milk, 1/2 cup	*			3 g
Benecol stanol smart chew (1)	850 mg			
SNACK				
Almonds, whole, 6	6 mg	0.5 g	7.5 g	
Shake: 1 cup soy milk				
1/2 cup strawberries	10 mg			6 g
LUNCH				
Vegetable soup, 1 cup		0.8 g		
Add to soup:				
1/4 cup cooked barley		0.7 g		
2 Tbsp. lentils	62 mg	0.3 g		
1/2 cup frozen veggies	12 mg	1.6 g		
Whole-wheat bread, 1 slice		0.5 g		
with 2 Tbsp. hummus		0.4 g		
1 pear	7 mg	0.8 g		
SNACK				
1 orange	17 mg	2 g		
Almonds, whole, 6	6 mg	0.5 g	7.5 g	
DINNER				
Broccoli, 1 cup		1.3 g		
Boca Burger (meatless)	*			10 g
Sweet potato fries (1/2 potato)	8mg	0.8 g		
1-1/2 tsp. olive oil				
1/2 cup baby carrots		1.3 g		
SNACK				
1/4 cup soy nuts	*	1 g		12 g
Benecol stanol smart chew (1)	850 mg			

Soy foods contain phytosterols but the amounts vary by processing methods used.

The Portfolio Diet included the following per 1,000 calories
- 9 grams soluble fiber
- 23 grams soy protein
- 14 grams almonds
- 1 gram plant phytosterols (stanols)

PORTFOLIO DIET

Including four healthy plant foods can be as effective as taking drugs.

NUTRITION NOTE

21 grams almond equals about
- 18 whole almonds
- 4 tsp. almond butter
- 3 Tbsp. sliced almonds

13

Fat

There are many types of fat. The diagram below illustrates how we classify types of fat.

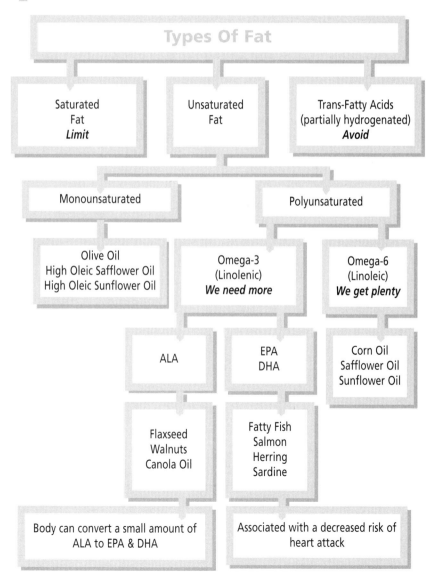

Types Of Fat

| Saturated Fat *Limit* | Unsaturated Fat | Trans-Fatty Acids (partially hydrogenated) *Avoid* |

Monounsaturated — Polyunsaturated

Olive Oil
High Oleic Safflower Oil
High Oleic Sunflower Oil

Omega-3
(Linolenic)
We need more

Omega-6
(Linoleic)
We get plenty

ALA

EPA
DHA

Corn Oil
Safflower Oil
Sunflower Oil

Flaxseed
Walnuts
Canola Oil

Fatty Fish
Salmon
Herring
Sardine

Body can convert a small amount of ALA to EPA & DHA

Associated with a decreased risk of heart attack

NUTRITION NOTE

For heart health, **limit** the amount of saturated fat, **eliminate** partially hydrogenated fats, and eat the correct **balance** of omega-3 and omega-6 essential fatty acids.

For years now, some "experts" have been telling us, "eat a low-fat diet to prevent heart disease." However, research has shown that this simple statement is incorrect. Restricting total fat does little to reduce cholesterol. The Women's Health Initiative, involving 48,000 postmenopausal women, ages 50 to 79, found that lowering fat to 20 percent or less did little to protect against heart disease and cancer.[33]

The Mediterranean diet is not low fat, yet in studies, those following it had a significantly lower overall death rate than those on the traditional, low-fat diet.

Determining the optimal amount of total fat and its link to diseases has not been established. It appears that the type of fat and the balance of fatty acids – not the amount of fat – are what provide the health benefits. What does have an impact is reducing bad fats and replacing them with healthy fats in the correct balance.

A certain amount of fat is necessary for health. Essential fats must come from foods since our body can't produce them.

We need to get re-acquainted with fat. It is time to move away from seeking low fat and focus on the type of fat we eat. All fats are not the same and only certain types of fats are linked to heart disease. There are good fats. Good fats lower your risk for heart disease and are essential to good health. Good fats to focus on that are often missing in a typical American diet are monounsaturated and omega-3 fats. There are also bad fats. These increase your risk for heart disease. For heart health, limit the amount of saturated fat, eliminate partially hydrogenated fats, and eat the correct balance of omega-3 and omega-6 essential fatty acids.

As you decrease saturated fat and eliminate trans fats, you might wonder what should replace those calories. Should it be carbohydrates as in low-fat diets? Should it be protein, such as the high-protein diets, or healthy fat as in the Mediterranean-type diet? The OmniHeart Study[35] looked at these questions to see how carbohydrate, protein and monounsaturated fat affected blood pressure and cholesterol. This study found that replacing saturated fat with either lean protein or healthy fat was even better than replacing saturated fat with carbohydrate.

The fats and oils in foods are combinations of saturated, polyunsaturated and monounsaturated fats. They are classified according to which fat exists in the highest amount. In the chart below, notice that both olive and canola oil have some saturated fat, but since they have more monounsaturated than saturated or polyunsaturated fats, they are classified as monounsaturated fats. Corn oil contains both polyunsaturated and monounsaturated fats but is classified as polyunsaturated which is the largest amount.

Types of Fat in Oils			
	Monounsaturated	Polyunsaturated	Saturated
Olive oil	10.7 grams	1.4 grams	1.9 grams
Canola oil	8.2 grams	4.1 grams	1 gram
Corn oil	3.4 grams	8.3 grams	1.8 grams
Coconut oil	0.08 grams	0.02 grams	12 grams

Fat Smart 4 Your Heart

TABLE 13.1
Fatty Acids In Various Oils and Fats

1 TABLESPOON	UNSATURATED FAT			SATURATED FAT
	Monounsaturated Fat	Polyunsaturated Fat		
		Omega-3	Omega-6	
Monounsaturated				
Avocado Oil	9.9	0.13	1.7	1.6
Almond Oil	9.5	0	2.4	1.1
Canola Oil	8.2	1.30	2.8	0.9
Hazelnut Oil	10.6	0	1.4	1.0
Macadamia Oil	11.0	0	0.3	2.2
Olive Oil	10.7	0.10	1.3	1.9
Peanut Oil	6.2	0	4.3	2.3
Rice Bran Oil	5.3	0.22	4.5	2.6
Sesame Oil	5.4	0.04	5.6	1.9
Sunflower Oil >70% oleic	11.7	0.03	0.5	1.3
Safflower Oil, high oleic, *Spectrum High Heat*	11.0	0	2.0	1.0
Tea Seed Oil	7.0	0.10	3.0	2.9
Omega-3				
Flax Oil	2.7	7.20	1.7	1.2
Polyunsaturated more omega-6 than omega-3				
Corn Oil	3.7	0.15	7.4	2.0
Cottonseed Oil	2.4	0.03	7.0	3.5
Grapeseed Oil	2.1	0.01	10.0	1.3
Hemp Oil	1.68	2.90	8.2	1.1
Poppyseed Oil	2.7	0	8.5	2.0
Pumpkin Seed	5	2.00	6.0	1.0
Safflower Oil	1.9	0	10.0	0.8
Sunflower Oil	2.6	0	9.0	1.4
Soybean Oil	3.1	0.90	6.9	1.9
Walnut Oil	3.1	1.40	7.2	1.2
Wheat Germ Oil	2.0	0.90	7.4	2.5
Saturated				
Butter	2.9	0.04	0.4	7.2
Coconut Oil	0.8	0	0.2	12.0
Lard	5.7	0.13	1.3	5.0
Palm Kernel Oil	1.5	0	0.22	11.0
Palm Oil	5.0	0.3	1.2	6.7

NUTRITION NOTE

Fats and oils are a mixture of monounsaturated, polyunsaturated and saturated fatty acids.

NUTRITION NOTE

Pumpkin seed and hemp oil provide some omega-3 but contain more omega-6 than omega-3

High-oleic safflower has more monounatuated than ordinary safflower oil.

Source: Nutritional information calculated using The Food Processor software by ESHA Research, Salem, OR., and product Web sites.

TABLE 13.2
THE TYPE OF FAT AND THE EFFECT IT HAS ON YOUR HEART

Type of Fat	Effect on Heart	Sources
Monounsaturated Healthy fats	Protects heart Lowers LDL, raises HDL when they replace saturated or trans fats	❍ Olive oil ❍ Canola oil ❍ Nuts, nut oils, natural peanut butter ❍ Avocado ❍ High-oleic safflower oil ❍ High-oleic sunflower oil
Polyunsaturated Omega-3 EPA, DHA	Protects heart, raises HDL, lowers LDL if replacing saturated fat or trans fats	❍ Fish – wild salmon, trout, herring, sardine ❍ Fish oil supplement
Polyunsaturated Omega-3 ALA	Protects heart, raise HDL and lower LDL Body converts small amount to EPA and DHA	❍ Flax ❍ Walnuts
Polyunsaturated Omega-6 needed but unhealthy when too high, must balance with Omega-3	Lowers HDL Lowers LDL	❍ Corn oil ❍ Safflower oil ❍ Sunflower oil ❍ Soybean oil ❍ Grapeseed oil
Saturated There are various types of saturated fat that differ in effects on cholesterol	Promotes heart disease Raises LDL, raises HDL, but not enough to offset the increase in LDL Lauric and myristic increase cholesterol more than palmitic	❍ Red meat, beef/pork, deli meats, sausage, hot dogs ❍ Butter, cheese ❍ Whole, 2% milk ❍ Coconut oil ❍ Palm oil ❍ Palm kernel oil
Saturated	Stearic acid neutral effect on cholesterol	❍ Cocoa butter
Trans-Fatty Acids **Trans Fats**	Promotes heart disease Lowers HDL Raises LDL	❍ Many packaged foods ❍ Any food that lists partially hydrogenated oil in ingredient list ❍ Margarine (unless it is non-hydrogenated) ❍ Shortening ❍ Fried foods in restaurants
Interesterified	Very little information available Chemically modified May have health risks more harmful than partially hydrogenated	❍ Oils listed as hydrogenated or fully hydrogenated may go through interesterification ❍ Some liquid oils are interesterified ❍ Some non-hydrogenated margarines and oils use it
Fractionated	Mechanically modified. Little information — same as saturated fat	❍ Oil is heated, cooled, separated ❍ Saturated fat increases

NUTRITION NOTE

1/3 of the saturated fat in cocoa butter is in a form that does not raise blood cholesterol.

TABLE 13.3
CHOOSING FATS

Best Choice (monounsaturated and omega-3)
Maintain portion control if you need to lose weight. These oils still have 120 calories per tablespoon!

- Liquid oils that have not been partially hydrogenated
  - Olive oil
  - Canola oil
  - Peanut oil
  - Avocado oil
  - Rice bran oil
  - High-oleic sunflower oil
  - High-oleic safflower oil
  - Almond oil
  - Hazelnut oil
  - Macadamia oil
  - Tea seed oil
- Avocado
- Canola oil mayonnaise
- Fish fat (but not fat in breaded or fried fish)
- Flaxseed
- Flax oil (not for use in cooking with heat)
- Natural peanut butter, sunflower butter, almond butter
- Nuts, raw or dry roasted, unsalted
- Olives (go easy, contain sodium)

Good Choice (foods rich in Omega-6 oil)

- Soy foods, such as tofu, roasted soy nuts, canned soybeans, tempeh, soy milk
- Sesame seeds
- Sunflower seeds

Replace these Omega-6 oils with healthier monounsaturated when possible.
(These may increase inflammation and most people get more than they need. Balance of omega-6 and omega-3 is the key.)

- Corn oil
- Soybean oil
- Grapeseed oil
- Sunflower oil
- Safflower oil
- Cottonseed oil
- Sesame oil
- Mayonnaise and salad dressings made with omega-6 oils

Moderation (saturated) to fit within your saturated fat allowance

- Butter and butter canola oil blends
- Palm oil, red palm oil, palm kernel oil and coconut oil (if saturated fat is less than 3 grams for the amount you will eat)
- Lean cuts of pork, beef, lamb, goat, sheep (choose 100% grass fed)
- Wild game, buffalo, emu, ostrich
- Poultry, choose free range or poultry fed omega-3 rich diets
- Eggs, enriched with omega-3
- Cheese, reduced-fat cottage cheese, reduced-fat yogurt
- Dark chocolate (choose 70% cocoa or higher or those that have processed to maintain flavanols)
- Coconut

Limit These (saturated)

- Dairy full-fat milk, cream, full-fat yogurt, regular cottage cheese, full-fat cream cheese, processed cheese,
- Fatty, marbled cuts of beef, pork, lamb and beef that is angus, prime, chuck
- Poultry skin, meat fat
- Sausage, hot dogs, bacon, fatty ground meat

AVOID the following. No amount of trans fat is healthy.

- Interesterified, hydrogenated or fully hydrogenated fats
- Partially hydrogenated listed by any fat. Avoid, even if one of the "good" fats, such as partially hydrogenated olive oil
- Shortening
- Deep-fried foods or oils that are used more than once
- Foods that state no trans fats but contain partially hydrogenated in the ingredient list

NUTRITION NOTE

No amount of trans fat is healthy.

CHOOSING OILS

In the oil section of the supermarket, you will find a wide selection of liquid oils. Liquid oils all contain small amounts of saturated fat and no trans fats. Oils are not required by law to list the grams of monounsaturated and polyunsaturated fats, although many will provide this information. None are required to list the amount of omega-3 or omega-6, and few will provide that information. Refer to the table 13.1 (Page 59) if you want that information.

Olive Oil

Olive oil is recognized for its many health benefits. It is considered by many as the healthiest oil you can buy. The FDA has allowed the qualified health claim that states:

> *"Limited and not conclusive scientific evidence suggests that eating about 2 tablespoons (23 grams) of olive oil daily may reduce the risk of coronary heart disease due to the monounsaturated fat in olive oil. To achieve this possible benefit, olive oil is to replace a similar amount of saturated fat and not increase the total number of calories you eat in a day. ...."*

NUTRITION NOTE

Replace 2 tablespoons of butter *(or other saturated fat)* with 2 tablespoons of olive oil to reduce the risk of heart disease.

What's The Best Olive Oil?

There is much confusion and mystery as to which olive oil to buy, how to cook with them, and how to store them. You will find conflicting recommendations if you ask several different experts. With so many bottles, a wide range of prices, and so many claims, how do you choose?

All types of olive oil contain heart healthy monounsaturated fat. However, only the extra-virgin varieties have the unique health benefits from the many components, such as tocopherols with vitamin E activity, hydrocarbons like squalene that are thought to have anti-cancer properties, sterols which may lower cholesterol, and plant phenols that are powerful antioxidants. To obtain the most health benefits, use extra-virgin olive oil. Avoid using extra-virgin olive oil with high-heat cooking since it will lose some of the benefits when heated to high temperatures.

Good, quality extra-virgin olive oil is not inexpensive to produce, but you don't have to purchase the most expensive. The best is the one you enjoy since we all have different tastes.

Since pure olive oil has a higher smoke point than extra-virgin and is high oleic (monounsaturated) and low in omega-6 linoleic acid, it would be a good choice for high-heat sautéing. Another option for higher heat is using canola oil or high oleic sunflower oil, designed for high heat. Even better is not to cook at high heat which will be discussed later.

NUTRITION NOTE

Choose extra-virgin olive oil for the most health benefits.

"Extra Light" or "Light" olive oil is refined oil. It is not lower in fat or calories.

Storage of olive oil

❖ For best flavor, use within three months after opening; however, it will be okay for 12 to 18 months. Choose the size bottle that you can use within this period of time. Extra-virgin olive oil has the least acidity.
As the oil is exposed to heat, air and light, it becomes more acidic and shelf life is shortened.

❖ Original bottles should be dark green or brown glass or wrapped in foil to keep out light. If you want to put the oil in a container for ease in pouring, choose a container that is dark glass, terra cotta or nonreactive metal (copper and iron are reactive) to protect the oil from the light. Do not use plastic as the oil may taste like plastic.

❖ Keep bottles tightly capped to decrease exposure to air.

❖ Store it in a pantry that is cool and dark. The cupboard you choose should be away from the heat of appliances or direct sunlight.

❖ Refrigeration causes condensation that will drip back into the oil and diminish the flavor of extra-virgin olive oil. Do not refrigerate unless you are instructed to do so on the bottle, as some dipping oils suggest.

Canola oil

Canola oil, like olive oil, is high in monounsaturated fat and one of the lowest in saturated fat, making it heart healthy. Like olive oil, it has been allowed to use an FDA health claim statement. It has a neutral flavor making it an all-purpose oil, especially when the strong flavor of extra-virgin olive oil is not desired. Look for expeller-pressed canola oil.

There is no current scientific evidence that canola is harmful to humans. These statements are based on misinformation and unsubstantiated rumors about rapeseed oils; an oil used long ago which is not related to the canola oil you buy in the store today. Canola oil was developed from natural cross-breeding (hybridization) from the rapeseed plant and does not contain euric acid.

High oleic oils

High oleic sunflower and high oleic safflower oils are higher in monounsaturated oils than standard safflower and sunflower which are high in linoleic or polyunsaturated fat.

What about heating oils at home?

Frying foods at home is not recommended since heat destroys nutrients and high heat may release HNE (4-hydroxy-trans-2-nonenal) a highly toxic compound. Polyunsaturated oils rich in omega-6 linoleic fatty acids, such as corn, soybean, sunflower and cottonseed, release especially high amounts of this toxin. It is then absorbed by foods in the same concentration as found in the oils. HNE is related to several diseases such a heart disease, stroke, Parkinson's, Alzheimer's and liver diseases. Saturated fats, which are low in linoleic (omega-6), do not release HNE; however, saturated fats are not heart healthy. Oils high in oleic or monounsaturated fats and low in linoleic,

NUTRITION NOTE

"Cold pressed," seen on some olive oils is a largely unregulated description in the U.S. This may change as the California Olive Oil Council has petitioned the USDA to revise current standards for olive oils to reflect those used by the International Olive Oil Council (IOOC).

Extra-virgin olive oil is cold pressed.

expeller-pressed

Oil is extracted mechanically by crushing rather than using chemicals.

such as macadamia oil, do not release HNE but are expensive.

Keep oils at a moderate temperature when cooking at home. In general, the less you heat oils or foods with oils, the healthier they are. If the oil starts to smoke, throw it away and start over.

Oils subjected to high heat become oxidized. These oxidized fats are absorbed in the intestines packaged as chylomicrons and transported to the liver where they are repackaged as VLDL cholesterol particles. As oxidized fats are increased in the diet, it alters lipid metabolism, increases the amount of oxidized LDL, and raises the risk of heart disease. It is best to add the oil for flavor at the end of the cooking process. Use a quarter cup of liquid, broth or water in your pan to cook food, add a small amount of extra virgin oil when done, stir and serve.

Tips For Eating A Healthy Balance Of Fats

❖ Limit saturated fat.

❖ Eliminate partially hydrogenated/trans fats.

◆ Cut back on processed foods in packages, bakery items, fried, snack and fast foods.

❖ Choose extra virgin olive oil, high-oleic safflower oil and canola oil as your primary cooking oil instead of corn, soybean or vegetable oil.

◆ Choose a mayonnaise made with olive or canola oil.

Spectrum Essentials, Kraft Mayo With Olive Oil and Smart Balance Omega Plus contain canola oil. Sometimes these healthier products are in the natural food sections of the grocery store. Some may also be found in health food stores.

◆ Switch to a margarine without partially hydrogenated fat made with canola oil. (*Spectrum Spread* is located in the health food sections of the grocery store or in health food stores.)

◆ Combine butter with olive or canola oil in a 50:50 ratio, blend and store in the refrigerator. You may find this combination in the store as *Spreadable Butter* with canola oil by *Land O'Lakes*.

◆ If you eat the yolk of eggs, choose eggs from chickens that were fed special diets of flax or algae to increase the omega-3. (*Eggland* is one such brand).

◆ Make your own vinaigrette dressing using extra-virgin olive oil or canola oil. See Page 371 for a recipe.

Fat Smart 4 Your Heart

❖ Eat fish more often.

- ◆ Have canned, wild salmon on your salad. Make it into a spread, put it on pizza, or try smoked salmon (lox) for breakfast (go easy on lox due to sodium content).

- ◆ Have a snack of sardines served on whole-wheat toast. (There are low-sodium varieties available.)

- ◆ Eat herring for an appetizer.

- ◆ When eating out for lunch, have tuna salad. At home, when making tuna salad, use canned wild salmon instead of tuna. It is richer in omega-3. Use canola or olive oil mayonnaise.

- ◆ Order grilled salmon when dining out.

- ◆ Substitute canned, wild salmon whenever tuna is suggested in a recipe or buy troll-caught albacore tuna. Both of these are lower in mercury than traditional canned tuna.

- ◆ Try anchovies on a veggie pizza. Ask for half the amount of cheese, try it with no cheese, or use a light sprinkle of Parmesan.

- ◆ Sprinkle ground flax on your breakfast cereal, salad or yogurt.

❖ Include ground flaxseed. See Page 116 for more ideas on including flax, the plant source of omega-3.

❖ When choosing nuts, walnuts are highest in omega-3.

❖ Eat more dark green vegetables such as kale, romaine, rapini, cabbage, brussel sprouts, bok choy and broccoli. These have small amounts of omega-3, but it all adds up.

❖ Add avocado and walnuts to your salad.

Fat Quiz

1. Pick the two oils that are best to use in cooking for heart health.
   - ❏ olive
   - ❏ peanut
   - ❏ canola
   - ❏ soybean

2. Most Americans get too much omega-6 and not enough omega-3 fats.
   - ❏ T   ❏ F

3. Very low-fat diets are the best choice for a healthy heart.
   - ❏ T   ❏ F

4. Frying foods is healthy if the right oils are used.
   - ❏ T   ❏ F

5. Extra-virgin olive oil is best kept:
   - ❏ refrigerated
   - ❏ in the cupboard
   - ❏ above the stovetop

6. Saturated fat occurs in foods naturally and, therefore, can never be completely avoided.
   - ❏ T   ❏ F

7. Some trans fat from partially hydrogenated oils may be included in a heart healthy diet.
   - ❏ T   ❏ F

8. Which oils are polyunsaturated?
   - ❏ corn
   - ❏ olive
   - ❏ sunflower
   - ❏ soybean
   - ❏ safflower
   - ❏ canola
   - ❏ grapeseed

9. Butter is:
   - ❏ saturated   ❏ monounsaturated   ❏ polyunsaturated

10. Olive oil is:
    - ❏ saturated   ❏ monounsaturated   ❏ polyunsaturated

ANSWERS
On Page 279.

Saturated Fat

14

Eating too much saturated fat may raise your LDL cholesterol. Saturated fat raises your blood cholesterol more than eating cholesterol-rich foods. On Page 16 you can calculate your daily allowance of saturated fat. Cutting saturated fat by 5 percent of total calories (11 grams less for a 2,000-calorie diet) and replacing it with the same amount of unsaturated fat may reduce LDL by about 7percent. Men eating the least saturated fat, according to the Health Professionals Follow-Up Study,[37] cut their risk of heart attack by more than 40 percent over those who ate the most saturated fat.

If your cholesterol is only slightly elevated, a reduction in saturated fat may lower LDL enough with diet alone. Even if diet is not enough to reduce your cholesterol to the desired goal, limiting saturated fat means you need less drugs. Saturated fat is found in beef, poultry, pork, lamb, veal, fish, milk and other dairy products such as cheese, unless they are skim or nonfat dairy. The leaner the cut of meat, the less saturated fat it contains.

Estimating Saturated Fat In Food
(Meat, Poultry, Fish, Cheese)

When you purchase foods without a nutrition facts label, it is difficult to determine how much saturated fat you are getting. Use these guidelines to estimate saturated fat when they do not have a nutrition facts label.

One-half (0.5) gram or less saturated fat per ounce cooked

- ❖ Lean fish, baked or broiled, not breaded
- ❖ Shellfish, not fried
- ❖ Poultry (breast, no skin)
- ❖ Ground turkey breast, all white meat
- ❖ 96% or higher lean ground meat
- ❖ Deli meats 96% or higher lean (high in sodium and nitrates)
- ❖ Wild game, venison, elk, rabbit

NUTRITION NOTE

How much fat is saturated fat?
- 2/3 of fat in cheese
- almost 1/2 of the fat in ground beef
- 1/3 of fat in beef and pork
- 1/4 of fat in poultry
- 1/5 of fat in fish

One gram saturated fat per ounce cooked

- ❖ Beef and pork, round and loin cuts (trim all visible fat before cooking), USDA choice or select grade
- ❖ 90-93% lean ground meat
- ❖ Ground buffalo burgers in restaurants
- ❖ Goose, domestic duck, pheasant with skin, raccoon, bear
- ❖ Salmon
- ❖ Sardines, herring

Two grams saturated fat per ounce cooked

- ❖ Beef and pork, USDA prime grade meat or certified angus
- ❖ Restaurant steaks (USDA prime grade)
- ❖ Beef and pork (most cuts other than round and loin such as chuck)
- ❖ Dark meat poultry
- ❖ Ground chuck
- ❖ Ground turkey (not from the breast)
- ❖ Deli meats (high in sodium and nitrates)
- ❖ 80-85% lean ground meat

Three grams saturated fat per ounce cooked

- ❖ Ribs
- ❖ Sausage, venison, bratwurst, bologna, liverwurst
- ❖ Regular ground beef, hamburger
- ❖ Hot dogs (high in sodium and nitrates)
- ❖ Fried fish
- ❖ Fried poultry
- ❖ Reduced-fat cheese (part-skim mozzarella, 2% reduced-fat)

Six grams saturated fat per ounce

- ❖ Regular cheese (cheddar, Swiss, colby, etc.)

NUTRITION NOTE

It takes ten pounds of whole milk to make one pound of regular cheese.

Coconut Oil

Recently, extra-virgin coconut oil has been promoted as a weight loss aid because it is a source of medium-chain triglycerides and a source of lauric acid. Lauric acid is transformed into monolaurin in the body and may have some health benefits such as slowing the growth of bacteria, viruses or parasites. In lab studies, it seems to protect against liver damage. Lauric acid is a saturated fat that does raise blood cholesterol. Until there is conclusive evidence of benefits, it should be treated as other saturated fats in the diet. Diets rich in omega-3 fats and low in processed carbohydrates can contain more saturated fat without adverse effects on health. Small amounts of coconut oil may be useful as a replacement in processed foods for partially hydrogenated oils. If saturated fat per serving is not more than three grams, these can usually be a part of a healthy diet in moderation.

15

Meat

I f you don't eat red meat, skip this chapter. If you are thinking about cutting red meat from your diet, you can be assured that it is possible to get all the nutrients necessary for good health without it. There have been studies that link red meat with an increased risk for heart disease, rheumatoid arthritis and several cancers, such as colorectal cancer. Some studies have found a risk between the type of iron found in meat and heart disease.[38, 39] One of the healthiest ways of eating is the Mediterranean diet. It includes red meat only a few times per month.

Lean Red Meat and Cancer Risk

Choosing lean cuts of red meat, which have less saturated fat, is heart healthier but may not change the cancer risk. Recent research indicates it may be the heme iron and myoglobin from red meat that are the potential factors linking red meat and cancer.

If you choose to include small amounts of red meat in your diet, you may also want to consider where the meat came from, how it was raised, and how the animals and the environment were treated when making your choices.

Is White Meat Healthier Than Red Meat?

Chicken and fish are "white" meat because they have less myoglobin. The amount of myoglobin varies with the amount of use the animal's muscles get. For example, chickens have darker meat in their legs and thighs but not their breasts because they do very little flying. Wild birds and ducks that fly often have darker breast meat.

"The other white meat" is an advertising claim used by the National Pork Board to position leaner cuts of pork as more desirable with the perception that white meat is healthier. The fact is that pork is classified as red meat along with all livestock, such as veal, lamb and beef. Venison, buffalo, caribou, wild boar and "100%" grass-fed beef are also classified as red meat but eat natural diets of grass instead of grains. What animals eat affects the fatty acids and amount of saturated fat in the meat, which is more important than whether it is red or white meat.

NUTRITION NOTE

Pork is classified as red meat along with all livestock, such as veal, lamb and beef.

What About Bison?

Bison farmers often feel that it is unnatural to grain-feed animals and prefer to feed their animals a diet of grass. However, some do grain feed, defending it as necessary to produce a consistent quality year around. This process of grain finishing decreases the nutritional benefits as discussed in chapter 16 and would make it no different than eating grain-fed beef. Seek out bison that is fed absolutely no grain if you want the nutritional advantage.

Bison, 3-1/2 oz. cooked lean meat has . . .		
Fat	**Saturated fat**	**Calories**
2.42 g	0.91 g	143 kcal

Grilling and Broiling Health Risks

Grilling, broiling and pan-fried meat, poultry or fish may produce cancer causing compounds called HCAs (heterocyclic amines). The amino acids in animal protein form HCAs; there are no issues with grilling fruits, vegetables or plant proteins. To decrease amounts, meat can be marinated or partially cooked before grilling to shorten the time exposed to high heat.

Another problem arises when fat drips onto the heat source and cancer causing compounds PAHs (polycyclic aromatic hydrocarbons) are deposited back on the food from smoke and flare-ups. By trimming meat and choosing lean cuts, the amount of these substances may be reduced.

AGEs (Advanced Glycation End Products) are formed when meat is exposed to high heat when grilled, broiled or fried. The concern is that they increase inflammation and have been linked to insulin resistance, diabetes and heart disease. If meat is steamed, boiled or stewed where the heat is lower and plenty of water is used, the AGE level is reduced.

Portions

Even the very leanest cuts of meat provide too much saturated fat if portions are large. Typical servings of meat tend to be much larger than the recommended three ounces; therefore, what appears reasonable on labels or nutrition charts for 3-ounce servings quickly becomes too much in the amounts typically consumed. Large portions of meat on your plate crowd out the inflammation fighting plant foods such as vegetables and fruits.

A typical 8-ounce restaurant serving of prime-cut beef rib steak has 830 calories, 66 grams of fat and 28 grams of saturated fat. The smallest steak at most restaurants is the tenderloin or fillet, but it is still larger than a 3-ounce serving. An average size 6-ounce beef tenderloin steak (prime cut) has 524 calories, 28 grams of fat and 15 grams of saturated fat.

NUTRITION NOTE

Meat cooked with high heat forms compounds (AGEs) which increase inflammation.

NUTRITION NOTE

A typical 8-ounce restaurant serving of prime-cut beef rib steak has 830 calories, 66 grams of fat and 28 grams of saturated fat.

Meat Smart 4 Your Heart

Definitions Of Lean and Extra Lean

Lean

When used on meat labels, lean means a 3.5-ounce serving that has no more than 10 grams of total fat, 4.5 grams or less of saturated fat, and less than 95 milligrams of cholesterol.

Extra Lean

When used on meat labels, extra lean means a 3.5-ounce serving that cannot have more than 5 grams total fat, no more than 2 grams of saturated fat, and less than 95 milligrams cholesterol.

Beef Grades Typically Found In Stores

Prime

These grades are more marbled with many flecks of white fat. They are higher in fat and saturated fat.

Choice

This grade is what is typically found in supermarkets and has less fat than prime or certified angus.

Select

This grade has the least amount of marbling and is tender but less juicy because it has less fat.

Certified Angus Beef

Angus is a breed of cattle. *Certified Angus Beef* is a branding program approved by the USDA to signify quality. Angus or black angus doesn't mean the same thing. Certification is based on the degree of marbling, which is the network of small streaks of fat that runs throughout the meat. It has less marbling than prime but more than choice. The marbling has a finer texture in *certified angus beef*. The fine marbling means the meat is more tender.

Remember that marbled fat equals flavor and tenderness in meats; the more marbling the more tender the meat. If you ask the butcher what the best cut of meat is, he will direct you from a taste standpoint and suggest the higher marbled, higher fat cut rather than a heart healthy choice. The heart healthy options are leaner, but tougher cuts that require moist cooking methods.

Lean Meat Cooking

Meat, poultry and fish traditionally have been cooked with added fat. Your goal in altering meat recipes is to choose your cuts wisely, and then cook and serve them without adding saturated fats, using a healthy fat if needed. Portion control is key. Even lean cuts have saturated fat and when eaten in large servings, it adds up. Too often we think if it is a lean cut, we can eat as much as we want! Tips to guide you:

Beef and pork

1. Buy lean cuts. Look for "round" and "loin." Top round, bottom round, eye of round, sirloin, top loin, tenderloin or filet mignon are lean cuts. Chuck and certified Angus are fattier.
2. PORK: Tenderloin, loin chops, low-fat ham (note sodium in ham is high). Pork that is "moisture enhanced" or "tender" has added water, sodium phosphate and salt, which may increase the sodium in 3 ounces from the 40 milligrams it contains naturally to 300 to 500 milligrams.
3. GROUND MEAT: Choose 95 percent lean or greater (the higher the percent of lean the lower the saturated fat)
4. Trim all visible fat before cooking. You lose two-thirds of the fat when you trim before cooking. If you trim after cooking, only one-third of the fat is lost. If a cut is more marbled, it may be impossible to trim all separable fat because to do so would result in pieces that are smaller than desired.
5. Bake, broil or roast meat on a rack so fat can drip away. However, if a cut is well trimmed, there will be little fat to drain and use of a rack is less important.
6. Broil, grill or stir-fry steaks and chops instead of frying in fat.
7. Pan broil in a dry skillet. Heat the pan over medium, not high heat, for three to four minutes. Rub or brush the food with a little oil. Add the items and allow them to cook undisturbed for four minutes, then turn. They will stick initially but as they cook they will release from the pan. If fat accumulates, remove fat with a paper towel as needed.
8. When browning stew meat or roasts, do not coat with flour or add oil to the pan. The flour coating absorbs fat. Use the same method as #7 above. If the flour is important for thickening the recipe, such as a stew, simply add it with the other ingredients after the meat has browned.
9. Learn to recognize a 3-ounce serving of meat as similar in size to a deck of cards or the palm of your hand. Even lean cuts have saturated fat, so again, portion control is the key. The protein portion of your plate should fill only one-quarter of the plate.

Ground Meat

To remove fat from ground beef and pork, the following technique can be used. Note that it is not helpful to do this to ground meat that is lean, such as ground round or ground sirloin, since it has very little fat. It is effective for ground beef, ground chuck or regular hamburger meat. It does not work for poultry, which instead of releasing fat simply absorbs it.

1. Place ground meat (no salt) in a skillet over medium heat and brown, breaking apart with a spoon. You may also do this in a microwave by placing the meat in a colander set above a dish to collect fat. Remove and break apart several times during the cooking process. (One pound raw yields 12 ounces cooked)
2. Drain fat from the skillet or remove colander and spread on several layers of white, nonrecycled paper towels. Blot the top with more paper towels. Place in strainer set above a dish to collect liquid.
3. Heat about 3 cups of water for a pound of ground meat until hot, but not boiling. (160°F)
4. Pour hot water over the beef to rinse off any remaining fat. Drain and then use de-fatted meat in recipes or freeze for future use. The liquid may also be de-fatted and added to the recipe if liquid is needed.
5. Add spices and seasonings after ground beef has been rinsed.

TABLE 15.1 Ground Meat			
4 ounces raw ground meat	Cal	Fat grams	Sat Fat grams
Ground Beef:			
95% lean ground beef	148	5.7	2.3
93% lean ground beef	160	8	3
90% lean ground beef	194	11	4.5
85% lean ground beef	239	17	6.8
80% lean ground beef	286	23	9.1
73% lean ground beef	350	31	12.4
Ground Poultry			
99% lean ground turkey or turkey breast	114	1	0
93% lean ground turkey	150	7	2.3
90% lean ground turkey	182	11.4	3.5
85% lean ground turkey	220	16	5.0
Ground Pork			
Fresh ground pork	300	24	9
Italian sausage	390	35	13

Information provided in part by the National Cattlemen's Beef Association and the Cattleman's Beef Board.

Nutritional information calculated using The Food Processor software by ESHA Research, Salem, OR and product packages.

Making Soups That Include Meat Or Poultry

When making soup, use a two-step process. Cook the meat, poultry or bones in liquid. Remove the meat and separate and discard any bone and fat. Set meat aside to add later. Refrigerate liquid overnight and then remove and discard hardened fat from the top. Use this de-fatted broth to make the soup, adding fresh vegetables and the cooked meat. You may also use a fat separator as described below.

Gravy

Use a fat separator to make gravy without all the fat. This handy gadget, available at any kitchen supply store, allows you to make gravy without having to chill it first. The fat rises to the top and you can pour off the liquid from the bottom which does not contain the fat. Thicken with a mixture of cornstarch or flour and water.

TABLE 15.2 BEEF CHOICE CUTS

3 oz. cooked	Calories	Total Fat (grams)	Saturated Fat (grams)
Eye round, roast	143	4.0	1.4
Chuck mock tender* steak, broiled	137	4.8	1.4
Chuck blade, roasted	296	21.9	8.7
Chuck clod roast, roasted	184	10.4	3.6
Arm pot roast, braised	263	16.9	6.7
Top blade, broiled	193	10.9	3.5
Bottom round, roasted	169	7.9	2.8
Top sirloin, broiled	186	8.9	3.4
Round tip, roasted	167	7.5	2.7
Sirloin tip, grilled	148	4.8	1.8
Top round, broiled	170	6.0	2.1
95% lean ground beef, pan browned	164	6.4	2.9
Short ribs, braised	400	35.6	15
Rib roast, prime rib, roasted	311	24.7	10.5
T-bone steak short loin, broiled	219	14.6	5.4
Porterhouse steak, broiled	241	17.1	6.3
Tenderloin, or filet mignon choice cut, broiled	196	10.5	4.0
Tenderloin prime cut, broil lean only 1/8" fat	262	18.8	7.5
Value cut shoulder tender petite roast, roasted	154	6.5	2.3
Value cut shoulder center steak, grilled	156	6.9	2.6
Value cut shoulder top lade or flat iron steak, broiled	194	11.5	4.6

*Chuck mock tender also known as chuck eye steak, fish steak, chuck fillet steak, and chuck tender steak.
*Choice cuts trimmed of all visible fat, includes seam and fat marbled within the muscle of the meat.
Source: www.nal.usda.gov/fnic/foodcomp/search/

TABLE 15.3 PORK CUTS

3 oz. cooked	Calories	Total Fat (grams)	Saturated Fat (grams)
Pork tenderloin, broiled	171	6.9	2.5
Boneless sirloin chop, broiled	177	7.3	2.4
Boneless center rib roast, roasted	214	12.8	4.5
Boneless top loin chop, broiled	152	5.2	1.8
Pork center loin chop, broiled	204	11.1	4.0
Sirloin roast, roasted	176	8.0	2.9
Pork center rib chop, broiled	221	13.4	4.9
Top loin roast, roasted	192	9.7	3.5
Blade chop, braised	272	21.1	7.9
Country ribs, braised	279	21.5	7.8

Separable lean and fat, 0" fat on outside, boneless

TABLE 15.4 LAMB

3 oz. cooked	Calories Fat	Total Fat (grams)	Saturated Fat (grams)
Leg	162	6.6	2.3
Arm chops	170	7.7	2.9
Loin chops	184	8.3	3.0
Blade chops	179	9.6	3.4
Rib roast	197	11.3	4.0

TABLE 15.5 VEAL

3 oz. cooked	Calories	Total Fat (grams)	Saturated Fat (grams)
Leg (top round)	100	2.5	1
Loin chop	100	3	1
Shank (fore & hind)	100	3	1
Rib	100	3.5	1
Blade shoulder steak	110	4.5	1.5
Arm shoulder	110	4.5	2
Arm/shoulder steak	110	4.5	2
Sirloin	130	7	3
Patty, breaded	210	12	3.5
Breast	180	13	5

16

Organic Vs. Grass Fed

Claims About How Animals Are Raised and Fed

Many of the claims made on meat and poultry labels are confusing. The only term that is third-party verified is "organic." Other terms such as antibiotic free are defined by the USDA, must be applied for and approved, but do not have a verification system in place. The USDA relies on testimonials and affidavits in the approval process so terms may be used incorrectly. To create even more confusion, there are marketing claims that vary in meaning among different brands and are not defined by the USDA.

"100%" grass-fed

100-percent grass fed means that the animal is fed a lifelong diet consisting of grass/forage. They are raised by rotating through pastures instead of feed lots. In winter, they may eat hay and silage but not grains such as corn and soybeans. They are not grain finished. Grazing is healthier for animals and the environment. Grass-fed animals are leaner, have less marbling and have a "meatier" taste. The amount of saturated fat within the muscle of the animal is two to three times less than that found in the muscle portion of grain-fed animals. The animals tend to be healthier and often do not require antibiotics. They gain weight much more slowly than grain-fed animals. Animals that are 100-percent grass fed and grass finished are difficult to find since many of the animals are fed grain such as corn, flax and oats to "finish" the meat. There is a very small amount of certified organic, grass-fed beef available, probably due to the unavailability of organic grasses. To find 100-percent grass-fed beef, visit your local farmers' markets where you can ask questions about how the animals are raised directly from the farmer or you can search internet sources, checking Web sites such as www.alderspring.com or www.texasgrassfedbeef.com.

NUTRITION NOTE

To find sustainably raised meat, poultry, dairy or eggs, visit www.eatwellguide.org

NUTRITION NOTE

To find 100% grass-fed beef, visit your local farmers' markets where you can ask questions about how the animals are raised directly from the farmer.

Nutritional Advantage Of "100% Grass fed"

Animals that eat only grass will be nutritionally superior. Grass-fed animals are lower in saturated fat, higher in heart healthy omega-3 fatty acids, and higher in conjugated linoleic acid (CLA). One percent of the total fat in grain-fed beef is in the form of omega-3. Grass-fed beef has 7 percent of the total fat as omega-3 (higher is better). These beneficial omega-3 fats are found almost exclusively in the muscle portion of the meat; and therefore, the excess fat should be trimmed from grass-fed animals before cooking. The ratio of omega-3 to omega-6 is also better when animals are eating only grass. Grass fed has an omega-6 to omega-3 ratio of 0.89:1 compared to traditional grain fed with a ratio of 13:1.[41] A ratio closest to 1:1 is most desirable.

Grass feeding not only affects the nutrition of the meat but the milk as well; it is higher in vitamin E.

100% organic

Grass-fed animals that range freely on open land that is not treated with herbicides or pesticides are often not specifically labeled organic, yet it is the most natural way of raising animals.

Organic meat and poultry is raised according to strict guidelines. No antibiotic or hormones are used and the animals must have access to the outdoors but that does not have to be open pastures. They are fed only 100-percent organic-certified grain. Organic grain-fed animals do not have the nutritional benefits found in 100-percent grass-fed animals.

Antibiotic free

Antibiotics are often mixed in animals feed at low levels. Seventy percent of the antibiotics in the U.S. are fed to animals to promote faster growth and to compensate for unhealthy conditions in which the animals live. A human health concern is that the number of antibiotic-resistant bacteria may increase when low doses are used in feed.

Meat that comes from animals that have never been administered antibiotics and that can provide that documentation to the USDA, may carry the label *"no antibiotics administered."* The USDA does not have a system in place to verify the claims about antibiotic use, so it must rely on documents submitted.

In recent years, several large poultry producers claim to have decreased their use of antibiotics. They say they use them only to treat sick birds; or that they no longer use the same antibiotics that are used to treat human diseases.

Choose poultry that states no antibiotics.

NUTRITION NOTE

Organic grain-fed animals do not have the nutritional benefits found in 100% grass-fed animals.

NUTRITION NOTE

Choose poultry that states no antibiotics.

Hormone use in poultry is illegal. Stating no hormones is meaningless.

Meat Smart 4 Your Heart

Hormone Free

The use of hormones in chickens, turkeys and pork is illegal, so stating a product has no hormones is meaningless. However, the statement *"no hormones added, federal regulations prohibit the use of hormones"* may be used. What you really want to know is if they were given antibiotics, and this statement does not answer that question.

Beef is different. There is no such thing as hormone-free beef because the animals produce hormones naturally. However the statement *"no hormones administered"* may appear if enough documentation can be provided to the USDA showing that the animals were never treated with hormones.

What Is Natural Meat Or No Additives?

The term *"natural"* has nothing to do with how an animal was raised or what it was fed. Animals that are fed antibiotics or given hormones may carry a natural label. According to the USDA definition, all fresh meat qualifies as "natural" as long as it does not have any artificial ingredients added to it after processing and is minimally processed.

Game and Exotic Meats

Game meat will have less saturated fat and higher heart healthy fats, such as omega-3 and conjugated linolenic acid (CLA). See Page 78 for nutritional information on wild game.

If you find game on a restaurant menu or in a store, it is ranched or farmed game. The diet they are fed can be free-range grasses but more often it is grain. Grain-fed domesticated game animals will have little of the nutritional benefits of wild game. One source to purchase game-raised, free-range meat is www.wildgame.com.

NUTRITION NOTE

There is no such thing as hormone-free beef because the animals produce hormones naturally.

TABLE 16.1   Game Meat

3 oz. Cooked, Baked, Broiled Unless Noted	Calories	Total Fat (grams)	Saturated Fat (grams)
Antelope	130	2.5	1
Alligator	148	3.0	nd
Bear	220	11.0	3
Bison	120	2.0	1
Beaver	180	5.9	1.7
Buffalo, water	110	1.5	0.5
Deer	130	2.5	1
Venison sausage (1 ounce)	90	8.0	3.5
Duck, domestic, skinless	170	10.0	3.5
Duck, wild, no skin	100	3.5	1
Elk	120	1.5	0.5
Emu, fillet	131	1.9	0.5
Frog legs, fried	290	20	nd
Goose, no skin	200	11.0	4
Goat	120	2.5	1
Moose	110	1.0	0
Ostrich, tenderloin	110	3.0	1
Ostrich, ground	120	2.5	0.9
Pheasant breast, skinless	110	3.0	1
Pheasant, with skin	150	8.0	2.5
Quail, with skin	199	12.0	3.3
Quail, no skin, raw	114	3.3	1.1
Rabbit, stewed, domesticated	170	7.0	2
Rabbit, stewed, wild	150	3.0	1
Raccoon	220	12.0	3.5
Squirrel	150	4.0	0.5
Turkey, wild	160	8.0	nd
Turtle	110	3.0	0.5

nd = no data

Source: www.nal.usda.gov/fnic/foodcomp/search

Game Meat Smart 4 Your Heart

17

Poultry

Poultry usually has less total fat and saturated fat than red meat, especially when the skin is removed prior to eating. Dark meat has more fat than the white meat, but most poultry fat is in the skin. Removing skin is more important than whether the meat is white or dark. How it is prepared is also important. Add a cheese sauce or heavy cream to the poultry and you have increased the saturated fat.

Poultry Facts			
3-1/2 oz. Cooked Roasted	Calories	Total Fat (grams)	Saturated Fat (grams)
Chicken breast no skin	165	3.5	1.0
Chicken breast with skin	197	7.8	2.2
Chicken dark meat, thigh no skin	178	9.2	2.6
Chicken dark meat, thigh with skin	247	15.5	4.3

Source: www.nal.usda.gov/fnic/foodcomp/search

Poultry Terms

Natural

Natural means no artificial ingredients are added during processing. It has nothing to do with how the poultry was raised or if it was fed antibiotics unless specifically stated otherwise.

Cage Free

Chickens raised outside of cages but may still be confined to an enclosed building. Most egg-laying chickens are in cages.

Free Range

Use of this term requires an application and approval from the USDA before adding it on poultry labels, but is not third-party verified. The term *free range* only applies to poultry – not eggs or beef.

For poultry, the USDA states that a free-range animal must be given some access to outdoors but does not specify for how long or what they eat when outdoors. For example, chickens could live in a crowded building that opens onto a concrete slab, hardly the same as chickens allowed to roam the outdoors freely on grass and soil.

Free roaming is used by some to mean that cages are not used; however, it does not mean access to outdoors.

POULTRY

1. Rotisserie chicken is available in many supermarkets. If you remove the skin, you reduce calories and fat since most of the fat is in the skin. Sodium is a problem since poultry is brined with a sodium solution before it reaches the store where someone puts it on the racks to grill. The sodium solution ensures juiciness and helps the skin turn a golden color. It is difficult to know how much sodium is added since the chickens do not come with labels. The chart below indicates the average amount.

1/4 Chicken (White)	Calories	Fat	Saturated Fat	Sodium
With skin	332	18 g	5 g	520-882 mg
Without skin	226	3.3 g	1 g	480-749 mg

Source: Average of company Web sites

2. Broasted is a cooking process that was trademarked by the Broaster Company of Beloit, Wis., in 1954. Chicken is marinated, then seasoned and cooked in a high-pressure fryer which the company claims produces moist chicken with 40 to 70 percent less fat than traditionally fried. The company Web site lists these nutrition facts:

TABLE 17.1 **Broasted Chicken**					
Genuine Broaster Chicken					
	Calories	Fat	Trans Fat	Saturated Fat	Sodium
Breast 6 oz.	315 w/skin	9 g w/skin	0.17 g	2 g	1,360 mg
If skin is removed from breast, calories are 215 and fat is 1.6 grams					
Thigh 4 oz.	289 w/skin	16 g w/skin	0.32 g	4 g	703 mg
If skin removed from thigh, calories are 179 and fat is 6 grams					

Source www.broaster.com

3. Ground turkey *breast* or ground chicken *breast* is only the meat from the breast, no skin. If it does not specify "breast" or "white meat only" and is labeled as ground turkey or ground chicken, it can contain the amount of skin in proportion to what is typically found on poultry.

While they can't legally add additional amounts of skin, the fat content will be higher than ground poultry that is only made from breast meat.

4. Remove skin and visible fat before eating to reduce saturated fat intake. Skin can be removed after cooking. If cooking at home, use a rack or grill where fat can drip off. Don't let the fat drip onto other food. For example, if you place chicken with skin on top of rice, as it bakes the fat in the skin will drip into the rice and be absorbed, defeating the process.

5. There are ways to cook without additional fat. You can bake, roast, broil, microwave, poach, stir-fry or oven-fry. Use these methods instead of deep-frying.

6. Season with herbs and spices instead of salt.

7. If you enjoy crispy breaded chicken, check out the recipe for Oven-Fried Parmesan Chicken Nuggets (Page 404).

TABLE 17.2 **POULTRY**			
3-1/2 oz. cooked	Calories	Total Fat (grams)	Saturated Fat (grams)
Chicken breast, raw	110	1	0
Chicken breast, skinless, roasted	165	3.5	1.0
Chicken thigh, skinless, roasted	178	9.2	2.6
Chicken, fried with skin, dark and light portions	229	13	3.5
Chicken, roasted and skinless, includes dark and light portions	161	6	1.7
Turkey breast, skinless and roasted	100	1.84	0.59
Turkey, dark, skinless and roasted	101	3.8	1.28
Turkey, light and dark, skinless	133	2.82	0.94
Turkey, light and dark, with skin	137	6.16	1.8

Source: www.nal.usda.gov/fnic/foodcomp/search

Saturated Fat, Meat, Poultry Quiz

1. Which has more saturated fat?
   - ❏ ounce of prime rib of beef
   - ❏ ounce of shrimp
   - ❏ ounce of cheddar cheese

2. Salmon is high in saturated fat. ❏ T ❏ F

3. Which are nutritionally red meat?
   - ❏ beef ❏ pork ❏ chicken
   - ❏ veal ❏ turkey ❏ lamb

4. Lean meats may have up to 10 grams of fat and 1-1/2 grams saturated fat in a 3-1/2 ounce serving.
   ❏ T ❏ F

5. Select the leanest ground beef varieties. (2 are correct)
   - ❏ angus ❏ round ❏ sirloin ❏ chuck

6. A large serving of meat is heart healthy if it is a lean cut that is well trimmed and cooked without added fats.
   ❏ T ❏ F

7. Organic beef is 100% grass-fed. ❏ T ❏ F

8. It is illegal to give poultry:
   - ❏ antibiotics ❏ hormones

9. If a chicken is labeled "natural," it is your guarantee that it has not been fed antibiotics. ❏ T ❏ F

10. Game meats are lower in saturated fat. ❏ T ❏ F

11. Rotisserie chickens are low in fat and low in sodium if eaten without the skin. ❏ T ❏ F

12. Ground turkey may contain dark meat and skin unless the package states "breast" or "all white meat."
    ❏ T ❏ F

ANSWERS
On Page 279.

13. The term "free range" is FDA regulated for use on:
    - ❏ poultry ❏ eggs ❏ both poultry and eggs

18

Harmful Fat – Trans Fats

As of January 1, 2006, food labels are required to list the amount of trans fat on the nutrition facts label because of the harmful effects of trans fats on our health. You will find the information right below saturated fat on the food label. Trans fats increase the risk of heart disease more than saturated fat. They raise triglycerides and also increase inflammation.[42, 43] Trans fats act like a switch to turn on the liver's production of cholesterol in the form of VLDL which becomes the bad LDL cholesterol, especially the small dense particles and Lp(a).

What Are Trans Fats?

Trans fats are a type of fat created in one of three ways. The first two are man-made and harmful, unlike the third which is natural and protective.

1. When oils are partially hydrogenated, which is stated on ingredient lists.
2. When vegetable oils are refined during a process called deodorization, low levels of trans fat, less than 2 percent, may be created. Only extra-virgin olive oil or vegetable oil that states "unrefined" will not go through the deodorization process. Look for brands such as *Spectrum Naturals* and *Rapunzel* which make some unrefined oils.
3. There is a small amount of natural trans fat which occurs in meat and dairy. Animals (beef, sheep, goat, deer, buffalo, etc.) have micro-organisms in their rumen (stomach) that create trans fat. Studies have found that the effect of naturally occurring ruminant trans fats is not harmful. Rather, this natural trans fat is protective. There is a need to differentiate between naturally occurring trans fats that do not have harmful properties and provide benefits, and synthetically created trans fats that do harm our health.

What Are The Major Sources Of Trans Fats?

About 34 percent of trans fats come from bakery items: muffins, croissants, donuts, cakes, flour tortillas, cookies and brownies. Restaurants, both carry-out and fast-food type, are a source of 12 percent of the trans fats in our diets. These come from foods such as fried chicken and French fries. Another 11 percent are in snack foods such as crackers, granola bars, microwave popcorn and chips. Margarine and shortening supply 7 percent.

NUTRITION NOTE

There is a small amount of natural trans fat found in meat and dairy.

Studies have found that the effect of naturally occurring ruminant trans fats do not have a harmful effect.

This natural trans fat is protective rather than harmful.

You might wonder if it is possible to find foods without trans fats. *Whole Foods,* a national chain health food store, does not sell any foods that contain trans fats from partially hydrogenated oils. Check your local health food store's policy. An example is a local health food store in Waukesha, Wis., *Good Harvest Market* (www.goodharvestmarket.com), which does not carry any foods that contain partially hydrogenated oils, high fructose corn syrup or artificial sweeteners. Check to see if you have a store near you that has a similar policy.

Look Beyond The Claim Of "No Trans Fats"

Some labels declare they are trans fat free and will boast in large print *"NO TRANS FAT,"* yet hidden in tiny print in the ingredients they list "partially hydrogenated," which means trans fats are in the product. How is that possible? If the amount per serving is less than a half (0.5) gram, FDA labeling rules allow the products to list trans fats as "zero." This is misleading, as consumers believe when it says "NO," there are none.

Get in the habit of checking ingredient lists for the words "partially hydrogenated" if you want to avoid trans fats.

Why Don't All The Fats Listed On The Label Add Up To The Total?

Total fat, saturated fat and trans fat are required on the label. The FDA has determined that mono and diglycerides, which are fats, do not have to be listed on the label and polyunsaturated and monounsaturated fats are optional. So, if only the required saturated and trans fat are listed, what are missing may be the other types of fats that do not have to be listed.

To further explain why they don't add up, it is important to know that all fats and fatty acids are rounded to the nearest 0.5 increment up to 5 grams and then to the nearest whole gram if greater than 5 grams. These rounding rules could result in up to a 1.5 gram difference between the total fat and what you get by adding up the listed fats.

How Much Is Safe?

The Institute of Medicine concluded that there is no safe level of trans fats in the diet. You might think these small amounts of trans fats are not important, but they can add up.

The Nurses' Health Study found that replacing only 30 calories of carbohydrates every day with 30 calories of trans fats, the amount found in a teaspoon of stick margarine, nearly doubled the risk for heart disease.[43]

The Institute of Medicine concluded that any amount of trans fats increases the risk of heart disease. Trans-fatty acids raise the ratio of LDL cholesterol to HDL cholesterol significantly more than saturated fat does.

The FDA has estimated that with trans fat labeling and the decrease in intake expected, thousands of cases of fatal and nonfatal coronary heart disease will be prevented annually.

> Ounce for ounce, trans fats are even more unhealthy for your cholesterol level than saturated fat. Trans fats nearly double your risk for heart disease. It is important to limit your intake of saturated fat. However, it is essential to eliminate partially hydrogenated oils from your diet.

Are Foods Without Trans Fats Healthy?

A cookie without trans fat may still be mostly white sugars and white flour, making it a poor choice. Or, a food free of trans fat could be very high in saturated fat. It is important to remember that many of the foods that are changing oils to remove trans fats are packaged, processed foods; sweets; desserts; or deep-fried and are not magically changed into health foods equal to vegetables and fruits when they get an oil change. Foods with naturally good fats such as salmon, almonds and avocado don't need an oil change since they never had trans fats and are low in saturated fat. The focus should be on consuming healthy foods with naturally good fats, eating less processed and junk foods, and eating more fruits and vegetables.

When Oils Are Heated, Do They Become Trans Fat?

You cannot convert oils to trans fat in your kitchen at home. To do that, you would need professional equipment, which includes a metal catalyst, along with a vacuum under high heat. You can, however, break down fats and create rancid fat and other unhealthy compounds.

Margarine Vs. Butter

For years it was believed that margarine was healthier than butter. It now appears that neither butter nor margarine are ideal choices. Butter has 7 grams of saturated fat per tablespoon. Saturated fat raises the harmful LDL cholesterol while it also slightly raises the good HDL cholesterol, yet not enough to compensate for the increase in bad LDL.

Most margarine contains Trans fats from partially hydrogenated oils. A National Academy of Sciences study concluded that Trans fats raise the bad LDL cholesterol, but they also lower the good HDL cholesterol.[44] This increases the risk of coronary heart disease more than saturated fat.

Some margarines use the process of interesterification which may be just as harmful. This process is difficult to identify on food labels. *Smart Balance* specifically states on their Web site that their product is free of trans fat and without the use of hydrogenation or esterification. Instead a patented process of blending oils is used.

Is it better to eat butter instead of margarine to avoid trans fat? How much can I have a day?

The best choice would be to substitute liquid oil, such as extra-virgin olive oil or expeller-pressed canola oil, instead of either butter or margarine. Using butter in limited amounts to stay within your saturated fat allowance may be difficult. One tablespoon is half the day's allowance for the average person. Butters that are light, whipped or mixed with canola oil have less saturated fat. The amount you can have depends upon what other saturated fats are in your diet, like meat, cheese and dairy, If you choose to use butter as part of your saturated fat allowance, you may wish to choose a butter that is organic to avoid pesticides and antibiotic residues.

Is tub margarine okay?

Tub margarine is not guaranteed to be free of trans fat. Check the ingredients to be sure. Some tub margarines that make the claim in bold letters, "No Trans Fats," list partially hydrogenated oil in the ingredients. Because the trans fat is less than one-half gram per serving they qualify to claim zero trans fats. When you finish that tub, all those small amounts have added up, and you could have consumed as much as 32 grams of trans fat.

What about olive oil margarine?

No matter what the oil, if is partially hydrogenated, it contains the harmful trans fats. If you want the benefits of olive oil, purchase it in the liquid form. Brush or spray it on foods instead of using margarine or butter.

Non-hydrogenated margarine?

These will not have partially hydrogenated oils listed in the ingredients. In most cases, the saturated fat, palm oil, is added. However, the amount is small – usually less than 1.5 grams of saturated fat per tablespoon. Some may use interesterification.

Is Palm Oil Okay?

It depends upon how much is used in a food and if interesterification was used. When palm oil appears in the ingredients, check the amount of saturated fat to determine how the item fits within your daily allowance. Choosing foods that replace trans fats with palm oil may be acceptable in some cases when the saturated fat remains within your daily allowance. In most cases, if the saturated fat is 3 grams or less for the amount you typically have for a serving, it can fit into your saturated fat allowance.

Interesterification

Interesterification combines fully hydrogenated oil with a liquid oil using heat with a metal catalyst. The process of interesterification has raised concerns in some studies, indicating that it may be even more harmful than partially hydrogenated fats. Like partially hydrogenated, interesterified fats raised the bad LDL cholesterol and lowered the good HDL cholesterol but went further to raise blood glucose and increase insulin resistance.[44] If further research agrees with these studies, removing trans fats and replacing them with interesterified fats may be as or more harmful. Currently the use of interesterification is not required to be indicated on labels, but may appear in the ingredients lists of some foods.

What Is Hydrogenated Or Fully Hydrogenated?

When oil is fully hydrogenated, it becomes a saturated fat. Fully hydrogenated vegetable oils are free of trans fats. They are too hard to be used alone, so they are combined with liquid oils to soften them slightly. This may, or may not be via interesterification. They are not the same as naturally occurring saturated fat, having been artificially saturated. It is not known if a fully hydrogenated fat acts differently or if there are any health issues that exist when using them.

Tips For Using Less Solid Fats Such As Butter Or Margarine:

❖ Use liquid oils to sauté, brown or stir-fry over medium heat.
❖ Put oil in a refillable bottle to spray foods. Spritz flavorful oils, such as walnut, macadamia or olive oil, instead of spreading a solid fat.
❖ Substitute nut butters, peanut, almond or sunflower, on toast or use in recipes that call for toppings made with butter or margarine.
❖ If butter is a key ingredient, as in butter cookies, use butter but make the cookies smaller. Use half butter and half oil to make a sauce. Don't drown food in sauces. Drizzle 1 or 2 tablespoons of sauce on your food. How often you eat these foods and in what amounts is also important. A small indulgence can be a part of a heart healthy diet when balanced with other healthy foods.
❖ Use half canola or nut oils, such as walnut, almond or macadamia, with half butter for baking when you can.
❖ Retrain your taste buds to appreciate foods without added fats. Is it a habit to put that glob of butter or margarine on your food? Try to enjoy foods without any added butter. Use herbs or lemon. You may discover new flavors you like better without butter.

Trans Fat Quiz

1. If a food package states "no trans fats" you can be confident that there are no trans fats in that item.
   ❏ T ❏ F

2. If partially hydrogenated is found in the ingredient list, the food has trans fats.
   ❏ T ❏ F

3. No amount of trans fat is desirable.
   ❏ T ❏ F

4. Saturated fats are more harmful than trans fats.
   ❏ T ❏ F

5. Tub margarines are a good choice because they are trans fat free.
   ❏ T ❏ F

6. Non-hydrogenated margarine which do not have trans fats may be eaten in unlimited amounts.
   ❏ T ❏ F

7. The best choice is oil instead of either butter or non-hydrogenated margarine.
   ❏ T ❏ F

8. Foods that are free of trans fat are low in saturated fat.
   ❏ T ❏ F

9. Trans fats are double trouble; they lower good cholesterol and raise the bad cholesterol.
   ❏ T ❏ F

10. Check the foods that may contain trans fat from partially hydrogenated oils.

    ❏ canned black beans   ❏ wheat crackers
    ❏ oat bran muffin   ❏ granola bars
    ❏ donuts   ❏ eggs
    ❏ fish sticks   ❏ whole-wheat bread
    ❏ cashews   ❏ popcorn
    ❏ oatmeal cookies

ANSWERS
On Page 279.

Smart 4 Your Heart

19

Cholesterol In Foods

A common, though incorrect, belief is that cholesterol in food is what raises cholesterol in your blood. Limit cholesterol, so the thinking goes, and you lower blood cholesterol. The liver makes 75 percent of the cholesterol we have in our bodies. Cholesterol, a waxy, fat-like substance, is found in the cell membrane of every cell of the body. Cholesterol is important to our health; it is used to make hormones and vitamin D. When there is too much of the wrong kind of cholesterol circulating in the blood, it increases your risk for heart disease.

The amount of cholesterol eaten has less influence on your blood cholesterol levels compared to the effect saturated and trans fats have on your cholesterol.

NUTRITION NOTE

The amount of cholesterol in foods has little effect on your blood cholesterol compared to the amount of cholesterol made in your liver.

Shrimp and Cholesterol

Shrimp is low in saturated fat, but many people avoid eating it because of its high cholesterol content. A study[45] at Rockefeller University in New York found that a diet with 300 grams (about 10 ounces) of shrimp per day, which provided 590 mg of dietary cholesterol, increased bad cholesterol LDL about 7 percent. However, good HDL cholesterol also increased about 12 percent. The shrimp diet improved the cholesterol to HDL ratio, which means shrimp did not increase the risk for heart disease. In addition, the shrimp diet decreased triglyceride by 13 percent, probably from the omega-3 fats found in seafood. Thus, most people may eat shrimp as a part of a balanced diet. However, if the shrimp is battered, breaded, deep-fried or drenched in butter, the saturated and partially hydrogenated oils would impact blood cholesterol levels.

BOTTOM LINE
Choose broiled and grilled shrimp.

Eggs and Cholesterol

One of the first foods people often give up when they want to eat heart healthy is eggs. This is due, in part, to the cholesterol scare of the 90s. Studies of moderate intake of eggs, up to one a day, did not increase the risk of heart disease in healthy individuals.[46] For those who had diabetes, however, having eggs on a daily basis did increase their risk of heart disease.

What you choose to eat with eggs, such as the bacon, sausage and fried potatoes loaded with saturated fat, is the real problem. A better choice is to have a bowl of steel-cut oatmeal with your egg.

In 2000, the American Heart Association (AHA) revised its dietary guidelines regarding eggs. Rather than singling out eggs, the guidelines were stated in daily dietary cholesterol limits, recognizing that all animal foods, including meats, poultry and dairy, contain cholesterol. The daily total cholesterol guidelines from the AHA are less than 200 mg for those with heart disease, diabetes or high LDL cholesterol. It is 300 milligrams for others. If portions of meat are not more than one-fourth of your plate (Page 51), and cheese is limited, eggs can fit within the cholesterol guidelines.

Cholesterol in Eggs	
Size of Egg	Cholesterol (mg)
Small	155
Medium	185
Large	210
Eggland brand large	180

Eggs are a source of many nutrients, including protein; lecithin; vitamin and the B vitamins, riboflavin, B_{12} and folate. Eggs also contain the phytochemicals lutein and zeaxanthin, which promote good eye health, along with choline, which is important for brain development of the fetus.

Omega-3 Enhanced Eggs

Some chickens are fed special diets that include flax or are allowed to roam free, eating grass and other plants. When you choose to eat eggs, check to ensure they are a good source of omega-3.

Egg Whites and Egg Substitutes

There is no cholesterol in egg whites. A large egg white has only 17 calories. Two egg whites can replace a whole egg. Using only egg whites will make an omelet or scrambled eggs with a tougher texture. Replacing half the eggs with egg whites, such as using one egg and two or three egg whites, will give good results. Egg substitutes are simply egg whites that may have coloring and preservatives added. In general, one-fourth cup of egg substitute is equal to one whole egg.

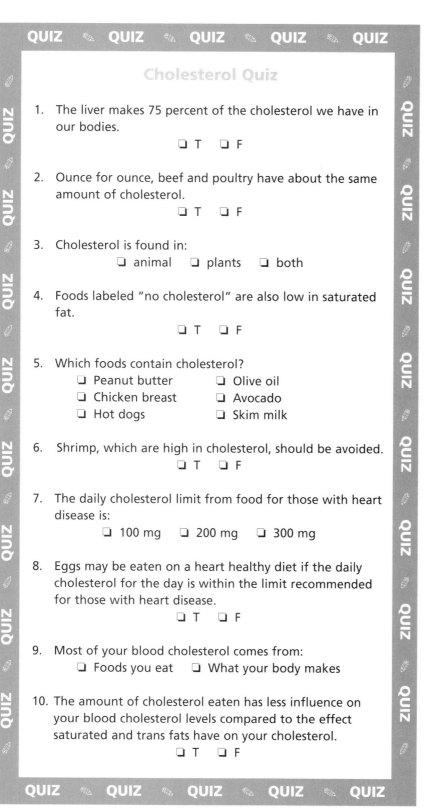

Cholesterol Quiz

1. The liver makes 75 percent of the cholesterol we have in our bodies.

   ❏ T   ❏ F

2. Ounce for ounce, beef and poultry have about the same amount of cholesterol.

   ❏ T   ❏ F

3. Cholesterol is found in:

   ❏ animal   ❏ plants   ❏ both

4. Foods labeled "no cholesterol" are also low in saturated fat.

   ❏ T   ❏ F

5. Which foods contain cholesterol?

   ❏ Peanut butter   ❏ Olive oil
   ❏ Chicken breast   ❏ Avocado
   ❏ Hot dogs   ❏ Skim milk

6. Shrimp, which are high in cholesterol, should be avoided.

   ❏ T   ❏ F

7. The daily cholesterol limit from food for those with heart disease is:

   ❏ 100 mg   ❏ 200 mg   ❏ 300 mg

8. Eggs may be eaten on a heart healthy diet if the daily cholesterol for the day is within the limit recommended for those with heart disease.

   ❏ T   ❏ F

9. Most of your blood cholesterol comes from:

   ❏ Foods you eat   ❏ What your body makes

10. The amount of cholesterol eaten has less influence on your blood cholesterol levels compared to the effect saturated and trans fats have on your cholesterol.

    ❏ T   ❏ F

ANSWERS
On Page 279.

TABLE 19.1 Amount Of Omega-3 (EPA + DHA) In 3.5 Oz. Of Fish
Does not include fish that have more than 0.5 ppm mercury since they exceed the EPA advisory level for safe consumption.

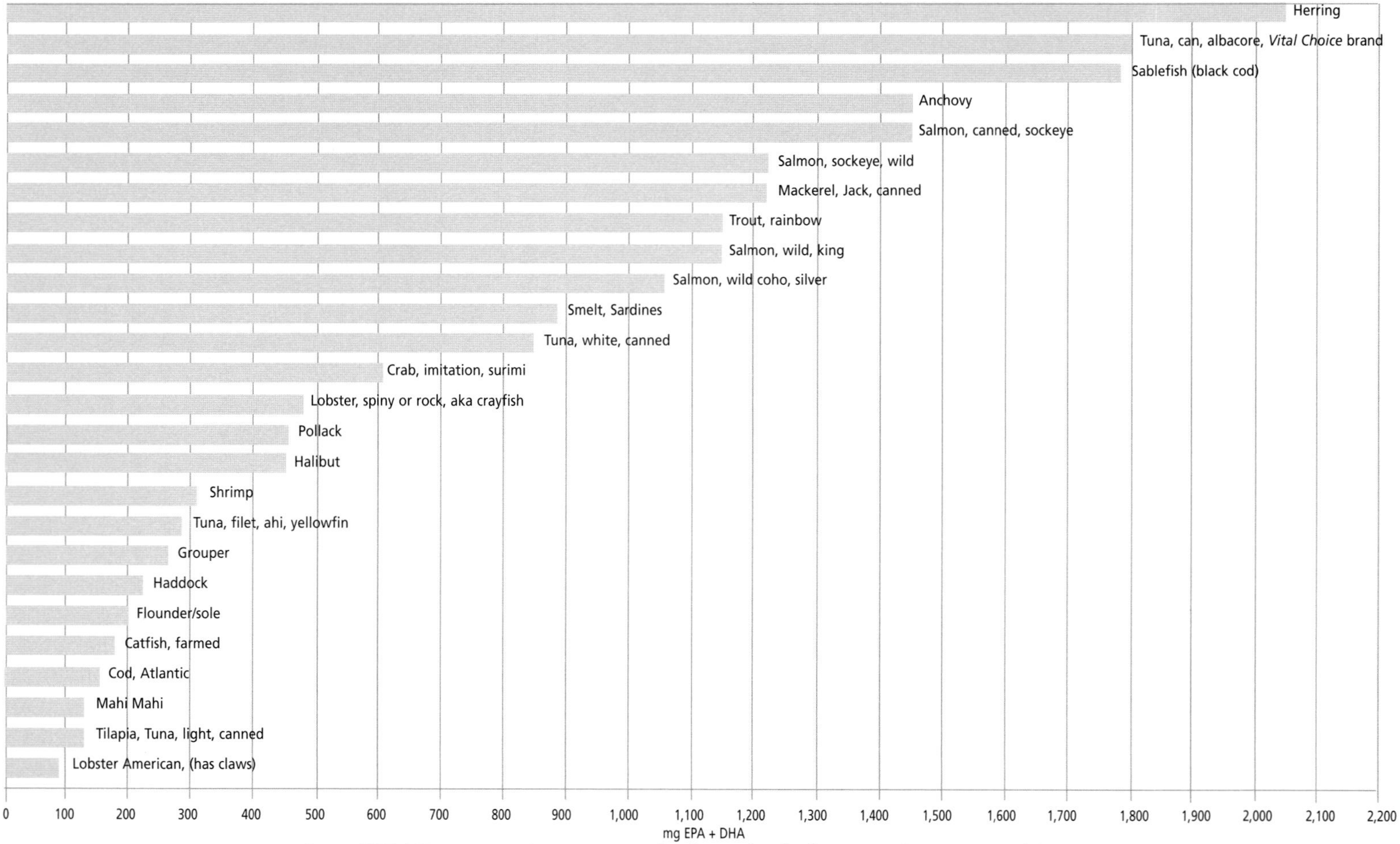

Bar chart labels (highest to lowest):

- Herring
- Tuna, can, albacore, *Vital Choice brand*
- Sablefish (black cod)
- Anchovy
- Salmon, canned, sockeye
- Salmon, sockeye, wild
- Mackerel, Jack, canned
- Trout, rainbow
- Salmon, wild, king
- Salmon, wild coho, silver
- Smelt, Sardines
- Tuna, white, canned
- Crab, imitation, surimi
- Lobster, spiny or rock, aka crayfish
- Pollack
- Halibut
- Shrimp
- Tuna, filet, ahi, yellowfin
- Grouper
- Haddock
- Flounder/sole
- Catfish, farmed
- Cod, Atlantic
- Mahi Mahi
- Tilapia, Tuna, light, canned
- Lobster American, (has claws)

x-axis: 0, 100, 200, 300, 400, 500, 600, 700, 800, 900, 1,000, 1,100, 1,200, 1,300, 1,400, 1,500, 1,600, 1,700, 1,800, 1,900, 2,000, 2,100, 2,200

mg EPA + DHA

Source USDA Nutrient Database • www.nal.usda.gov/fnic/foodcomp/search/ • www.vitalchoice.com

Smart 4 Your Heart

20

Fish
Omega-3 (EPA and DHA)

Eating fish is good for your heart, brain and immune system. Even your joints may feel better. Eating seafood regularly may cut the risk of death from heart disease by 20 percent and the risk of sudden death by 90 percent.

The benefits are linked to a good fat called omega-3 fatty acids and the evidence is strongest for two important omega-3 fatty acids called EPA (eicosapentaenoic acid) and DHA (docosahexaenoic acid), both found in fish.

Some of the benefits seen in studies for EPA and DHA are that they:
- ❖ May reduce the fat in the blood (triglycerides) and reduce VLDL a type of cholesterol that becomes LDL. They may also increase HDL.
- ❖ Reduce fatty plaque in the walls of the arteries and improve blood flow.
- ❖ Prevent irregular heart beats, a cause of sudden cardiac death.
- ❖ Have a small but beneficial affect on lowering blood pressure.
- ❖ Reduce the tendency to form blood clots that could lead to a stroke or heart attack.
- ❖ Reduce inflammation, thereby improving symptoms of certain inflammatory diseases such as rheumatoid arthritis, asthma, psoriasis and other skin conditions.
- ❖ May decrease depression and improve emotional well-being.
- ❖ Are important for the proper development of infants' brain, nerve and eye tissues.

Are All Omega-3 Fats The Same?

There is a third omega-3 fatty acid found in some plants and seeds, such as flaxseed, walnut and canola oil. It is called ALA, alpha-linolenic acid. ALA is a healthy fat which functions differently than EPA and DHA. It is possible to convert some ALA into EPA and DHA, but humans do not do this very efficiently. Only 2 to 5 percent of ALA is converted on average, with up to 10 percent in some cases. It may require 20 to 50 grams of ALA to get 1 gram of EPA and DHA, depending upon the individual and his or her diet.

TWO TYPES OF OMEGA-3

1. Plant (flax) alpha-linolenic (ALA)

2. Marine derived (seafood or marine algae)
   - eicosapentaenoic acid (EPA) and
   - docosahexaenoic acid (DHA).

Having a direct source from fatty, cold water fish, such as wild Alaskan salmon, Atlantic mackerel, herring, sardines, anchovies or a fish oil supplement, is the most effective way to get adequate amounts of EPA and DHA with low risk of mercury or other contaminants.

NUTRITION NOTE

For heart health, EPA and DHA are the omega-3 fatty acids that reduce risk of coronary artery disease.

Two government agencies, the FDA and the Agency for Healthcare Research and Quality (AHRQ), as well as the American Heart Association, reviewed the evidence and reached the conclusion that fish oil is what is needed for heart health. For heart health, EPA and DHA are the omega-3 fatty acids that reduce risk of coronary artery disease.

In September 2004, the FDA approved a qualified health claim for the omega-3 fatty acids, EPA and DHA, found in fish. An FDA-qualified health claim is also allowed on fish oil supplements, which states:

"Supportive but not conclusive research shows that consumption of EPA and DHA omega-3 fatty acids may reduce the risk of coronary heart disease."

How Much Omega-3 Fatty Acids Do You Need?

The National Academy of Sciences Institute of Medicine set guidelines for ALA, but did not specify amounts for EPA and DHA. However, the American Heart Association (AHA) and the National Institute of Health (NIH) recommend 650 mg of EPA and DHA for healthy individuals. The AHA also advises a higher level of 1,000 mg for those with heart disease and 2,000 to 4,000 mg for those with high triglycerides.

TABLE 20.1	Daily Amounts Of Omega-3 For Healthy Adults		
	ALA***	EPA/DHA	EPA/DHA for those with heart disease*
Adult Men	1,600 mg	650 mg**	1,000 mg
Adult Women	1,100 mg	650 mg**	1,000 mg
Pregnancy	1,400 mg	250-300 mg DHA	
Children 0-12 months	500 mg		
Children 1-3 yr.	700 mg	No guidelines have been specifically established for children, but suggestions range from 100-200 mg DHA.	
Children 4-8 yr.	900 mg		
Boys 9-13 yr.	1,200 mg		
Boys 14-18 yr.	1,600 mg		
Girls 9-12 yr.	1,000 mg		
Girls 14-18	1,100 mg		

*Note: 2,000 to 4,000 milligrams EPA + DHA for triglyceride lowering.
**AHA and NIH guidelines
***IOM is a nonprofit organization that operates under the umbrella of the **U.S. National Academy of Sciences.** Adequate Intake was set only for ALA. Adequate Intakes were not set for EPA and DHA.

What About Mercury and PCBs In Fish?

Mercury is a heavy metal that, when consumed in excess, may damage the brain and kidneys and harm a developing fetus. PCBs (polychlorinated biphenyls) are man-made pollutants that were banned in 1979. They remain in the environment because they break down very slowly. They are believed to cause cancer.

The concern about mercury and pollutants does not mean you should avoid fish, as you would miss out on all the health benefits. However, it is better, especially for young children or women who are pregnant, nursing or trying to get pregnant, to avoid those fish that are highest in mercury. Others should eat them infrequently, if at all.

AVOID High-Mercury Fish

❖ Shark
❖ Swordfish
❖ Tilefish (golden bass, golden snapper, golden mackerel)

❖ King Mackerel (but not smaller species of mackerel such as Pacific, Jack, Atlantic, etc., which are used for canning.)

The *Environmental Working Group* (EWG) advises the avoidance of nine species in addition to those above.

❖ Tuna Steaks
❖ Sea Bass
❖ Oysters from the Gulf Coast

❖ Marlin
❖ Halibut
❖ Northern Pike

❖ Walleye
❖ White Croaker
❖ Largemouth Bass

Source: EWG Brain Report (with permission to reprint granted) www.ewg.org/reports/BrainFood/pr.html

Choose Low-Mercury Fish and Seafood
(from highest in omega-3 to lowest)

❖ Herring
❖ Troll-Caught Albacore Tuna*
❖ Salmon
❖ Barramundi
❖ Farmed Trout
❖ Sardines
❖ Crab Mid-Atlantic Blue
❖ Scallops
❖ Oysters
❖ Pollock

❖ Perch
❖ Shrimp
❖ Light Canned Tuna
❖ Haddock
❖ Flounder
❖ Farmed Catfish
❖ Cod
❖ Tilapia

*Troll-caught albacore mercury levels are lower (0.14 ppm vs. 0.353 ppm) because they are younger and smaller than longline-caught albacore.

Tips To Reduce Mercury and Pollutants When Choosing Fish:

❖ Visit www.gotmercury.org to calculate your individual mercury intake level based on the seafood type and amount consumed.
❖ Choose younger and smaller fish, such as sardines, herring, smelt.
❖ Eat a variety of low-mercury fish from a variety of bodies of water, rather than a single species, as they all accumulate contaminates at different rates. Different waters have varying amounts of pollutants.
❖ Shrimp, mussels and oysters are low-mercury, moderate omega-3 sources of shellfish.
❖ Remove fish skin and dark muscle tissue and fat where chemical toxins such as PCBs collect. Mercury accumulates in the muscle of the fish; therefore removing skin does not remove mercury. An exception to removing fat and skin is on wild salmon, which is low in PCBs.
❖ Do not eat the internal organs of fish, which may contain high levels of contaminants.
❖ Cook fish, allowing the fatty liquid to drain away. Bake, broil or boil/poach to reduce pollutants. This also reduces the beneficial omega-3. It does not reduce mercury.
❖ Cut back on the amount of canned tuna. Albacore canned white tuna is higher in omega-3, but also higher in mercury than canned light tuna (0.358 vs. 0.118 ppm.).

NUTRITION NOTE

Troll-caught, canned albacore tuna is higher in omega-3. These smaller tuna are lower in mercury.

Yellowfin tuna may be marketed as "Ahi" tuna.

Fish Smart 4 Your Heart

- Choose canned, troll-caught, albacore tuna. Troll-caught, canned albacore tuna is higher in omega-3. These smaller tuna are lower in mercury. Sources for troll-caught, canned tuna are: www.vitalchoice.com or www.marylouseafoods.com/marketplace.
- Substitute canned wild salmon for canned tuna as it is lower in mercury.
- Fresh tuna steaks most often are Yellowfin (Ahi). While lower in mercury than Bigeye or Bluefin, they are still considered high in mercury.
- If you fish or eat locally caught fish, check local advisories about its safety. Predatory fish such as Northern Pike, Largemouth Bass and Walleye are consistently high in mercury. Bottom feeders, such as Carp and locally caught Catfish, are also very high in other contaminants and many advisories suggest avoiding them.

How Much Fish Do I Have To Eat?

The American Heart Association (AHA) recommends we eat fish twice a week for a total of 7 ounces of fish weekly. In 2004, Americans ate 12 pounds of fresh and frozen fish a year. This was an increase of 20 percent from the previous decade but still not enough to meet the AHA recommendation, which would require almost 23 pounds a year.

The amount of EPA and DHA varies according to the type of fish. The fish richest in omega-3 requires smaller amounts than those that are lower in omega-3. A weekly serving of 7.5 ounces of herring, which is rich in omega-3, would provide the AHA recommended amounts of 650 milligrams EPA and DHA needed for healthy individuals. Eating 11 ounces a week of canned, red sockeye salmon, another good source of omega-3, would provide an average of 650 milligrams per day. Tilapia, a fish lower in EPA and DHA, would require more than 7 pounds per week to provide that same amount. Tilapia is farm raised and is higher in omega-6 than omega-3. If you have heart disease, the recommended amount of EPA and DHA is higher, which would require 20 ounces of wild sockeye salmon a week to obtain the daily average of 1,000 milligrams.

See Table 20.2 on next page to locate the type of fish you are eating. Then find how much you need to eat per day or within a week to obtain a daily average of 1,000 milligrams EPA plus DHA. If you are not eating enough fish, you may increase the amount or supplement with fish oil capsules.

Tuna: Either buy canned light tuna (which is lower in mercury) or purchase water-packed Albacore (troll-caught).

Choose water packed (oil and water don't mix) The oil packed lose some omega-3 when drained.

Canned light tuna is yellowfin and/or skipjack tuna.

One ounce Barramundi, Australis has 167 mg total omega-3. The amount that is EPA and DHA is not available.

Source USDA Nutrient Database www.nal.usda.gov/fnic /foodcomp/search www.vitalchoice.com

TABLE 20.2 Approximate Ounces Of Fish Per Week To Provide A Daily Average Of 1,000 mg EPA/DHA			
Fish, cooked unless noted otherwise	EPA/DHA per ounce (can vary)	Ounces per day for 1,000 mg (1 gram)	Amount to eat per week
1,200 mg or more per 3.5 oz. serving			
Herring, kippered	607	1.6	11.5 oz.
Troll-caught Albacore Tuna, canned *Papa George's,* www.papageorge.com	550	2	14 oz.
Troll-caught, Albacore Tuna, canned *Vital Choice* www.vitalchoice.com	514	2	14 oz.
Sablefish (Black Cod)	510	2	14 oz.
Herring, pickled	416	2.4	17 oz.
Anchovy	414	2.4	17 oz.
Salmon, Sockeye, canned	413	2.4	17 oz.
Salmon, Sockeye, wild	351	2.8	20 oz.
Mackerel, Jack, canned	351	2.8	20 oz.
700-1,200mg per 3.5 oz. serving			
Trout	330	3	21 oz.
Salmon, Wild King, raw	329	3	21 oz.
Salmon, Wild Coho/Silver	302	3.3	23 oz.
Sardines	278	3.6	25 oz.
Tuna, Albacore, canned	246	4	28 oz.
400-700 mg per 3.5 oz. serving			
Crab, imitation, (Surimi)	174	5.7	2.5 pounds
Lobster, Spiny or Rock, aka crayfish (no claws)	137	7.3	3 pounds
Halibut	133	7.5	3.25 pounds
Pollock	134	7.5	3.25 pounds
Less than 400 mg per 3.5 oz. serving			
Shrimp	90	11	4.75 pounds
Tuna, Ahi or Yellowfin	80	12	5.5 pounds
Grouper	71	14	6 pounds
Haddock	68	15	6.4 pounds
Flounder/Sole, raw	57	17.5	7.6 pounds
Catfish, farmed	50	20 (1.25 pounds)	8.75 pounds
Cod, Atlantic	45	22 (1.4 pounds)	10 pounds
Mahi Mahi	40	25	11 pounds
Tilapia	38	26	11.5 pounds
Tuna, Light, canned (may include Skipjack, Bluefin, Yellowfin, or Tongol)	35	28	12.4 pounds
Lobster, American (has claws)	24	2.6 pounds	18 pounds
Orange Roughy	9	111 (7 pounds)	48 pounds

Is Fried Fish Okay?

Poached, broiled, baked and steamed fish are healthier options than fried fish. Frying adds additional, often unwanted, calories. Usually, the oils used for frying in restaurants contain trans fats; therefore the benefits from eating fish are cancelled out by the bad effects of the oils. (See the recipe for "Oven - Fried" fish Page 412.)

Smoked Fish

When fish are smoked they lose some of the good omega-3 fats. Salt is added during the processing so sodium levels rise. Chinook salmon has 39 percent less omega-3 and 61 percent more sodium when smoked.

Canned Salmon

It is often believed that all canned salmon is wild, but that is no longer true. You are advised to check the label for a statement that the salmon is wild. Canned is an economical source that is available all year. Salmon is available canned without added salt.

The liquids found in canned salmon are oil and juices from the salmon since no water is added to the can. It can be saved in a jar, kept in your freezer, and used instead of water in a recipe such as the seafood stew (Page 421) or to poach fish. Choose the traditional varieties with the bones and skin as they are more flavorful and richer in heart healthy omega-3. The bones are soft enough to mash and safe to eat, also providing you with a good source of calcium. The skin and the gray flesh just below the skin are rich in omega-3 fatty acids. Do not remove the dark flesh since as much as two-thirds of the omega-3 may be concentrated in this tissue. Wild salmon tends to be lower in PCBs than farmed, so you may safely eat it.

Canned pink and chum salmon are rosy colored and have a soft texture and mild flavor. Sockeye has a deeper red color, firmer texture and is higher priced. Farmed canned salmon is softer in texture. The omega-3 amount for 3.5 ounces of red sockeye is 1,230 milligrams; for pink it is 1,288 milligrams. It is a small enough difference so that you can use personal preference or cost to make a buying decision.

Farmed Salmon vs. Wild Salmon

Salmon labeled "Atlantic" is farmed, since wild Atlantic salmon is currently protected as an endangered species. All salmon from Alaska is wild since fish-farming is not allowed.

Atlantic salmon refers to the species and could be farmed or pen-raised in the Pacific, Maine, Canada, Norway, Iceland, Scotland, Ireland, the Shetlands, China or Chile.

Omega-3 in farmed vs. wild salmon

Looking only at the total amount of omega-3 may be misleading. Nineteen percent of the total fat in farmed salmon is the heart healthy omega-3 while 22 percent of the fat in wild salmon is from omega-3. A gram of omega-3 in farmed salmon has more calories than a gram of omega-3 in wild salmon. Farmed also has more pro-inflammatory omega-6.

Fish (3.5 ounces)	Calories	Total Fat	Omega-6	Omega-3 Percent of fat as Omega-3	Calories Per Gram of Omega-3
Atlantic farmed salmon	206	12.3 g	580 mg	2,147 mg 17%	96
Atlantic wild salmon	124	8.1 g	170 mg	1,840 mg 23%	67

Colored Salmon

Wild salmon get their reddish color from their diet of lobster, shrimp, krill, plankton and algae. Farmed salmon have naturally gray-colored flesh but get their red color as a result of coloring pellets in their feed. This practice makes people think they are getting wild – which they are not. The pellets contain chemically synthesized artificial astaxanthin and canthaxanthin.

Sablefish

Another underutilized fish rich in omega-3 that may meet some of the demand is Sablefish, also known as Black Cod or Butterfish. Its flesh is white and mild flavored, making it a fish that is well liked. Much of the sablefish that is caught is not used in this country but exported. It has more mercury than salmon but smaller sablefish are quite low in mercury, with nearly as much omega-3 as that found in wild salmon. See table below.

Fish (3.5 oz.)	Mercury Parts per million (ppm)	Omega-3 (EPA + DHA) milligrams (mg)
Sablefish	0.07 to 0.22 ppm	1,787 mg
Salmon	0.014 ppm	1,230 to 1,840 mg

FISHING METHODS FOR TUNA

Troll-/pole-caught: Hooks and shorter lines catch smaller, low-mercury tuna.

Long-Line: Lines can be 50 miles long and catch larger, higher-mercury tuna from deeper water.

Troll-Caught Albacore Tuna

Another option for omega-3 fish that is low in mercury is troll-caught Albacore tuna. It is smaller in size, higher in omega-3 and lower in mercury than larger Albacore (0.14 parts per million vs 0.38 ppm) used in most of the canned white tuna and served as fresh tuna steaks.

Fish Smart 4 Your Heart

Australis Barramundi Fish

Similar to farmed trout, an environmentally sound indoor farming system in the U.S is raising barramundi, a white, firm-fleshed fish that because of its unique evolutionary history, makes its own beneficial omega-3 fatty acids, without consuming significant quantities of fish oil. It has been awarded a "best choice" selection by Monterey Bay Aquarium Seafood Watch. A 5-ounce serving has 195 caolories and 833 milligrams of omega-3 and no mercury.

www.seafoodwatch.org

Farmed Trout

The U.S. Trout Farmers Association is an example of a farmed fish that provides a healthy and safe supply of fish through the use of good management practices. Nearly all the rainbow trout you find in the U.S. market, or on restaurant menus, is farm raised. Research has shown that farm-raised trout has a minimal effect on the wild population. The farmed trout are slightly higher in fat, but the percent of fat that is in the form of EPA and DHA is almost the same.

Fish (3.5 oz.)	Calories	Total Fat	Omega-3 (EPA + DHA)	Percent of Fat as Omega-3
Wild Trout	150	5.8 g	988 mg	17%
Farmed Trout	169	7.2 g	1,154 mg	16%

Don't Like Fish, Allergic To Fish Or Vegetarian?

If you don't like fish, you could meet your dietary needs with the use of fish oil supplements containing EPA and DHA.

If you are allergic to fish, you may be able to take fish oil. Allergens in foods including fish are usually the protein component. Because fish oils are essentially void of protein, people who would react to eating fish generally can consume fish oil. However, it is advised that you consult your allergist or health care practitioner first. There are also marine algae supplements.

Marine algae, a good source of DHA, are produced and used in some microalgae-based supplements. The algae may be grown in land-based tanks. Some of the brands available are: DHA Neuromins, made from microalgae oil sold at health food stores; or O-Mega-Zen3 available at www.nutru.com; and v-pure omega-3 available at www.water4net; and DEVA omega-3 DHA available at www.devanutrition.com.

Is It Safe To Eat Fish With All The Concerns About Mercury and PCBs?

To obtain the benefits of omega-3 with the least amount of risk, include a variety of fish that are low in mercury and prepared to minimize PCBs.

Fish Quiz

1. The American Heart Association recommends two fish meals per week; therefore, fried fish is a good choice for heart health.

    ❏ T   ❏ F

2. The omega-3 found in fish which may reduce the risk of heart disease are EPA and DHA.

    ❏ T   ❏ F

3. ALA, the omega-3 found in flax, is FDA approved for use in lowering triglycerides.

    ❏ T   ❏ F

4. Check the fish that are high in mercury and should be avoided by some individuals.

    ❏ Swordfish   ❏ Grouper
    ❏ Salmon   ❏ King Mackerel
    ❏ Tilefish   ❏ Shark

5. While fish have mercury and PCBs the benefits of omega-3 outweigh the risks, and low-mercury fish should be included in a heart healthy diet.

    ❏ T   ❏ F

6. Smoked fish are a good source of omega-3.

    ❏ T   ❏ F

7. Canned wild salmon is a good source of omega-3, and since it is low in mercury, it is a good substitute for canned tuna.

    ❏ T   ❏ F

8. Farmed salmon are high in mercury.

    ❏ T   ❏ F

9. Light tuna has less mercury and less omega-3 than white tuna.

    ❏ T   ❏ F

10. There are plant DHA fish oils from marine algae for those who are allergic to fish.

    ❏ T   ❏ F

ANSWERS
On Page 279.

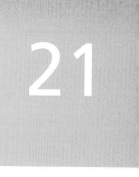

21

Fish Oil Supplements

The benefits of fish oils are many. The best way to obtain fish oil is directly from the foods you eat, primarily from low mercury, high omega-3 fish (such as anchovies, herring, sardines and wild salmon).

What if you don't like fish or you don't have it often enough? What if you prefer low-fat fish such as tilapia or cod? Or, what if you need fish oil in therapeutic amounts for triglyceride lowering that would require eating unrealistic amounts of fish? When it is not possible to get the amounts needed from foods, a dietary supplement containing fish oils is the next best thing to eating fish. But often those taking a fish oil supplement do not take enough, thinking one capsule a day is all that is needed.

TABLE 21.1
The American Heart Association's Recommendations
For Omega-3 Fatty Acid Intake (EPA + DHA) [51]

Group	Recommendation
No coronary heart disease	650 mg of EPA + DHA. Eat a variety of LOW-mercury fish at least twice a week.
Individuals with a diagnosis of heart disease	Consume about 1 g (1,000 mg) of EPA + DHA per day, preferably from fatty fish. EPA + DHA supplements with physician approval.
Individuals who need to lower triglycerides	2 to 4 grams (2,000-4,000 mg) of EPA + DHA per day provided as supplements with physician approval.

A typical over-the-counter, 1,000-mg fish oil capsule contains 300 milligrams of EPA and DHA. There are some brands that are more concentrated with 500 to 1,000 milligrams EPA and DHA in one capsule. Prescription fish oil has 850 milligrams per capsule. Fish oil is also available as a liquid.

How To Read A Fish Oil Supplement Label

Below is a fish oil supplement label. The numbers can vary for different brands. This requires you to follow a couple of steps to determine how many capsules you should take. The number of pills required can range from one to eight, depending on the concentration of EPA/DHA in each brand.

First: find the EPA and DHA; ignore the total amount of fish oil stated on the front, since the heart protective guidelines are based on EPA and DHA. The 1,000 milligrams of natural fish oil concentrate on the example contains other fatty acids and only one-third (300 milligrams) is EPA and DHA.

Second: add EPA + DHA together and divide by serving size or number of pills per serving.

In the example, EPA is 180 and DHA is 120. Serving size is one softgel so it is not necessary to divide. Each softgel has 300 milligrams EPA + DHA.

Finally, determine how many pills are required to meet your requirements. For example, a healthy person without heart disease needs 650 milligrams EPA + DHA; therefore, taking two pills provides 600 milligrams (300 X 2). For an individual with heart disease who needs 1,000 milligrams, it requires taking three pills which provides 900 milligrams.

Fish Oil	1,000 mg natural fish oil
Supplement Facts	
Serving Size 1 Softgel	
Servings Per bottle 125	

Each Softgel Contains	
Calories 10	Calories From Fat 10
	% Daily Value
Total Fat 1 g	2%
Saturated Fat 0.5 g	3%**
Sodium 0 mg	0%**
Protein Less than 1 g	
Natural Fish Oil Concentrate 1000 mg	***
EPA (Eicosapentaenoic Acid) 180 mg	
DHA (Docosahexaenoic Acid) 120 mg	

**Percent Daily Value (DV) are based on a 2,000 calorie diet
***Daily Value (DV) not established

TABLE 21.2
Amount Of EPA/DHA Per Capsule Of Some Brands Of Fish Oil

Brand Fish Oil	EPA/DHA Per Capsule	Pills Per Day For 1,000 mg EPA/DHA
Vital Oils 1000 (enteric coated)	1000	1
GNC Triple Strength (enteric coated)	900	1
Lovaza prescription	850	1-2
Pharma Life Omega-3	700	1-2
Nordic Natural Ultimate Omega	600	2
Vitamin Shoppe 1,000 mg	500	2
Carlson Super Omega-3	500	2
Carlson Norwegian Salmon Oil	305	3
Vita Smart 1,000 mg (Kmart)	300	3-4
Walgreens Natural 1,000 mg	300	3-4
Member's Mark 1,000 mg (Sam's Club)	300	3-4
Spring Valley 1,000 mg (Walmart)	300	3-4
Eskimo-3, liquid	1,200/tsp.	1 tsp.
Carlson Meg Omega liquid fish oil	2,400/tsp.	1 tsp.
Liquid fish oil	1,000-1,300/tsp.	1 tsp.
Liquid cod liver oil	1,000/tsp.	1 tsp.

Can Mercury Or Toxins Be Found In Fish Oil Supplements?

An independent lab that tested for mercury, PCB and dioxins found that there were no detectable levels in any of the 41 different brands they tested. To find out what brands they looked at, visit their site at www.consumerlab.com *Consumer Reports* tested 16 different brands and a Harvard study that reported on fish oils also found no detectable levels of carcinogens, mercury, dioxin or PCBs in any of the tested samples.[52] Most companies use molecular distillation and steam deodorization to remove environmental pollutants from their fish oil supplements. These purification processes are highly effective at separating pollutants from omega-3 fatty acids.

What About Flax Oil Supplements?

The type of omega-3 found in flaxseed is **NOT** the same as that found in fish. Plant sources lack the beneficial longer-chain omega-3 fatty acids (EPA and DHA) of fish oil. For heart protection, the recommendations are for the type of omega-3 found in fish. Flaxseed oil contains the plant source of omega-3 called (alpha linolenic) ALA. The body has to convert ALA to EPA and DHA but only converts a small amount. Currently, flax oil supplements are not allowed to carry the health claim about being beneficial for heart health that fish oils are able to use. Flax oil is not a substitute for fish oils for cholesterol lowering.

NUTRITION NOTE

Flax oil is not a substitute for fish oils for cholesterol lowering.

Fish Oil Supplements' Effect On Lipids and Risk For Heart Disease

Fish oil increases the good HDL cholesterol by 1 to 9 percent and lowers triglycerides. Fish oil is not used to lower LDL cholesterol. It may slightly increase LDL. Several studies have shown fish oil raises LDL by 5-10 mg/dl but could be as much as 20-30 mg/dl.[53] If LDL rises significantly when you take fish oil, you may want to have lipoprotein testing to determine if there is an abnormality that is not identified in standard lipid tests when LDL is calculated. When triglycerides are very high (over 500), the conversion of VLDL to LDL is decreased, which is partially responsible for the high triglycerides. Taking fish oil corrects this problem, allowing the conversion which then lowers the triglycerides but at the same time increases LDL. If LDL rises above the desired goal, it would require treatment.

When taken in large doses of 3 to 5 grams, fish oil has produced a 30 to 45 percent reduction in triglycerides.[54] In most studies, using a low dose, *1 gram or less, was not enough* to improve triglycerides.

Some studies with fish oil showed significant reduction in lipoprotein Lp(a), an independent genetic marker correlated with increased risk of heart disease.[55]

Continued on next page

The most dramatic results seen in several major trials, GISSI-Prevenzione and DART, was the decrease in sudden cardiac death.[56, 57]

There is strong evidence that fish oil reduces arrhythmia (irregular heart beat) and slightly lowers blood pressure.[58]

The benefits of taking fish oil seems to increase with time, so after six months, triglycerides and diastolic blood pressure levels were better than they were after one to three months of taking fish oil.

Prescription Fish Oil

In 2005, the FDA approved a fish oil product, Lovaza, for lowering triglycerides, which your doctor may prescribe. It is more concentrated, with 84 percent of the fish oil in the form of EPA and DHA compared to the usual 20 to 30 percent in over-the-counter fish oil. One capsule has 375 mg DHA and 465 mg EPA for a total of 840 mg. This may be especially helpful when taking amounts necessary for triglyceride lowering. There are some over-the-counter fish oils that contain as much or more, see Page 104.

Only one drug interaction has been documented with Lovaza, and that occurred when a large dose of four pills (3,360 mg EPA + DHA) was combined with the blood-thinning drug warfarin sold as *Coumadin*. It is recommended that when adding fish oil with warfarin, your prothrombin time is checked and your dosage adjusted by your doctor, if necessary.

What To Check When Buying Fish Oil

❖ Before you go shopping:
   a. Check www.consumerlab.com to see what brands they tested. No brands tested had detectable levels of mercury. All contained the claimed amount of EPA and DHA.

❖ At the store:
   a. Do you prefer liquid or pill?
   b. How much of the fish oil is in the form of EPA and DHA?
   c. If in pill form, how many do you have to take to get the dose required. More concentrated allows you to take less pills.
   d. Choose enteric coated if you experience fishy burps.
   e. If buying a liquid fish oil, choose the size you will use in a couple of weeks for optimal freshness. When exposed to air they start to break down and could become rancid.

What Is The Difference Between Fish Oil, Salmon Oil and Cod Liver Oil?

Fish oil is obtained from the muscle and fat tissue of oily fish, but cod liver oil is obtained from the livers of cod fish. Cod liver oil contains a higher ratio of DHA to EPA than fish oil. Fish oil has more EPA than DHA. Salmon oil is naturally higher in DHA than EPA. Some supplements contain only DHA. EPA is important to heart health, and DHA supports brain and nervous system functions.

Cod liver oil was given in previous times as a means to get vitamins A and D. Those who had to take it remember its unpleasant taste. The amounts of vitamin A may be toxic if cod liver is taken in the large amounts required for triglyceride lowering. Some brands remove vitamin A from their cod liver oil to avoid these concerns. Taste has also improved.

NUTRITION NOTE

Do not confuse fish oil with cod liver oil.

Fish oil comes from the body of the fish.

Cod liver oil comes from the liver of fish.

Taking Fish Oil Pills

❖ Take with food to avoid fishy burps and to minimize side effects of loose stools. Enteric-coated fish pills lessens "fishy burps." If taking more than one pill, take in divided doses, two or three times daily if you experience any side effects from taking them all at one time. Store and take refrigerated or frozen.

❖ To minimize side effects, start with a small dose and gradually increase if you need to take more than 1,000 milligrams a day. An example of how to increase to reach 2,000 milligram is below.

Softgel 300 mg EPA/DHA	Breakfast	Lunch	Dinner
Week 1	1 softgel		1 softgel
Week 2	1 softgel	1 softgel	2 softgel
Week 3	2 softgel	2 softgel	2 softgel
Week 4	2 softgel	2 softgel	3 softgel

If you still need to increase the amount, continue to do so gradually in the same manner.

❖ Keep your fish oils in the refrigerator after they are opened to retain freshness. Small amounts can be kept at room temperature such as a daily pill box or when traveling.

Fish Oil Supplement Quiz

1. One fish oil capsule with 1,000 mg daily is all that is needed.
   ☐ T   ☐ F

2. To lower triglycerides, you need at least 2,000 mg of EPA and DHA combined.
   ☐ T   ☐ F

3. You may substitute flax oil capsules for fish oil to obtain the omega-3 beneficial for heart health.
   ☐ T   ☐ F

4. Fish oil supplements use a purification process that effectively removes mercury, dioxin and PCB.
   ☐ T   ☐ F

5. Cod liver oil is the same as fish oil.
   ☐ T   ☐ F

6. If fish oil causes "burps," it is recommended to use enteric-coated pills.
   ☐ T   ☐ F

7. Fish oil may interfere with cholesterol-lowering prescription drugs and should not be taken with these medications.
   ☐ T   ☐ F

8. It is not safe to take fish oil pills if you also eat fish that are high in omega-3.
   ☐ T   ☐ F

9. The American Heart Association recommends using fish oils supplements if not eating enough fish to provide 1,000 mg of fish oil in the form of EPA and DHA.
   ☐ T   ☐ F

10. Fish oil has a strong bitter smell and taste when it is rancid.
    ☐ T   ☐ F

ANSWERS
On Page 279.

Smart 4 Your Heart

TABLE 21.3
Seafood Nutrition
Cooked with dry heat unless otherwise indicated

3-1/2 OUNCES COOKED, 100 gm	CALORIE	PROTEIN (gm)	TOTAL FAT (gm)	OMEGA-3 (mg) DHA+EPA	SATURATED FAT (gm)	CHOL. (mg)	SODIUM (mg)
FINFISH							
Anchovy, fresh, raw	130	20	5	1,449	1.3	60	10
Anchovy (one piece, 4 gram) canned, oil drained	8	1	0.4	54	0.08	3	147
Anchovy, canned, oil drained	879	29	9.7	2,055	2.2	85	3,668
Bass, freshwater	146	24	5	763	1	70	90
Bass, striped	124	23	2.9	967	0.65	103	88
Sea Bass, Chilean	124	24	2.5	762	0.6	53	87
Bluefish	159	26	5.4	988	1.2	76	77
Bluegill/Sunfish	114	25	0.9	139	0.2	86	103
Catfish, farmed	152	19	8	177	1.8	64	80
Catfish, wild	105	18	2.8	237	0.7	72	50
Cod, Atlantic	105	23	0.8	158	0.16	55	78
Cod, Pacific	105	23	0.8	276	0.1	47	91
Croaker, raw	104	18	3.1	220	1.0	61	56
Flounder/Sole, raw	91	19	1.2	199	0.3	48	81
Grouper	118	25	1.3	248	0.3	47	53
Haddock	112	24	0.9	238	0.2	74	87
Halibut	140	27	2.9	465	0.4	41	69
Herring, Atlantic	203	23	11.5	2,014	2.6	77	115
Herring, Atlantic, kippered, 1 filet 7"X 2-1/4" (2.3 oz.)	141	16	8	1,396	1.8	53	597
Herring, Atlantic, pickled, 1 piece, 15 g (1/2 oz.)	39	2	2.7	208	0.3	2	130
Herring, Pacific	250	21	17.7	2,125	4.1	99	95
Lingcod	109	23	1.3	263	0.2	67	76
Mackerel, Atlantic	262	24	17.8	1,203	4.1	75	83
Mackerel, Jack, canned	156	23	6.3	1,230	1.8	79	379
Mahi Mahi	109	24	0.9	139	0.2	94	113

3-1/2 OUNCES COOKED, 100 gm	CALORIE	PROTEIN (gm)	TOTAL FAT (gm)	OMEGA-3 (mg) DHA+EPA	SATURATED FAT (gm)	CHOL (mg)	SODIUM (mg)
Monkfish	97	18	1.9	610	0.3	32	23
Northern Pike	113	25	0.8	1,370	0.2	50	49
Orange Roughy	105	23	0.9	31	.03	80	69
Perch, Ocean, Atlantic	121	24	2	374	0.3	54	96
Perch, Yellow	117	25	1.2	324	0.3	115	79
Pollock, Alaska	113	23	1.1	468	0.2	96	116
Pollock, Atlantic	118	25	1.3	542	0.2	91	110
Pompano, Florida	211	24	12	728	4.5	64	76
Red Snapper	128	26	1.7	321	0.4	47	57
Rockfish, Pacific	121	24	2	443	0.5	44	77
Sardines, (2) 1 oz., Atlantic, canned, oil, drained, with bone	59	7	3	278	0.4	40	143
Sablefish (Black Cod)	250	17	19.6	1,787	4.0	63	72
Salmon, raw, Wild King (Chinook)	190	20	12	1,150	1.9	61	48
Salmon, Lox, smoked Chinook	117	18	4.3	450	0.9	23	784-2,000
Salmon, Wild Chum, Chum, Dog, Keta	154	26	5	804	1.0	95	64
Salmon, canned, Dog, Keta	141	21	5.5	1,175	1.5	39	379
Salmon, Wild Coho, Silver	139	23	4.3	1,059	1.0	55	58
Salmon, farmed Coho, Silver	178	24	8	1,279	1.9	63	52
Salmon, Wild Pink, Humpback	149	25	4.4	1,288	0.7	67	86
Salmon, canned, drained, with bone, Pink, Humpback	136	23	4.8	1,052	0.8	82	399
Salmon, canned, drained, with bone, Sockeye, Red	166	23	7.3	1,445	1.5	44	360
Salmon, Wild Sockeye, Red	216	27	11	1,230	1.9	87	66

3-1/2 OUNCES COOKED, 100 gm	CALORIE	PROTEIN (gm)	TOTAL FAT (gm)	OMEGA-3 (mg) DHA+EPA	SATURATED FAT (gm)	CHOL (mg)	SODIUM (mg)
Salmon, Atlantic, farmed	206	22	12.3	2,147	2.5	63	61
Salmon, Atlantic,	182	25	8.1	1,840	1.2	71	56
Wild Shark, raw	130	21	4.5	843	0.9	51	160
Smelt	124	23	3	889	0.6	90	77
Sole/Flounder, raw	91	19	1.2	199	0.3	48	81
Sturgeon	135	21	5	368	1.1	77	69
Swordfish	155	25	5	819	1.4	50	115
Tilapia	128	26	2.6	135	0.9	57	56
Tilefish	147	24	4.7	905	0.8	64	59
Trout, Wild, Rainbow	150	23	5.8	988	1.6	69	56
Trout, Rainbow, farmed	169	24	7.2	1,154	2.1	68	42
Tuna, Bluefin	184	30	6.3	1,504	1.6	49	50
Tuna, Skipjack	132	28	1.3	328	0.4	60	47
Tuna, Ahi/Yellowfin	139	30	1.2	279	0.3	58	47
Tuna, Light, canned in water, 3.2 oz.	96	21	0.7	123	0.2	25	279 (41 no salt)
Tuna, Light, canned in oil, 3.2 oz.	169	25	7	109	1.3	15	303 (43 no salt)
Tuna, Albacore, canned in water, 3.2 oz.	110	20	2.5	741	0.7	36	324 (43 no salt)
Tuna, Albacore, troll-caught, canned 3.2 oz, *Vital Choice*	175	24	7.9	1,602 total includes DPA	1.5	24	99 no salt
Tuna, Albacore, troll-caught, fresh filet *Vital Choice* brand 3.5 oz.	198	29	8.2	1,800 total includes DPA	1.5	18	225
Tuna, Albacore, canned in oil	166	24	7.2	217	1.1	28	352 (44 no salt)
Tilefish, Gulf of Mexico	147	24	4.7	905	0.8	64	59
Walleye Pike	119	25	1.5	398	0.3	110	65
Whiting	116	23	1.7	518	0.4	84	132
Whitefish	172	24	7.5	1,612	1.2	77	65

3-1/2 OUNCES COOKED, 100 gm	CALORIE	PROTEIN (gm)	TOTAL FAT (gm)	OMEGA-3 (mg) DHA+EPA	SATURATED FAT (gm)	CHOL (mg)	SODIUM (mg)
SHELLFISH							
Crab, Alaska King	97	19	1.5	413	0.1	53	1,072
Crab, Dungeness	110	22	1.2	394	0.2	76	378
Crab, Blue	102	20	1.8	474	0.2	100	279
Crab, Imitation, Surimi	102	12	1.3	605	0.3	20	841
Crab, Snow/Queen	115	24	1.5	477	0.2	71	691
Crayfish, farm	87	17	1.3	100	0.2	137	97
Lobster, American/ Northern	98	20	0.6	84	0.1	72	380
Lobster, Spiny or Rock	143	26	1.9	480	0.3	90	227
Shrimp, all varieties	99	21	1.1	315	0.3	195	224
MOLLUSKS							
Abalone, raw	105	17	0.7	49	0.2	85	301
Clams	148	25	1.9	284	0.2	67	112
Mussels, Blue	172	24	4.5	782	0.8	5.6	369
Octopus	164	30	2	314	0.4	96	460
Oysters, farmed, Eastern U.S.	79	7	2	440	0.7	38	163
Oysters, Pacific	163	19	4.6	1,376	1	100	212
Scallops, Bay and Sea	112	23	1.4	365	0.1	53	265
Squid, raw	92	15	1.4	488	0.3	233	44

Source: www.nal.usda.gov/fnic/foodcomp/search; The Food Processor software by ESHA Research, Salem, Ore., version 8.5; and www.vitalchoice.com

Note: Seafood varies by where it is caught and the diet it ate (whether farmed or wild.)
It is not unusual to find different values depending upon the fish used to obtain the data.
Canned fish varies greatly depending on manufacturer and fishing methods.

22

Flaxseed
Omega-3 (ALA)

Cold water fatty fish and fish oil are the most effective ways to obtain omega-3 for heart health. There are also plant sources of omega-3. The body converts about 2 to 5 percent of the omega-3 found in plants into the type of omega-3 found in fish. The plant source is important because it contains linolenic, a fatty acid, which we must obtain from foods since our body cannot make it.

Flax is one of the richest sources of the plant omega-3, alpha linolenic acid (ALA). Flaxseeds are small brown or golden colored seeds with a nutty taste that are grown worldwide. Much of the flax in the U.S. comes from Canada and North Dakota.

It is recommended that men obtain 1,600 milligrams, and women get 1,100 milligrams of ALA daily. A half-ounce of walnuts (seven halves) has 1,300 milligrams and a tablespoon of ground flax has 1,600 milligrams. See Table 22.1 on Page 117 for amounts in other foods.

Plant Sources Of Omega-3 (ALA)

- Flaxseed, flax oil
- Canola oil
- Hempseed oil and hempseed
- Pumpkinseed oil and pumpkinseeds
- Walnuts and walnut oil
- Chia seeds
- Foods made with canola oil (mayonnaise, etc.)
- Foods with flax added (breads, cereals)
- Soybeans and soy foods

How To Get Flax

If you aren't already eating flaxseed, you might be wondering how to add it to your diet. There are several forms of flax: whole, ground or milled, liquid oil and softgels. The most benefit is from the whole seed that has been ground or milled. If the seeds are eaten whole, you don't get as much benefit because the seed has a tough covering that passes through your body as roughage without being digested. More omega-3 is available when eating flax that is ground or crushed than eating the whole seed.

NUTRITION NOTE

Whole or Ground Flax?
For the most benefit, grind or buy it pre-ground or milled since little of the omega-3 (ALA) can be digested from whole seeds.

What About Flax Oil Vs. Fish Oil To Lower Blood Cholesterol?

Flax oil, unlike fish oil, does not have an FDA approved health claim as being beneficial for lowering cholesterol. Flaxseed oil contains ALA, the parent oil that must be converted by the body to the cholesterol-lowering EPA and DHA found in fish. But typically, little is converted, ranging from as little as 0.2 percent to as much as 10 percent under ideal situations. It would take 3 tablespoons of flax oil a day if you converted 10 percent of the ALA in flax to get the amount of EPA and DHA found in 1 teaspoon of fish oil. The cost and amount of calories to take flax oil for lowering cholesterol makes fish oil the better choice.

In some studies ALA improved heart health even though it did not lower triglycerides.[59, 60] Like fish oil, ALA increases flexibility of cell membranes, allowing arteries to be more pliable, and reduces inflammation. Several studies have shown that eating ground flaxseed lowered Apo B, which is a measure of the LDL particle number. When Apo B levels are high, there is increased risk for heart disease.

Flax and Prostate Cancer

There was a concern raised about prostate cancer and ALA, the type of omega-3 found in flax. The source of ALA in the study was beef, which has a small amount, and those men eating the large amounts of beef had the highest intakes of ALA and prostate cancer. The majority of evidence at this time suggests there is little concern that flax increases the risk of prostate cancer.

Packaged Foods With Flax Or Added Omega-3

When choosing these foods, check the ingredient list to determine if the flax is whole or has been ground or milled. Cereals and bars, which are typically not refrigerated, often use whole, not milled, flaxseed to give them a longer shelf life. The amount of omega-3 claimed on the packages is not easily used by your body since it is not ground. The whole flax does add a nice crunchy texture. If you enjoy some of these products, add ground flax when eating them.

Some products, such as cereal bars by *Zoe* and products by *Hodgson Mill*, grind or mill the flax. These are good choices, but use them quickly once opened to prevent them from becoming rancid.

Baking Effects On Milled Or Whole Flax

NUTRITION NOTE

FLAX OIL
Do not heat, bake or cook with flax oil. The liquid oil breaks down when heated.

FLAXSEED
Ground flaxseed may be used in baking as the other components protect the omega-3.

Studies found that when milled or ground flaxseed was added to baked goods such as muffins, the nutrient content remained intact, even after the heat from baking. However, liquid flax oil should not be heated.

How To Handle Flaxseed

❖ Whole seed is the most cost-effective way to buy flax. Store at room temperature for up to one year and grind it yourself as needed.

❖ A coffee grinder works great for grinding at home. Most food processors and blenders don't work as well; however, if you already have one, give it a try to see if it works. Pulse flax to get a cracked texture; the consistency you desire will be achieved based on how much you pulse. Continue to grind for a finer, flour-like texture.

❖ Ground or milled seeds are best stored in the freezer in an airtight, opaque container and used within three months. If refrigerated, use within a few days. Do not store at room temperature once ground.

❖ For the freshest ground flax, grind the whole seed as you need it. It is more convenient to grind what you expect to use in several days or a week and store it in the refrigerator or freezer. It does not freeze into a solid chunk, so you can take out the amount you need for immediate use.

❖ Flax is also sold already milled or ground. Check the "sell by" date and only buy ground seed sold in vacuum-sealed opaque bags. Once you open the vacuum-sealed package, store it in the freezer up to three months.

❖ If you buy milled flax in bulk bins or packages that are not vacuum sealed, it should be from stores where it is sold refrigerated, with a high rate of turnover to avoid rancidity.

❖ Nutrients in whole flax are not as available as ground, but whole can add a nice crunchy texture to foods. It is a good source of roughage or fiber.

❖ Golden flax is the same nutritionally as the more common brown flax. Some people like the golden variety because the lighter color is less noticeable when added to baked goods. The exception is a type of yellow flax called solin, which is very low in omega-3 and has a completely different oil profile.

❖ You can toast whole flaxseed. You may also add a bit of honey, brown sugar or maple syrup to it after toasting and use as a topping to sprinkle on cereal, yogurt and fruit. To toast whole flax, place in a dry pan over medium heat. Stir to prevent burning. It is ready when it is just starting to darken in color. It is best to consume immediately or freeze.

Tips To Include Flax In Your Daily Diet

❖ Start out slowly – 1 teaspoon per day, increasing each week by a teaspoon with a goal of 1 to 3 tablespoons (ground) per day. Give your body a chance to adjust to the extra fiber, which for some may cause loose stools.
  As with any high fiber food, don't forget to drink plenty of water.

❖ Sprinkle on hot or cold cereal – do not overmix, as the texture may become "gummy."

❖ You may need additional milk to thin cereal that is thickened from the flax.

❖ Sprinkle on top of yogurt. If you're eating a single serving container of yogurt, sprinkle on a small amount, as you eat more, add more flax rather than stirring it into the yogurt, which has less eye appeal.

❖ Sprinkle it on salad after you have tossed it with dressing. It can also be incorporated into salad dressing that will be used right away. Leftover dressing thickens upon standing.

❖ Sprinkle flax on celery sticks spread with peanut butter or other nut butters.

❖ Spread light or soy cream cheese or nut butter on whole-grain bread (toast if desired) and sprinkle with ground flaxseed.

❖ Sprinkle coarsely ground, cracked or toasted flax into soup just before serving. Cooking in soup is not recommended.

❖ Replace part of the crumbs used in meatloaf with flax.

❖ Add a couple tablespoons to ground meat before shaping into hamburgers or meatballs.

❖ Add it to any breading mixture.

❖ Add it to toppings for fruit crumbles.

❖ Replace a couple of tablespoons of each cup of flour in a recipe with an equal amount of ground flax.

Two helpful sources for more information

❖ Flax Council of Canada www.flaxcouncil.ca (204) 982-2115

❖ *Flax Your Way To Better Health* by Reinhardt-Martin www.flaxrd.com

TABLE 22.1   Omega-3 — ALA (Alpha Linolenic Acid) In Foods

FOOD	Omega-3 (mg) ALA (18:3)
OILS	
Avocado oil, 1 Tbsp.	130
Canola oil, 1 Tbsp.	1,300
Coconut oil, 1Tbsp.	none
Flaxseed oil, 1 Tbsp. (13 g)	7,249
Hazelnut oil, 1 Tbsp.**	272
Hempseed oil, 1 Tbsp. **	2,700
Macadamia nut oil, 1 Tbsp. **	500
Olive oil, 1 Tbsp.	100
Pumpkinseed oil, 1 Tbsp.**	2,240
Rice Bran oil, 1 Tbsp.	220
Soybean oil, 1 Tbsp.	920
Tea seed oil, 1 Tbsp.	100
Walnut oil, 1 Tbsp.	1,410
Wheat germ oil, 1 Tbsp.	900

NUT AND SEEDS (see nut chart for additional nuts on Page 125)	
Chia seeds, whole, 1 Tbsp.**	3,510
Flaxseeds, whole, 1 Tbsp. (9.7 g)	1,760
Flaxseeds, ground, 1 Tbsp. (7 g)	1,595
Hempseeds, 1 Tbsp.	800
Walnuts, 1 Tbsp. chopped (0.25 oz.)	643
Pecans, 1 Tbsp. chopped (0.25 oz.)	70

SOY FOODS	
Green soybeans, edamame, shelled 1/2 cup	480
Soybeans, 1/2 cup cooked	510
Soy milk, 1 cup	210
Tempeh, 4 oz.	250
Tofu, 4 oz. firm	360
Tofu, silken style, 3 oz.	187

MAYONNAISE	
Spectrum Omega-3 soy mayo with flax oil, 1 Tbsp.	2,000
Mayonnaise, 1 Tbsp. w/canola oil	1,021
Smart Balance mayonnaise, 1 Tbsp.**	500
Mayonnaise, 1 Tbsp. w/soybean oil	690
Mayonnaise, 1 Tbsp. light	250

MARGARINE, BUTTER, SPREADS (1 TBSP.)	
Spectrum Spread	2,000
Smart Balance buttery spread	400
Canola Harvest, non-hydrogenated margarine with flax oil**	1,500
Butter	.05

OTHER FOODS	
Eggland eggs**	100
Broccoli raab, 1/2 cup cooked	111
Broccoli, 1/2 cup cooked	90
Black beans, 1/2 cup cooked	90
Spinach, 2 oz. raw	80
Kale, green leafy, 1/2 cup cooked	70
Kidney beans, 1/2 cup	60
Avocado, 1/4	60
Romaine lettuce, 1 cup raw	53
Turnip greens, 1/2 cup cooked	46
Kiwi, 3 oz.	40
Green Peas, frozen 1/2 cup	20
Arugula, 1/2 cup raw	17
Mustard greens, 1/2 cup cooked	15
Watercress, 1 cup raw	8
Beet greens, 1/2 cup cooked	4

CEREALS AND GRAINS	
Zoe's Flax & Soy Granola Cereal, 1/2 cup**	2,200
Nature's Path Hemp Plus Granola, 1/2 cup**	400
Barilla Plus pasta, 1/2 cup uncooked**	180
Wheat germ, 1 Tbsp.	50
Oat bran, 1 Tbsp.	10
Wheat bran, 1 Tbsp.	10

OTHER FOODS enriched with omega-3 in form of EPA + DHA (mg)	
Smart Balance Omega Plus, 1 Tbsp.**	75 EPA+ 75 DHA
Gold Circle Farms DHA eggs**	150 DHA
Gold Circle Farms liquid whites (60 g) **	50 DHA
Silk Plus Soymilk with omega-3 **	370 ALA + 32 DHA
Horizon Organic Low-fat 1% Milk Plus DHA **	32 DHA
Eggland eggs	2 EPA + 50 DHA

**data from manufacturers' Web sites
Source: www.nal.usda.gov/fnic/foodcomp/search

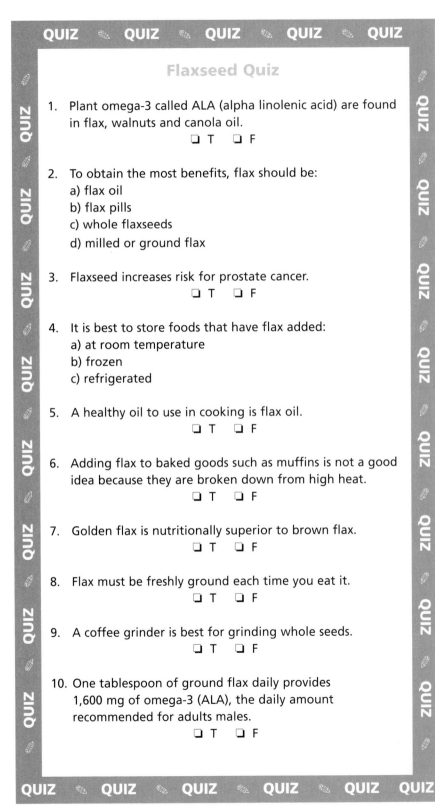

Flaxseed Quiz

1. Plant omega-3 called ALA (alpha linolenic acid) are found in flax, walnuts and canola oil.
   ❑ T ❑ F

2. To obtain the most benefits, flax should be:
   a) flax oil
   b) flax pills
   c) whole flaxseeds
   d) milled or ground flax

3. Flaxseed increases risk for prostate cancer.
   ❑ T ❑ F

4. It is best to store foods that have flax added:
   a) at room temperature
   b) frozen
   c) refrigerated

5. A healthy oil to use in cooking is flax oil.
   ❑ T ❑ F

6. Adding flax to baked goods such as muffins is not a good idea because they are broken down from high heat.
   ❑ T ❑ F

7. Golden flax is nutritionally superior to brown flax.
   ❑ T ❑ F

8. Flax must be freshly ground each time you eat it.
   ❑ T ❑ F

9. A coffee grinder is best for grinding whole seeds.
   ❑ T ❑ F

10. One tablespoon of ground flax daily provides 1,600 mg of omega-3 (ALA), the daily amount recommended for adults males.
    ❑ T ❑ F

ANSWERS
On Page 279
and Page 280.

Smart 4 Your Heart

23

Nuts

Nuts may reduce the risk of heart disease. It has been found that those who ate nuts more than four times a week had fewer fatal heart events than those who ate nuts less than once a week. It only takes 1 to 2 ounces of nuts to see this benefit. Beyond that, no further benefit is seen.

Evidence of the benefits from eating nuts led to FDA authorization of a qualified health claim for some nuts.

Nuts Able To Make A Health Claim
❤ Almonds   ❤ Hazelnuts   ❤ Peanuts
❤ Pecans   ❤ Pistachios   ❤ Walnuts   ❤ Some Pine Nuts

The FDA claim states, "Scientific evidence suggests, but does not prove, that eating 1.5 ounces per day of most nuts, as part of a diet low in saturated fat and cholesterol, may reduce the risk of heart disease."

One and one-half ounces is approximately one-fourth to one-third of a cup. See the table below for determining how many nuts are in an ounce.

TABLE 23.1
Number Of Nuts and Seeds In 1 Ounce
Size varies so weigh for accuracy

❖ Almonds (24)	❖ Pecans (20 halves)
❖ Brazil Nuts (6-8)	❖ Pistachios (49 whole)
❖ Cashews (18)	❖ Pumpkin Seed or pepitas (142 or scant 1/4 cup)
❖ Hazelnuts/Filberts (20)	❖ Pine Nuts (158 scant 1/4 cup)
❖ Macadamia Nuts (10-12)	❖ Soy Nuts, roasted (6 Tablespoons)
❖ Peanuts (28 whole)	❖ Walnuts (14 halves)

Adapted from International Tree Nut Council Nutrition Research & Education Foundation, Nutrition In Every Handful, www.nuthealth.org.

Although nuts are high in fat, it is good fat – mostly unsaturated fat which improves your blood lipid levels when they replace less healthy saturated or trans fats. People who traditionally eat nuts generally have reduced inflammation and less risk of heart disease and Type 2 diabetes.[62]

Nuts are rich in the amino acid arginine which protects the lining of the artery walls. Arginine is used by the artery walls to produce nitric oxide. Nitric oxide is a blood dilating substance that helps to widen and relax the inside diameter of the artery so that blood flow is not restricted. Nitric oxide also makes it less likely that blood will become sticky and form clots.

Nuts and seeds contain compounds known as phytosterols. Phytosterols block absorption of cholesterol. Phytosterols also enhance immune function and exhibit anticancer effects.

Pistachios and sunflower kernels are the highest in phytosterols, but phytosterols are only one of the components in nuts that improve heart health. Nuts are rich in magnesium, calcium, copper, folic acid, potassium, vitamin E and fiber. Plant chemicals with antioxidant benefits are in nuts. Pecans have the highest level of antioxidants for nuts.

Omega-3 In Nuts

Walnuts are the nuts with the highest omega-3 content of 2,574 milligrams ALA per ounce.

Vitamin E In Nuts

Nuts and seeds are good sources of vitamin E. Almonds are richest in vitamin E and were used in the Dietary Portfolio studies that were effective in lowering cholesterol.[15, 16, 25]

What About Peanuts?

Peanuts are not technically nuts. They are legumes. However, they have been linked to the same health benefits as tree nuts in studies. Peanuts cannot be eaten raw because they are legumes. Choose dry roasted, unsalted. Some dry roasted peanuts have sugar and other flavor enhancing ingredients added, making them less healthy.

What About Seeds?

Currently, there is not a health claim for seeds; however, seeds such as flax, sunflower and pumpkin have healthy monounsaturated fats, vitamin E, minerals and phytochemicals found in nuts. They may be used along with nuts for heart healthy eating. Flax and chia seeds are rich in omega-3 in the form of ALA (Page 125).

NUTRITION NOTE

Nut Facts:
- Almonds – highest in Vitamin E
- Walnuts – highest in Omega-3
- Pecans – highest in antioxidants
- Pistachios – highest in phytosterols
- Brazil – high in selenium
- Cashews – rich in copper

Will Nuts Make Me Fat?

It has not been proven that nuts cause weight gain any more than other foods.[63] In fact, eating nuts may prevent hunger and overeating since they provide satiety or the feeling of fullness. When a food is determined to be healthy, the assumption is that we are allowed to eat unlimited amounts without any consequences. Calories still count, even in healthy food options.

The amount of nuts needed for heart health benefits is 1 to 2 ounces daily. Beyond that, you are only adding extra calories when one handful is enough to reap the benefits. Adding a few nuts to a salad or to your bowl of oatmeal will not cause weight gain. Mindlessly eating handfuls of salted, roasted nuts that are irresistible due to the added salt and flavorings, along with several cans of soda or beer, will contribute to weight gain. By the time your brain registers that you are full, you have consumed several hundred calories.

To avoid weight gain and still get the health benefits of nuts, eat them in place of less healthy foods that would provide similar amounts of calories.

Substitute One-Quarter Cup Of Nuts For Any One Of The Following For The Same Calories:

- ❖ 2 tablespoons of butter
- ❖ 4 tablespoons of cream cheese
- ❖ 32 pretzels
- ❖ 2 ounces of cheese
- ❖ 15 baked potato chips
- ❖ 11 saltine crackers
- ❖ 2 small chocolate chip cookies
- ❖ 1 brownie (2" X 2-1/2")

Roasted Or Raw

When nuts are roasted at temperatures higher than 170°F, their fats break down. There is also a loss of some nutrients such as thiamin and vitamin E.

Raw nuts are not subjected to any heat and are minimally processed. Raw nuts have the advantage of no added fat, sweeteners or salt. When nuts are eaten in their natural state, you are less likely to eat too many of them. When they are roasted, salted, chocolate covered, sugar coated, spiced or flavored, it is tempting to overeat them to satisfy our salt and sweet cravings. In addition, all the added fat, sodium or sweeteners may harm rather than help your heart health. Learn to enjoy nuts for their own flavors. Check the baking section or the health food section rather than the snack section when you shop for nuts.

Storing Nuts

Raw nuts in the shell may be stored for six to 12 months in a cool, dry place such as the cupboard in an air-conditioned home.

Once nuts are shelled, they may be stored unopened for about three months at room temperature, in a cool, dry place. Some vacuum-sealed packages have dates stamped on the package that refer to how long they will last if unopened.

After opening nuts, transfer them to heavy plastic bags, glass jars or other airtight containers and refrigerate for six months or freeze up to 12 months.

If you buy nuts in bulk, go to a busy store that has a high turnover. Look for bins that are refilled from the top and dispensed from the bottom to make sure the nuts are fresh.

Do not leave nuts in a hot car. While it may seem like a handy snack to keep in your car, the inside of your car may quickly reach temperatures over 170°F on a hot, sunny day.

Nut Butters

Spreads made from nuts and seeds are produced by grinding the nuts into a paste. Be sure to check the ingredient list when you shop for various nut butters. The best choices are those that list only the nut or seed from which they are made — nothing else. If partially hydrogenated oil is listed, it is not recommended. If salt, sweeteners, starches or palm oil have been added, they are less desirable choices.

Look for "natural" versions which have the oil separated on the top. When opened, stir the oil in and store in the refrigerator to prevent rancidity and future oil separation. Do not pour off the oil or you will end up with a dry, hard product that is difficult to get out of the jar. Some natural peanut butters use palm oil, a saturated fat, to prevent separation, allowing the nut butter to be stored at room temperature. However, this adds unnecessary saturated fat and is not the best choice.

Nut Butter Tip

Before you open the jar of natural nut butter, turn the jar upside down and let it stand overnight. The oil will rise and then when opened, it will be on the bottom, making it easier to stir the oil into the nut butter without a mess.

You may find natural nut butters in the refrigerated section of the grocery store. They will not have the oil on top or will only have a very thin layer because they have been kept chilled after they were packaged. Be sure to check the ingredient list to make sure partially hydrogenated is not listed.

Ways To Use Nut Butters

❖ Before drizzling over hot vegetables, thin almond or cashew butter with a little bit of warm water, reduced-sodium soy sauce, or *Bragg's Liquid Amines*.

❖ Dip broccolini, or broccoli stalks and stems (peel if they are too tough), into almond butter. At room temperature, it should be the right consistency for dipping.

❖ Sunflower butter is a great substitute for those with peanut allergies.

❖ Combine equal amounts of mashed beans and nut or seed butters for a sandwich spread.

❖ Toast whole-grain bread and spread with almond butter; sprinkle with ground flaxseeds and a touch of cinnamon.

❖ Spread macadamia nut butter or your favorite nut butter on apples.

❖ When making hummus, substitute peanut butter or almond butter for the tahini typically called for. Tahini is a ground seed butter made from sesame seeds. This works if you cannot find tahini or do not care for its taste.

❖ Replace the butter, margarine or shortening in a cookie recipe with an equal amount of macadamia nut butter or any other nut butter.

❖ Substitute cashew, almond or sunflower butter for the peanut butter in any of your recipes, such as cookies, for a change or if allergic to peanut butter.

❖ Substitute almond butter for half of the fat in the topping used for fruit crumbles or when making a graham cracker crust.

❖ Add a spoonful to your hot, steel-cut oatmeal or to a breakfast smoothie.

❖ Top your hot, whole-grain pancakes or waffles with nut butter. Add a few dark chocolate chips and top with another pancake or waffle for an on-the-go sandwich.

❖ Spread thinly on a small square of dark chocolate.

❖ Cashew butter goes well with sauces. Add it to barbeque sauce or make a dip or sauce (see recipe Page 336).

❖ Dip fresh fruit into macadamia butter or another favorite nut butter.

Nut Quiz

1. Nuts are high in healthy fats and may be eaten in unlimited amounts.
   ❏ T   ❏ F

2. The FDA health claim for nuts states _____ of nuts may reduce the risk of heart disease.
   a) 3/4 cup
   b) 2 handfuls
   c) 1-1/2 ounces
   d) 3 ounces

3. Arginine in nuts protect the lining of the artery walls.
   ❏ T   ❏ F

4. The nut which is highest in omega-3 is:
   a) almonds   b) peanuts   c) walnuts

5. Nuts richest in vitamin E:
   a) almonds   b) peanuts   c) walnuts

6. The best way to store shelled nuts:
   a) at room temperature up to a year
   b) refrigerated for a year
   c) frozen up to a year

7. Peanut butter and other nut butters that are natural and do not contain any partially hydrogenated oils are best.
   ❏ T   ❏ F

8. The best choice are nuts that are:
   a) dry roasted
   b) unsalted
   c) raw

9. Nuts that are allowed to carry a health claim are:
   a) almonds   b) Brazil nuts   c) hazelnuts   d) cashews
   e) peanuts   f) pecans   g) macadamia nuts
   h) pistachios   i) walnuts   j) some pine nuts

10. Nuts are more "fattening" than other foods and are best avoided when trying to lose weight.
    ❏ T   ❏ F

ANSWERS
On Page 280.

Smart 4 Your Heart

TABLE 23.2   Nuts and Seeds Nutrition

Nut (number of nuts in ounce)	Calories	Total fat (g)	Saturated fat (g)	Fiber grams	Omega-3 ALA mg	Calcium mg	Vitamin E IU % DV	Copper mg % DV	Magnesium mcg % DV	Iron mg % DV	Zinc mg % DV	Potassium mg
Almonds (24)	163	14	1.1	3	0	70	11 / 37%	.31 / 16%	78 / 19%	1.2 / 7%	.95 / 6%	200
Brazil Nuts (6)	186	19	4.6	2	10	50	3.2 / 11%	.5 / 25%	64 / 16%	.97 / 5%	1.3 / 9%	187
Cashews (18)	157	12	2.2	1	10	10	.38 / 1%	.62 / 31%	83 / 21%	2 / 11%	1.6 / 11%	187
Hazelnuts/Filberts (20)	178	17	1.3	3	25	32	6 / 21%	.5 / 24%	46 / 12%	1.3 / 7%	.69 / 5%	193
Macadamia Nuts (10-12)	203	22	3.4	2	58	20	.24 / 1%	.146 / 8%	.33 / 8%	.75 / 4%	.37 / 2%	104
Peanuts, (30 whole)	166	14	1.9	2	1	15	2.9 / 10%	.19 / 10%	50 / 12%	.64 / 4%	.94 / 6%	200
Pecans (20 halves)	196	20	1.7	3	282	19	1.5 / 5%	.34 / 17%	34 / 9%	.72 / 4%	1.2 / 9%	116
Pistachios (46 whole)	158	13	1.5	3	72	30	.97 / 3%	.37 / 18%	34 / 9%	1.1 / 7%	.62 / 4%	291
Pine Nuts (158/scant 1/4 cup)	191	19	1.4	1	46	4	3.9 / 11%	.38 / 19%	71 / 18%	1.6 / 9%	1.8 / 12%	169
Soy Nuts, roasted (1/3 cup)	132	6	.95	2.3	474	37	.82 / 3%	.3 / 15%	49 / 12%	1.4 / 8%	1 / 7%	382
Walnuts, English (14 halves)	185	18	1.7	2	2,574	28	.3 / 1%	.45 / 22%	45 / 11%	.82 / 5%	.88 / 6%	125
Seeds: 2 Tbsp.												
Flax/Linseeds 2 Tbsp. = 14 g (grd.)	75	5.9	.5	3.8	3,190	36	.08 / 0%	.17 / 8%	59 / 15%	1 / 6%	.68 / 5%	114
Pumpkin Seeds 2 Tbsp. = 14 g	77	6.5	1.2	0.6	30	6	.06 / 0%	1.0 / 50%	76 / 19%	2 / 12%	1 / 6%	113
Sunflower Seeds 2 Tbsp. = 18 g	103	9	.9	1.9	10	20	6.2 / 21%	0.3 / 15%	64 / 16%	4.2 / 7%	.9 / 6%	116
Sesame Seeds 2 Tbsp. = 18 g	103	9	1.2	2	70	175	.07 / 0%	.73 / 37%	63 / 16%	2.6 / 15%	1.4 / 9%	85
Poppy Seeds 2 Tbsp. = 17.6 g	94	7.8	.85	1.8	60	.255	.2 / 1%	.27 / 14%	55 / 14%	1.5 / 9%	1.7 / 11%	123
Chia Seed 2 Tbsp. = 20 g	98	6	0.6	7.5	3,509	126	--	0.04 / 2%	1.5 / .4 %	1.9 / 10%	.69 / 5%	32

Source: Food Processor Software by ESHA Research, Salem, Ore., and manufacturer Web sites.

Nut Butters

Natural nut butters that do not have added sweeteners, saturated fats or salt are best. They taste more like nuts and are less sweet. Many nuts are made into nut butters. For a wide variety of unusual nut and seed butters, check out www.futtersnutbutters.com or a well-stocked store.

- ❖ Almond butter
- ❖ Brazil nut butter
- ❖ Cashew butter
- ❖ Hazelnut butter
- ❖ Macadamia nut butter
- ❖ Pecan butter

- ❖ Pistachio butter
- ❖ Pumpkin seed butter
- ❖ Soy butter
- ❖ Sunflower seed butter
- ❖ Tahini
- ❖ Walnut butter

Peanut Butter

A reduced-fat peanut butter is not the healthiest choice. Sweeteners are used to replace some of the fat. The added sugars are not better than the healthy type of fat they replace. If you are concerned about calories eat a smaller portion of natural peanut butter.

Make Your Own Nut Butter

You can make your own nut butters. Use a food processor and blend until an oily mass forms. Nuts vary in their oiliness. Peanuts, macadamia nuts, Brazil nuts and cashews need little, if any, oil, while 2 cups almonds require 1 to 3 teaspoons added oil to form a creamy texture. For a neutral taste, use canola oil. If making almond butter, you can use almond oil, or if making walnut butter, use walnut oil.

You can also combine nuts to make a new variety, such as pistachio and almond, peanuts and sunflower seeds, or whatever combination appeals to you. Or, add a little cocoa powder to hazelnuts or peanuts.

Storing Natural Nut Butters

Store nut butters in the refrigerator to avoid becoming rancid. If too firm to spread, allow to stand at room temperature for a short time.

24

Soluble Fiber
(Viscous)

Not all fiber is the same. Clinical trials have found that soluble fiber, especially from oats, oat bran, barley and psyllium, decreases LDL blood cholesterol.[66] For every 1 to 2 grams of soluble fiber eaten per day, LDL cholesterol may decrease 1 percent or more.

Soluble fiber is also found in dried beans, lentils, fruits and vegetables. However, until more studies are done on specific foods, the only ones currently allowed to carry the FDA claim are oats and barley foods, if they contain enough beta-glucan per serving, and foods and supplements that contain psyllium.

Soluble Fiber That Lowers Cholesterol

❖ **Beta-Glucan:** found naturally in oats; barley; and in smaller amounts in mushrooms, yeast, bacteria and algae.

❖ **Psyllium:** derived from seed husks of the plant called Pantago ovata.

How Much Soluble Fiber?

The soluble fiber goal to aim for is 9 grams soluble fiber for every 1,000 calories, or about 10 to 25 grams daily, however, as little as 3 grams a day is effective in lowering cholesterol. To find the amount of soluble fiber in foods, see Page 132.

Two Types Of Fiber

Food labels are required to list total dietary fiber. Total fiber includes the two kinds of fiber, soluble and insoluble, both of which are important for health. Food labels are not required to list the types of fiber separately on the label, although some labels do provide that information.

Insoluble Fiber

Insoluble fiber is the type that keeps our digestive system working well. Think of it as the scrubbers or roughage that help regulate bowel movements.

Soluble Fiber

Soluble fiber becomes gummy in water forming a gel which helps to lower cholesterol, keep blood sugar levels stable and gives you a feeling of fullness. It is also referred to as viscous fiber. Soluble fiber slows the absorption of fats and carbohydrates into the bloodstream, which improves blood sugar control.

Sources Of Fiber

High In Soluble Fiber To Lower Cholesterol	High in Insoluble Fiber
Oats Barley Oat Bran Psyllium Legumes Rye Fruits (apples, berries)	Wheat Bran Millers Bran Bran Flakes Whole-Wheat Bread Skin and Peel of Fruits and Vegetables Nuts and Seeds

Nutrition Facts

Serving Size: **1/3 cup** (30 g)

Servings Per container 17

Amount Per Serving

Calories 70

Calories From Fat 10

	% Daily Value
Total Fat 1 g	2%
Saturated Fat 0 g	0%
Trans Fat 0 g	
Cholesterol 0 mg	0%
Sodium 200 mg	8%
Total Carbohydrate 24 gm	8%
Total Dietary Fiber 13 g	51%
Soluble Fiber 3 g	
Insoluble Fiber 10 g	
Sugars 8 g	
Protein 4 g	
Vitamin A 4% Vitamin C	0%
Calcium 8% Iron	1%

Finding Fiber on Food Labels

Total dietary fiber is listed under "Total Carbohydrates." Soluble is not required by food labeling laws to be listed. If you don't find soluble fiber listed, e-mail or call the company which may provide you with the necessary information.

On Page 17, you calculated your total fiber needs. Of your total fiber, 10 to 25 grams should be from soluble fiber.

If you have not been eating a high fiber diet, it takes time to adjust. You might wonder how you can add fiber without the bloating, abdominal cramping and gas that often accompanies high fiber diets. To begin adding fiber to your diet, you may find the four-month plan helpful.

Four-Month Plan To Start Adding Soluble Fiber To Your Diet

MONTH 1: For the first week, start out with <u>5 grams a day</u>. See "month 2" example below and add 3 grams at breakfast and 2 grams at dinner. Use Table 24.1 (Page 132) to find foods you like. If you find discomfort, cut back to 2 or 3 grams until you feel comfortable again. After a few days, increase to the 5 grams and maintain that for the month before you add more.

MONTH 2: Add 5 grams at lunch for a total of <u>**10 grams a day**</u>. This amount may give you a 5 to 10 percent lowering of LDL.

Breakfast: Aim for at least **3 grams** of soluble fiber
❖   Have one to two servings of a cereal that has soluble fiber such as oatmeal, steel-cut oats or rolled barley flakes. (Note: bran flakes or high wheat fiber types have insoluble fiber that does not lower cholesterol.) Alternatively, have a smoothie with dry rolled oats, rolled barley or oat bran added, or yogurt or low-fat cottage cheese with oat bran sprinkled on top. A little higher in carbohydrate is a homemade oat bran muffin (recipe Page 321), plus
❖   Piece of whole fruit such as an orange or pear (not juice).

Lunch: Aim for at least **5 grams** of soluble fiber
❖   Add legumes to your salad or canned soup; mash them into a bean spread such as hummus; or have a split pea, lentil or bean soup. If you're just starting, 1 tablespoon is enough, plus
❖   One-half cup cooked or 1 cup raw vegetables (not juice), plus
❖   One serving of fruit

Dinner: Aim for at least **2 grams** of soluble fiber
❖   One cup of cooked (or 2 cups raw) vegetables, plus
❖   One large green tossed salad

Snacks: Have a serving of fruit along with the peel rather than juice or canned fruit. Include some vegetables for even more soluble fiber or to make up for meals where you did not reach your goal.

After the second month, you can add a supplement with psyllium, such as *Metamucil*, on days when you find it difficult to include enough high soluble fiber foods, such as when traveling. Foods are the best way to lower cholesterol, so aim to eat food rather than supplements as often as possible.

MONTH 3: Add 5 more grams (15 grams total) for a 10 to 15 percent lowering of LDL

MONTH 4: Continue with 15 grams and add another 5 grams soluble fiber in foods or a psyllium supplement divided throughout the day for a total of 20 grams soluble fiber, which may result in a 15 to 20 percent lowering of LDL.

Sample Menu With 20 Grams Soluble Fiber

FOOD	SOLUBLE FIBER
Breakfast (4 grams)	
1 cup steel-cut oats	2
1/2 cup blackberries	0.88
1 Tbsp. ground flaxseed	0.65
1 cup soy milk, plain	0.49
Snack: (0.1 grams)	
6 almonds	0.1
Lunch (8 grams)	
2 cups dark green, leafy salad greens	0.9
1/2 cup kidney beans	2.9
1/2 avocado	2.0
1 Tbsp. vinegar and oil dressing	0
1 medium orange	2.06
Snack (4.6 grams)	
1/4 cup unsalted roasted soy nuts	1.5
6 baby carrots	1.4
1/2 cup jicama slices	1.7
Dinner (4 grams)	
4 oz. grilled salmon	0
1/2 cup barley pilaf	1.4
1 cup cooked broccoli	2.6
1 cup green tea	0
Total	20.58 grams

Drink Plenty Of Water

Fluids are important when you increase your fiber intake to avoid constipation. A good amount for you to drink is eight to 12 (8-ounce) glasses of fluid each day, including water and other beverages.

BEANO

If beans give you gas, this over-the-counter product that you take at the time of eating foods, not after, may help reduce gassiness.

Soluble Fiber and Statin Drugs

If you are taking a statin drug and need to lower you LDL even more, rather than increase the dose, ask your doctor if you could try adding psyllium for further reduction in cholesterol. See details of the study below.

Meta-Analysis

Eating a psyllium-supplemented cereal resulted in a 5 percent decrease in total cholesterol and a 9 percent decrease in LDL.[65] The amount used in the studies equaled 7 grams of soluble fiber from psyllium. A tablespoon of psyllium husk contains 8.5 grams of soluble fiber. Psyllium is what is found in over-the-counter fiber supplements such as *Metamucil*.

Statin Drugs Plus Fiber Study

The effect of combining psyllium fiber with the statin drug, simvastatin, was studied and the findings were reported in the Archives of Internal Medicine.[66] It was the first study that compared the use of a statin with soluble fiber in the diet. The study showed that adding dietary soluble fiber daily, or increasing the statin dose, produced the same amount of cholesterol-lowering effect.

The treatments, randomly assigned, were:

❖ Simvastatin (statin drug) 20 milligrams a day
❖ Simvastatin 10 milligrams a day
❖ Simvastatin 10 milligrams a day plus 2 grams of soluble fiber three times daily (about 1 teaspoon plain or 1 tablespoon orange flavored *Metamucil* three times a day).

Findings

Doubling the dose of a statin from 10 to 20 milligrams does not result in doubling the reduction in the LDL cholesterol. It only reduces it by an additional 6 percent. The same 6 percent reduction in this study was obtained by adding 18 grams *Metamucil* three times a day for a total of 6 grams of soluble fiber daily.

The authors of the study stated "Psyllium soluble fiber should be considered as a safe and well-tolerated dietary supplement."

In other words, *Metamucil* safely produced the same result as doubling the statin dose in reducing LDL blood cholesterol, total cholesterol and Apo B. Using this strategy will result in less cost and less risk of side effects since the drug dose is smaller.

Table 24.1
Soluble Fiber

GRAINS - Cereals	Serving Size	Total Fiber (grams)	Soluble Fiber (grams)
GRAINS - Cereal, Hot			
Oat bran, cooked	1/3 cup dry or 1 cup cooked	5	3
Oatmeal, (1/2 cup dry oats)	1 cup cooked	4	2
Oats, steel-cut, dry	1/4 cup dry	4	2
Heart Balance barley cereal	1/3 cup dry or 1 cup cooked	6	2.6
Rye, cream of	1/2 cup	2	0.8

GRAINS - Cereal, Ready To Eat First ingredient rolled oats or whole, intact grain	Serving Size	Total Fiber (grams)	Soluble Fiber (grams)
Uncle Sam's	1 3/4 cup	10	2
Zoe's granola	1/2 cup	7	2
Bear Naked granola	1/2 cup	6	2*
Food for Life Ezekiel 4:9	1/2 cup	6	1.2
Nature Path Optimum Power Blueberry	1 cup	10	2.5*
Nature Path Optimum Slim	1 cup	11	2.5*
Nature Path Smart Bran with psyllium and oat bran	2/3 cup	13	3
Kashi Go Lean Crunch	1 cup	8	3
Kashi Go Lean, high protein	3/4 cup	10	1

soluble fiber not on package, obtained from mfg.

GRAINS - Bread	Serving Size	Total Fiber (grams)	Soluble Fiber (grams)
White bread	1 slice	0.5	0
Whole-wheat bread	1 slice	2	0.5
Graham crackers	2-inch square	0.3	0.2

GRAINS - Oats	Serving Size	Total Fiber (grams)	Soluble Fiber (grams)
Oatmeal, dry rolled oats	1/2 cup	4	2
Oat bran	1/4 cup dry	3.6	1.5
Oat groats (whole)	1/2 cup dry	9	4.6

GRAINS - Barley, Rice, Pasta	Serving Size	Total Fiber (grams)	Soluble Fiber (grams)
Barley, cooked, pearled	1/2 cup	3	0.8
Barley, cooked, hulled	1/2 cup	7	1.4
Barley flakes, dry	1/2 cup	10	2
Couscous, whole-wheat, cooked	1/2 cup	1.3	0.3
Brown rice, long-grain, cooked	1/2 cup	2	0.2
Millet, cooked	1/2 cup	3.3	0.6
Spaghetti, cooked	1/2 cup	1.3	0.2
Spaghetti, whole-wheat, cooked	1/2 cup	3	0.4
White rice, cooked	1/2 cup	0.5	0.1
Whole-wheat kernels, cooked	1/2 cup (3 Tbsp. dry)	3.7	0.42
Wild rice, cooked	1/2 cup	1.5	0.2

FLOUR	Serving Size	Total Fiber (grams)	Soluble Fiber (grams)
Barley flour	1/2 cup	7.4	1.5
Whole-wheat flour	1/2 cup	7.3	1.24
All-purpose flour	1/2 cup	1.69	0.6
Brown rice flour	1/2 cup	3.63	0.4
Dark rye flour	1/2 cup	14.46	2.4
Medium rye flour	1/2 cup	7.45	1.58
Ultragrain whole-wheat	1/2 cup	7.3	1.2
Ultragrain all-purpose blend of white and *ultragrain*	1/2 cup	4	0.9

VEGETABLES	Serving Size	Total Fiber (grams)	Soluble Fiber (grams)
Artichoke, cooked	1 medium	4.7	1.8
Asparagus, cooked	6 spear	0.7	0.3
Avocado	1/2 medium	5.0	2.0
Bamboo shoots, canned	1/2 cup	2.0	1.7
Beans, green, cooked	1/2 cup	2	1.0
Bean sprouts, raw	1/2 cup	1.5	0.4
Beets, cooked	1/2 cup	1.5	0.7
Beet greens, raw	1 cup	1.4	0.6
Bok choy, cooked	1/2 cup	1.4	0.5
Bell pepper, red/green, cooked	1/2 cup	1.3	0.5
Bell pepper strips, raw	4 pieces (1-1/2 oz.)	0.7	0.08
Broccoli, cooked	1/2 cup	2.7	1.3
Broccoli, raw	1 cup	2.6	1.2
Broccoflower, cooked	1/2 cup	2.5	0.3
Brussels sprouts, cooked	1/2 cup	3	1.0
Cabbage, green, cooked	1/2 cup	1.8	0.8
Cabbage, nappa, cooked	1/2 cup	1.2	0.6
Cabbage, red, shred, raw	1/2 cup	0.8	0.3
Cabbage, savoy, cooked	1/2 cup	2.0	0.9
Carrots, baby, raw	6	2.8	1.4
Carrots, cooked	1/2 cup	2.5	1.3
Cauliflower, cooked	1/2 cup	1.7	0.5
Cauliflower, raw	1 cup	1.7	0.9
Celery, raw	1 stalk	1.1	0.4
Celery root, cooked	1/2 cup	1.2	0.5
Chives, raw	2 Tbsp.	0.6	0.04
Chiles, hot, raw	1 (1-1/2 oz.)	0.68	0.2
Collard greens, cooked	1/2 cup	2.6	1.2
Corn, cooked	1/2 cup	2	0.3
Cucumber, whole	1 medium 8"	0.5	0.06
Endive, curly, chopped	1/2 cup	0.8	0.3
Eggplant, cooked	1 cup	2.5	0.4
Jicama, raw	1/2 cup	3.2	1.7
Kale, cooked	1/2 cup	1.3	0.6
Leeks, cooked	1/2 cup	1.1	0.5
Kohlrabi, raw	1/2 cup	2.4	1.7
Lettuce, iceberg	1 cup	0.8	0.1
Lettuce, romaine	1 cup	0.9	0.3
Leafy salad, mixed greens	1 cup	1.2	0.4
Mixed vegetables, cooked	1/2 cup	4	1.6

Soluble Fiber

VEGETABLES (CONT.)	Serving Size	Total Fiber (grams)	Soluble Fiber (grams)
Combination vegetables, frozen:			
Varies by brand			
Broccoli, cauliflower	1/2 cup	1.5	0.6
Corn/green beans/carrots	1/2 cup	4.0	1.9
Broccoli/peppers/mushrooms	1/2 cup	1.8	0.7
Peas and carrots	1/2 cup	2.5	0.9
Mushrooms, cooked, sliced	1/2 cup	1.8	0.2
Mustard greens, cooked	1/2 cup	1.4	0.7
Onion	medium	1.98	0.8
Okra, cooked	1/2 cup	2.5	0.7
Parsnips, cooked	1/2 cup	3	1.4
Peas, sweet, cooked	1/2 cup	4.5	0.5
Pea pods, cooked	1/2 cup	3.0	1.7
Potato, with skin, baked	1 medium (6 oz.)	2.9	1.2
Potato, no skin, baked	1 medium (6 oz.)	2.5	0.5
Potato, mashed	1/2 cup	1.6	0.9
Pumpkin, cooked	1/2 cup	3.6	0.6
Radish, raw	7 medium	0.5	0.2
Rutabaga, cooked	1/2 cup	2.2	0.9
Soybeans, green, cooked	1/2 cup	4	1.5
Spinach, cooked	1/2 cup	2.7	0.5
Spinach, raw	1 cup	0.4	0.1
Squash, butternut, cooked	1/2 cup	1.5	0.5
Squash, spaghetti, cooked	1/2 cup	1.1	0.1
Squash, winter, cooked	1/2 cup	2.8	0.3
Sweet potato, baked, no skin	1 medium (4 oz.)	3.4	1.7
Swiss chard, cooked	1/2 cup	1.84	0.9
Water chestnuts	1/2 cup	1.2	0.9
Tomato, fresh	1/2 cup	1	0.2
Tomatoes, canned	1/2 cup	1.1	0.3
Turnip, cooked	1/2 cup	2.3	1.0
Turnip greens, cooked	1/2 cup	2.5	0.8
Zucchini, cooked	1/2 cup	1.2	0.5
Vegetable only soup	1 cup	2	0.8

BERRIES	Serving sizes (grams)	Total Fiber (grams)	Soluble Fiber
Blackberries	1 cup (144 g) (5 oz.)	7.6	1.76
Blueberries	1 cup raw (145 g) (5 oz.)	3.9	1.10
Cherries	21 each or; 1 cup (140g) (5oz.)	3.3	1.54
Cranberries	1 cup (110 g) (3.8 oz.)	4.6	1.53
Raspberries	1 cup (123 g) (4.3 oz.)	8.4	1.50
Strawberries	1 cup (144 g) (5 oz.)	3.3	1.20

MELONS	Serving sizes	Total Fiber (grams)	Soluble Fiber (grams)
Cantaloupe	1/4 medium (142g) (5 oz.)	1.06	0.3
Honeydew	1/10 medium (142g) (5 oz.)	0.8	0.2
Watermelon	2 cups diced pieces (280g) (10 oz.)	0.6	0.4

FRESH FRUIT	Serving Size	Total Fiber (grams)	Soluble Fiber (grams)
Cantaloupe	1/4 medium		
Apple, w/peel	1 medium (138 g) (4.8 oz.)	3.73	1.42
Apple, no peel	1 medium	2.5	0.9
Applesauce	1/2 cup	1.6	0.5
Apricot, fresh	1 (35 g) (1.2 oz.)	0.84	0.47
Banana	1 medium (118 g) (4 oz.)	2.83	0.91
Fig, fresh	1 (50 g) (1.7 oz.)	1.65	0.33
Guava	1 (90 g) (3.2 oz.)	4.86	2.43
Grapes, Thompson	1.5 cups (138 g) (4.8 oz.)	2.4	0.4
Grapefruit	1/2 medium (3.2 oz.)	1.41	1.04
Kiwifruit	1 large (74 g) (2.6 oz.)	3	1.03
Lemon	1 medium (58 g) (2 oz.)	1	-
Lime	1 medium (67 g) (2.4 oz.)	2	-
Mango	1/4 cup (85 g) (3 oz.)	1.53	0.88
Nectarine	1 medium (140 g) (5 oz.)	2	0.8
Orange	1 medium (131 g) (4.6 oz.)	3.13	2.06
Orange juice	4 oz.	0.23	0.07
Papaya	1 small (105 g) (3.7 oz.)	1.89	-
Passion Fruit	2 (36 g) (1.25 oz.)	3.74	1.87
Peach	1 medium (98 g) (3.5 oz.)	1.96	0.86
Pear	1 medium (166 g) (5.8 oz.)	3.98	0.83
Pineapple	2 slices, 3.5"diameter, 3/4" thick (168g) (6 oz.)	2.02	0.17
Plantain	1/2 cup cooked (77g) (2.7 oz.)	1.77	0.60
Plum	1 medium (66 g) (2.3 oz.)	1	0.5
Pomegranate	1 each, 3-3/8"diameter, (154g) (5.4 oz.)	0.92	0.18
Pomelo	1/2 cup (95 g) (3.4 oz.)	0.95	-
Quince	1 (92 g) (3.25 oz.)	1.75	0.41
Rhubarb	1 cup chopped (122g) (4 oz.)	2.20	0.68
Starfruit	1 (91 g) (3.2 oz.)	2.46	0.18
Tangerine	1 medium 2"diameter (109g) (3.8 oz.)	3	0.9

DRIED FRUIT	Serving size	Total Fiber (grams)	Soluble Fiber (grams)
Apricots	2 pieces (1/4 oz.)	0.6	0.3
Dates	2 each (1/2 oz.)	1.2	0.3
Fig	2 each (1.3 oz.)	4.6	1.9
Prunes	2 each (1/2 oz.)	1.19	0.5
Raisins, not packed	1/4 cup (1 oz.)	1.4	0.4

Soluble Fiber

DRIED BEANS, PEAS, LEGUMES, SOY FOODS	Serving Size	Total Fiber (grams)	Soluble Fiber (grams)
Black beans, cooked	1/2 cup	4.9	0.65
Chickpeas, garbanzo	1/2 cup	6	1.5
Kidney beans	1/2 cup	6	2.9
Lentils	1/2 cup	8	1.3
Navy beans, cooked	1/2 cup	5.8	2.2
Northern, Great, cooked	1/2 cup	5.6	1.4
Pinto beans	1/2 cup	5.5	2.1
Soybeans, cooked	1/2 cup	5.1	2.3
Split peas, cooked	1/4 cup	4	1.4
Hummus	2 Tbsp.	1.6	0.4
Soy milk	1 cup	3.2	0.47
Tempeh	4 oz.	6	2.6
Textured vegetable protein	1/4 cup or 24 g	4	0.2
Tofu	1/4 cup	1.4	0.9

SEEDS & NUTS	Serving size	Total Fiber (grams)	Soluble Fiber (grams)
Almonds, roasted w/skin	1/2 oz.	1.67	0.2
Brazil nuts	1/2 oz.	1.06	0.2
Cashews	1/2 oz.	0.47	0.23
Flaxseed, ground	2 Tbsp.	4	1.3
Hazelnuts	1/2 oz.	1.37	0.44
Macadamia nuts	1/2 oz.	1.22	0.44
Peanuts	1/2 oz.	0.98	0.27
Pecans	1/2 oz.	1.36	0.42
Pistachios	1/2 oz.	1.46	0.04
Pumpkin seeds	1/2 oz.	0.55	0.08
Soy nuts, roasted	1/4 cup	3.4	1.5
Sunflower seeds	2 Tbsp.	1.8	0.6
Walnuts	1/2 oz.	0.95	0.31

PSYLLIUM SUPPLEMENTS	Serving size	Total Fiber (grams)	Soluble Fiber (grams)
Metamucil, capsules	6	3	2
Metamucil, flavored**	1 round Tbsp.	3	2
Metamucil, powder, unflavored*	1 rounded tsp.	3	2
Metamucil, wafers	2 wafers	6	3
Dry psyllium husk powder	1 rounded tsp. (5 grams)	4.5	3.5

* 7 grams original coarse
**11 grams orange flavored coarse

Source: Food Processor Software by ESHA Research, Salem, Ore., and manufacturer Web sites.

25

Psyllium, Oats and Barley

Among the grains, oats and barley are rich in soluble fiber and contain the highest concentration of vitamin E, such as tocotrienols, which may also provide some heart benefits.

The FDA allows health claims for soluble fiber found in the following:
1. Psyllium seed husk, (7 grams per day)
2. Oats in the form of whole oats, rolled oats, oat bran and oatrim contain beta-glucan (β-glucan), a serving of at least 3 grams per day
3. Barley beta-glucan (3 grams per day)

What has 3 grams beta-glucan soluble fiber?
- ❖ 1-1/2 cup cooked oatmeal (old-fashioned)
- ❖ 3/4 cup dry rolled oats
- ❖ 1/3 cup of whole oat groats = 1 cup cooked
- ❖ 6 Tbsp. dry, steel-cut oats = 1 cup + 2 Tbsp. cooked
- ❖ 1 cup cooked, hulled barley
- ❖ 1/3 cup dry oat bran

Barley

Five clinical trials showed LDL cholesterol was lowered 6 percent with 3 grams of soluble fiber daily from barley flakes, barley flour and pearled barley when substituted for wheat and rice, which are low in soluble fiber. When soluble fiber from barley was increased to 6 grams daily, LDL cholesterol dropped. as much as 17 percent.[67] One cup of cooked, hulled barley would provide 3 grams. Since beta-glucan is found throughout the entire barley kernel, even if barley is refined, such as pearled barley, it will still contain some soluble fiber.

FDA Health Claim For Barley

"Soluble fiber from foods such as [name of food is inserted here], a part of a diet low in saturated fat and cholesterol, may reduce the risk of heart disease."

Products that provide at least 0.75 grams soluble fiber that are allowed to make a health claim include:

- ❖ Whole-grain barley, called kernels or berries
  - ✦ hulled barley, tough hull mechanically removed
  - ✦ hulless barley, a variety with hull so loose it falls off by itself
- ❖ Pearled barley, pot or scotch (some bran and germ is removed as it is polished)
- ❖ Barley bran
- ❖ Barley flakes
- ❖ Barley flour
- ❖ Barley meal

A waxy, hulless variety of barley, *Prowashonupana*, also known under the brand name *Sustagrain*, was developed through conventional plant breeding. It has two to three times more beta-glucan than other types of barley. It can be purchased as barley flakes, steel-cut or flour from www.kingarthur.com.

Try barley as a hot cereal. You can purchase barley flakes to use like rolled oats. The next time you make a side dish with pasta or rice, try substituting barley. Barley flour results in baked goods with a lighter texture than whole-wheat flour and is easily substituted for all-purpose flour. Barley flour works best in recipes that do not use yeast. Barley has less gluten than wheat. Gluten is what helps yeast-raised breads rise.

Oats

Oats are a good source of beta-glucan, the soluble fiber which reduces LDL cholesterol.

Antioxidants such as the phenol called avenanthramides are unique to oats and protect LDL cholesterol from being oxidized. It is only after cholesterol is oxidized that it is able to stick to artery walls. The antioxidants in oats include tocotrienols which have vitamin E activity and add additional protection. The amino acid ratio in oats of lysine to arginine may further protect the heart.

Oat Bran

The outer layer of the grain is removed to produce oat bran. Because oat bran is more concentrated in soluble fiber, you get more cholesterol-lowering soluble fiber compared to rolled oats for the same volume. Oat bran, which is one-half soluble fiber, lowers cholesterol more than wheat bran, which is only one-fifth soluble fiber.

In one study, 2 ounces (7 tablespoons uncooked) of oat bran per day lowered LDL 16 percent after three months and increased HDL by 15 percent.

Another study found 3.5 ounces (two-thirds cup) of dry oat bran daily, lowered LDL by 14 percent.

Add oat bran to already healthy foods such as your oatmeal or other cereal or to a smoothie. While manufacturers add oat bran to foods such as cookies or potato chips, you would have to eat too much of them to get the amount of soluble fiber required. Remember, oat bran does not magically transform unhealthy processed foods.

NUTRITION NOTE

Oat bran may lower LDL by 14-16%.

What About Instant Oats?

It is the least desirable form of oats. In many cases, instant oats have added sugars and salt, which makes them a much less healthy choice even though they have soluble fiber. Instant oats are more finely ground than steel-cut oats or rolled oats, which gives it a higher glycemic index. It is digested more quickly and raises blood glucose levels faster, potentially increasing damage to blood vessels and producing higher insulin levels, all promoting heart disease. It is best to obtain soluble fiber in less-processed forms of oats such as steel-cut and old-fashioned oats.

NUTRITION NOTE

Instant oats are the least desirable form of oats.

How Oat and Barley Fiber Works To Lower Cholesterol

The beta-glucan forms a gel that combines with bile acids. The fiber and bile acid are excreted. Your body needs bile acid to digest fat; therefore, the liver takes cholesterol from the blood to make more bile acid. The result is lower blood cholesterol.

Effect On LDL, Particle Number, Particle Size, Blood Pressure, Blood Sugars

The soluble fiber in oats and barley lowers LDL cholesterol, lowers the particle number and increases the LDL particle size. Small, dense particles are more common in people with heart disease.

Oat and barley fiber does more than help lower your cholesterol. Studies have found it helps to maintain healthy blood pressure, helps you to feel more satisfied after you eat, and it helps stabilize blood sugar in Type 2 diabetes.

Psyllium: Soluble Fiber In Supplements

If you decide to get part of your soluble fiber from a supplement, you should know that not all fiber supplements contain fibers that are effective in lowering cholesterol. Some methods of processing the raw fiber may weaken the gel that a soluble fiber forms and reduce or eliminate its ability to lower cholesterol.

Some fiber may be hydrolyzed to avoid a gummy mouth feel or avoid the gritty taste, resulting in a product that is clear when mixed in water. Nevertheless, as viscosity is lost, so is the cholesterol-reduction benefit.

Fiber supplements containing psyllium are currently the only ones allowed to carry the following FDA health claim: "Diets low in saturated fat and cholesterol that include 7 g/day of soluble fiber from psyllium may reduce the risk of heart disease."

A fiber supplement may promote regularity, but if you want to use it to lower cholesterol, check the ingredients for one that contains psyllium.

Psyllium

Psyllium is a grain similar to wheat, rye or oats. The husk of the plant is a rich source of soluble fiber. Instead of buying a fiber supplement, you can purchase psyllium in health food stores as a powder and add it to foods such as cereals and smoothies. This a more economical way to get the cholesterol-lowering benefits of psyllium.

Initially, when you add psyllium to your diet, you may experience a feeling of fullness as the psyllium expands in the intestine. This usually lasts only until you have a bowel movement.

Like any new food you add to your diet, start out slow. In extremely rare cases, some people have had an allergic reaction to psyllium.

Taking Medications and Vitamins With Psyllium Fiber Supplements

If possible, take medications two hours before or after you take your fiber supplement. Check with your pharmacist or health care provider for specific guidelines. Some drugs such as warfarin (*Coumadin*) or digoxin may have reduced absorption if you take them with your fiber supplement.

NUTRITION NOTE

Diets low in saturated fat and cholesterol that include 7 g/day of soluble fiber from psyllium may reduce the risk of heart disease.

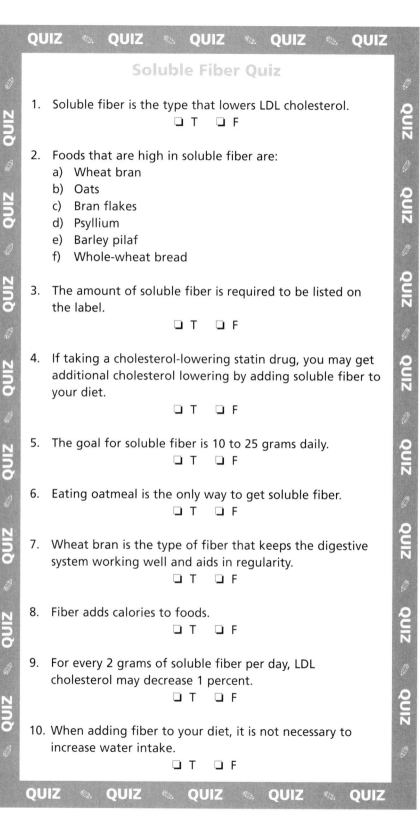

Soluble Fiber Quiz

1. Soluble fiber is the type that lowers LDL cholesterol.
   ❏ T   ❏ F

2. Foods that are high in soluble fiber are:
   a) Wheat bran
   b) Oats
   c) Bran flakes
   d) Psyllium
   e) Barley pilaf
   f) Whole-wheat bread

3. The amount of soluble fiber is required to be listed on the label.
   ❏ T   ❏ F

4. If taking a cholesterol-lowering statin drug, you may get additional cholesterol lowering by adding soluble fiber to your diet.
   ❏ T   ❏ F

5. The goal for soluble fiber is 10 to 25 grams daily.
   ❏ T   ❏ F

6. Eating oatmeal is the only way to get soluble fiber.
   ❏ T   ❏ F

7. Wheat bran is the type of fiber that keeps the digestive system working well and aids in regularity.
   ❏ T   ❏ F

8. Fiber adds calories to foods.
   ❏ T   ❏ F

9. For every 2 grams of soluble fiber per day, LDL cholesterol may decrease 1 percent.
   ❏ T   ❏ F

10. When adding fiber to your diet, it is not necessary to increase water intake.
    ❏ T   ❏ F

ANSWERS
On Page 280.

Smart 4 Your Heart

26

Whole Grain

I f you eat whole grains they will protect you against chronic diseases such as heart disease, diabetes and obesity. Whole-grain foods are also linked to a lower risk of insulin resistance and a decreased risk for developing metabolic syndrome.

FDA Claim For Whole-Grain Foods

Grain products that contain all portions of the grain kernel, including the bran, germ and endosperm and have at least 51 percent whole grain by weight, are allowed to carry the FDA claim, "a diet rich in whole-grain foods ... may reduce the risk of heart disease and certain cancers."

Whole grains are better for you, but how do you know if you are getting the whole grain in the foods you buy? When you prepare and eat whole, intact kernels of wheat, rye, quinoa, bulgur, brown rice and popcorn, you know you are getting whole grains. It is not as clear when you choose cereals, crackers, granola bars and breads. These foods are made from grains ground into flour. Many food labels contain statements such as "made with whole grain," "high in fiber," "wheat," "organic" or "multigrain." These statements could mean the food inside is 100 percent whole grain, or it could have very little or even no whole grain with some fiber added.

"Made With Whole Grain"

Adding even a tiny amount of whole grain allows the use of the phrase "made with whole grain." The amount of whole grain may vary from 100 percent to very little.

A whole grain consists of three parts: the bran, the germ and the endosperm. With modern grain mills, the most nutrient-rich portion, bran and germ, can be removed, leaving the starchy, low-nutrient endosperm.

After refining, foods may be enriched to add back some, but not all, of the nutrients and none of the phytochemicals. The importance of some of these chemicals, many which act as antioxidants in our diet, is only beginning to be discovered.

Nutrients That Are Still Missing Or Are At Lower Levels In Refined, Enriched Grains

❖ Copper
❖ Potassium
❖ Zinc
❖ Fiber
❖ Manganese
❖ Magnesium
❖ Vitamin E

❖ Lectins
❖ Phytochemicals (plant chemicals with health benefits) such as:
     ✦ Saponins
     ✦ Phenolic acids
     ✦ Lignans
     ✦ Phytic acid

Check The First Ingredient Listed

To determine how much whole grain is in a food, check the ingredient listing. Ingredients are listed by weight. The heaviest ingredient is listed first, and the rest follow in order. The ingredient listed last weighs the least. Therefore, if the first grain or flour listed is "whole," you know there is more whole grain by weight than the ingredients listed after it. The best choices only have whole grains listed.

> whole wheat

Less desirable are those with whole listed first, followed by refined flour.

> whole-wheat flour, enriched wheat flour

The least desirable are those with whole grains that appear <u>after</u> a refined grain.

> unbleached, enriched wheat flour; stone-ground whole-wheat flour

Three Steps For Choosing Foods Made From Flour

There are three steps to choosing foods made from flour (bread, crackers, cereals, granola bars). Find the list of ingredients and look for:

1. Does the first grain listed have "whole" describing it? For example, "whole wheat" or "whole rye."
2. What type of oil is used? Check to be sure there is no "partially hydrogenated" or "interesterified" listed. Fully hydrogenated oil may be interesterified.
3. What type of sweetener is used, if any? No high fructose corn syrup, fructose, corn syrup solids or corn syrup should be listed.

Once they pass the three steps, you are ready to look at the nutrition facts for how much sodium, fiber, calories, sugars and other nutrients a serving has as you decide what to buy.

Gluten-Free Whole Grain

If you are gluten intolerant, choose gluten-free whole grains. You may eat the following whole-grain choices:

❖ Amaranth
❖ Brown Rice
❖ Buckwheat
❖ Corn
❖ Millet
❖ Montina (Indian rice grass) www.montina.com
❖ Quinoa
❖ Sorghum grain www.glutenfreemall.com
❖ Teff
❖ Wild Rice
❖ Oats are also gluten-free, but are often contaminated with grains that do contain gluten. There are sources that offer oats free of gluten contamination.

NUTRITION NOTE

Some grains such as spelt and farro are lower in gluten but are not gluten-free.

What About Wheat Germ and Bran?

You can buy bran and germ separately. The bran and germ are not whole grain, but parts of a whole grain that are typically removed during refining. Do not be fooled into thinking that adding bran and germ to white flour is the same as being a whole grain. Breaking foods into components and putting them together is what processed food is all about. Eating the whole, intact grain provides a synergy of the whole food, providing more benefit than the sum of its parts.

NUTRITION NOTE

Adding bran and germ to white flour is not the same as being a whole grain.

Natural Or Organic Grains

Natural or organic does not mean that the item is whole grain. Organic grain may be either refined or whole grain. Organic means that the grain was grown without conventional pesticides, no artificial fertilizers or sewage sludge and does not include genetically modified foods. When choosing organic foods, you want to be sure they are also whole grain.

Dark Or Brown-Colored Bread

Color is not a guide to determine if a food is whole grain. Dark brown breads may have molasses or caramel food coloring and little if any whole grain. A whole grain may be light in color such as 100 percent white-whole wheat flour or oats.

High Fiber Is Not Whole Grain

The less processed and refined a grain is, the more dietary fiber of the whole grain remains; however, each grain varies as to how much natural fiber it has.

You may be fooled when a processed food with refined (white) flour adds fiber in the form of bran. Some high "fiber-added" foods do not list whole grain as the first ingredient yet they are high in fiber. High fiber is not a guarantee of whole grain. Check the ingredient list for "whole" instead of the grams of fiber on the nutrition facts label.

WHOLE, INTACT GRAINS
Excellent choices

❖ Amaranth
❖ Barley, hulled, hulless
❖ Brown rice
❖ Brown jasmine rice
❖ Brown basmati rice
❖ Buckwheat berries, unhulled groats
❖ Farro (emmer wheat)
❖ Grano (ancient durum wheat)
❖ Kamut (form of wheat)
❖ Millet
❖ Montina (Indian rice grass)

❖ Oat groats
❖ Popcorn
❖ Quinoa
❖ Rye berries
❖ Sorghum grain
❖ Spelt berries (type of wheat)
❖ Teff
❖ Triticale
❖ Wheat berries, red or white
❖ Wild rice

Groats or berries are the whole intact grain with only the inedible hulls removed.

NUTRITION NOTE

Eat whole, intact grain more often than foods made from ground grains and/or flour. Intact grains are digested more slowly.

Grains may be found as:
•groats
•berries
•steel-cut
•rolled
•grits
•cracked
•flakes
•puffed
•pearled
•flour

Whole Grain Smart 4 Your Heart

WHOLE GRAIN
Very good choices
Cut into pieces, rolled, cracked, hulled, pearled

❖ Bulgur (bran intact or whole kernel)
❖ Barley, rolled flakes
❖ Barley, steel-cut
❖ Barley, pearled, quick, medium
❖ Buckwheat grits
❖ Cracked whole wheat

❖ Kasha (toasted buckwheat)
❖ Rolled oats
❖ Steel-cut oats
❖ Scottish oatmeal
❖ Rye flakes
❖ Rolled wheat flakes

WHOLE GRAINS GROUND INTO WHOLE-GRAIN FLOUR/MEALS
Good choices when excellent or very good choices cannot be used

❖ Brown rice flour
❖ Cornmeal, stone-ground, nondegermed
❖ Enriched whole-wheat flour
❖ Graham flour
❖ Sorghum flour
❖ Stone-ground whole-wheat flour
❖ White whole-wheat flour
❖ Whole cornmeal and polenta

❖ Whole durum wheat flour
❖ Whole spelt flour
❖ Whole rye flour
❖ Whole rye meal
❖ Whole-wheat farina
❖ Whole-wheat flour
❖ Whole-wheat pastry flour
❖ 100% whole wheat flour

Organic grains are not always whole. Any organic whole grain flour would be a good choice.

NOT WHOLE GRAINS – LEAST DESIRABLE CHOICE
Missing one or more of the three parts that are found in whole grain – bran, germ and endosperm – unless the first ingredient is "whole"

❖ All-purpose flour
❖ Bleached flour
❖ Bran, wheat bran, millers bran, rice bran
❖ Bread flour
❖ Bulgur with bran removed
❖ Corn grits
❖ Cornmeal, degerminated
❖ Couscous
❖ Cream of wheat
❖ Cracked wheat
❖ Durum wheat
❖ Enriched flour
❖ Enriched wheat flour
❖ Farina or cream of wheat

❖ Gluten flour
❖ High gluten wheat flour
❖ Multigrain, rye, pumpernickel
❖ Oatmeal bread
❖ Organic wheat flour
❖ Polenta, degerminated
❖ Semolina – the starch part of the durum wheat without bran or germ
❖ Spelt flour
❖ Unbleached enriched flour
❖ Vital wheat gluten
❖ Wheat flour
❖ Wheat germ
❖ 100% wheat

NUTRITION NOTE

Packages do not identify flours or grains as "refined." If you don't see "*whole*," it is refined.

See Page 285 for types of wheat used in pasta.

Tips For Adding Whole Grain To Your Diet

❖ If you like hot cereals, choose steel-cut oats, steel-cut barley or cooked whole kernels of oats.

❖ Make your own granola or muesli. See recipe on Page 315.

❖ Use thick-cut, old-fashioned rolled oats or any other grain rolled into flakes such as barley flakes, rye flakes or wheat flakes instead of corn flakes or bread crumbs in recipes such as meatloaf.

❖ Use instant brown rice in place of instant white rice. Use regular brown rice for regular white rice. Cooking time increases slightly.

❖ Make a multigrain mixture. See recipe on Page 327. Use this instead of white rice. Make up several bags and store it in the freezer until needed. Cook in a rice cooker which cooks any grain perfect every time.

❖ Replace one-third ground meat in meatloaf, meatballs, chili, lasagna, etc., with cooked bulgur.

❖ If your store does not carry a good selection of whole grain, talk to the manager and tell him what you would like, or shop at stores that do carry whole grain. If sold in bulk bins, you may buy as much or little as you need.

❖ Serve dishes such as stroganoff, chili, pasta sauce, stew or stir-fry on brown rice, cooked barley, whole-wheat pasta, or another whole grain such as quinoa, bulgur, millet, etc.

❖ Add cooked grains (freeze leftover grain in small amounts for this purpose or keep some cooked refrigerated grains which last a week) to canned or homemade soups, or stews. Barley, brown rice and bulgur work well.

The following foods made from ground flour should be used in moderate amounts, especially on low-glycemic diets, for treating high triglycerides or metabolic syndrome.

❖ Use whole-grain pita pockets and whole-grain tortillas for sandwiches or pizza crusts.

❖ Buy whole-wheat pasta. Try the angel hair or spirals which are thinner and seem less chewy. Cook them about two-third of the suggested cooking time. Taste and then decide if the pasta needs a minute or two longer cooking. If you overcook, it gets mushy and raises blood sugars faster than when still firm but not hard (al dente.) Low-carb pasta has added fiber and protein but some are not whole grain.

❖ When baking, replace 2 tablespoons of the flour with tiny, raw whole grain such as teff, amaranth, millet or whole-grain cornmeal, for extra crunch.

❖ In recipes, substitute half of the all-purpose flour with whole-wheat pastry flour or barley flour. As your family gets used to whole grain, you may increase the amount of the whole-wheat pastry flour until you are no longer using any of the all-purpose white flour.

Tips For Adding Whole Grain To Your Diet
(continued)

❖ Replace up to one-third of the flour with rolled oats or rolled barley.

❖ In recipes that require flour to thicken sauces in casseroles or gravy, use whole-wheat flour or barley flour.

❖ Make oat or barley flour with a grain mill or by pulsing rolled oats or rolled barley in a food processor or coffee grinder for 60 seconds. One and one-half cups of rolled grain will make 1 cup flour. Substitute up to half of the all-purpose flour with the oat or barley flour. Store extra in the freezer, for up to six months.

❖ Switch to whole corn meal, instead of the degerminated variety. Look for it in the natural foods section and check the ingredients for "whole."

❖ Sprinkle whole-grain cereals, such as granola, or toasted rolled grain like rolled old-fashioned oats or rolled barley on yogurt, salads and soups or as a topping on frozen yogurt, fruit crumbles or cakes. You can make crunchy toasted topping from rolled oats (old-fashioned or thick-cut oats work best) or rolled barley by baking till golden, 350° F for 15 minutes. Store leftover toasted grains in refrigerator or freezer.

❖ To bread foods such as chicken, fish or eggplant, use crushed, whole-grain cereal such as bran flakes or oat flakes.

❖ Replace cornflakes with oat bran flakes.

❖ Replace crisp rice cereal with brown rice cereal.

❖ When preparing a graham cracker crumb crust, choose a brand of graham crackers that is whole grain and does not have any partially hydrogenated oils added. Try the *Midel* or *Health Valley* brand or replace one-fourth of the crumbs with finely crushed whole-grain cereal such as kamut flakes, or *Kashi 7 whole-grain flakes*.

❖ Choose a brand of pancake mix that is whole grain such as *Hodgson Mills* or *Nature Path's*.

❖ When preparing muffins and quick breads, stir in one-half cup whole-grain flaked cereal and add 2 to 3 tablespoons of extra liquid.

❖ Look for brands that make whole-grain mixes for muffins and brownies, such as *Bob's Red Mill* (www.bobsredmill.com), *Nature's Path* (www.naturespath.com), and *Hodgson Mills* (www.hodgsonmill.com).

❖ Replace refined flour baking mixes with *Arrowhead Mills* or *Bob's Red Mill*. Both are made with whole-wheat flour and do not contain any partially hydrogenated oils.

Whole-Grain Quiz

1. An FDA health claim for whole grains is allowed on foods with 51 percent or more whole grain by weight.
    ❏ T   ❏ F

2. The statement "made with whole grains" could appear on a food that is mostly refined "white" flour and a small amount of whole grains.
    ❏ T   ❏ F

3. Which ingredient list for a whole-grain bread would be the best choice?
    a) whole-wheat flour, unbleached, enriched wheat flour, water (5 grams fiber per slice)
    b) sprouted organic whole-wheat berries, filtered water, gluten (2 grams fiber per slice)
    c) cracked wheat, wheat flour (2 grams fiber per slice)

4. If you are on a gluten-free diet, you cannot eat whole grains.
    ❏ T   ❏ F

5. Which of the following are whole grains?
    a) bran cereal   d) seven-grain bread
    b) brown bread   e) wheat germ
    c) high-fiber bran muffin   f) steel-cut oats

6. Organic grains are whole.
    ❏ T   ❏ F

7. Adding bran or wheat germ to white flour makes it the same as a whole grain.
    ❏ T   ❏ F

8. Most rye bread is whole grain.
    ❏ T   ❏ F

9. Which cracker is the best whole-grain choice?
    a) low-sodium saltine (wheat flour)
    b) melba toast (wheat flour)
    c) multigrain saltines (wheat flour, whole-wheat flour)
    d) woven wheat cracker (whole-wheat flour)

10. A good substitute for white rice is?
    a) couscous
    b) quinoa
    c) low-carbohydrate, fiber-added pasta

ANSWERS
On Page 280.

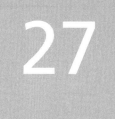

27

Beans and Legumes

Legumes are the dried seeds of plants that have double-seamed pods containing a single row of seeds. They include dry peas, dry beans and lentils (also called pulses or dals.) The use of the term dry beans is somewhat confusing. Beans may be purchased dry, which requires soaking and cooking. They are found cooked and canned and sometimes may be found freshly picked at farmers' markets or produce sections.

Legumes include black beans, black-eyed peas, cannellini or white kidney beans, chick peas or garbanzo, great northern beans, fava, lima, pinto, pink, red, turtle, navy beans, kidney beans, split peas, soybeans, lentils, etc.

Legumes are rich in soluble fiber, the type of fiber that lowers cholesterol. In one study, one-half cup of pinto beans lowered total cholesterol 19 percent and LDL 14 percent.[70]

For heart health, as little as one-half cup a day may reduce cholesterol by 8 percent. For every 1 percent you lower cholesterol, you lower your risk of heart disease by 2 percent. Therefore, a half cup of beans translates into a 16 percent lower risk of heart disease. Legumes may also help control blood sugars, lower blood pressure and prevent constipation.

Legumes are low in saturated fat; contain no cholesterol; are high in folate, B vitamins, calcium and potassium; contain plant phytosterols and lecithin; and in their natural state are low in sodium.

The folate in beans helps to lower the risk of heart disease and stroke. Folate, a B vitamin, works by decreasing levels of homocysteine, an amino acid that when elevated, is associated with higher risk of heart disease.

Legumes contain lecithin, a source of phosphatidylcholine that can be broken down into choline, a B vitamin important for fat metabolism, building brain cell membranes and treating memory loss.

NUTRITION NOTE

One-half cup of legumes per day may reduce cholesterol.

NUTRITION NOTE

Bean Tip: Start slow. Add a tablespoon or two each day to any food you already plan to eat – salad, soup, casserole, side dish.

Simple Ways To Add Beans and Lentils

❖ Instead of trying to make a daily bean dish, simply add beans to what you already eat:
  ✦ Add a spoonful of beans to canned or homemade soup.
  ✦ Puree the beans and add to soups.
  ✦ Add a tablespoon for each serving to your favorite recipes for casseroles, meat dishes or side dishes.
  ✦ Add mashed great northern beans to mashed potatoes.
❖ Make bean, lentil and split pea soups.
❖ Use beans to replace some or all of the ground meat in tacos, burritos and chili.
❖ Add mashed beans to ground meat burgers. (See Page 408)
❖ Add black beans to a pizza.
❖ Serve bean chili over a baked sweet potato.
❖ Heat spicy chili beans and spread on a whole-wheat tortilla, top with salsa, roll up and serve.
❖ Make bean spreads:
  ✦ Mash beans and use the spread when making a sandwich instead of the usual mayonnaise or butter. Top with lettuce, tomato, onion, sprouts.
❖ Make bean dip:
  ✦ Buy hummus or make your own (see recipe section).
  ✦ Serve with cut-up vegetables.
❖ Add beans to homemade or purchased salads:
  ✦ Add to leafy green tossed salad, pasta salad, potato salad or any others.
  ✦ Make a cold bean salad.
❖ Sauces:
  ✦ Puree the beans and add to sauces to thicken.
  ✦ Red lentils will blend well in pasta/spaghetti sauce. You may use less meat or no meat since they are a source of protein.
❖ Mash and put them in desserts such as spice cake, brownies or cookies.
❖ Explore soybeans, green soybeans (edamame), and all the products made from the soybean such as tofu and tempeh. See Chapter 28 (Page 157) on soy.
❖ Bean flours. Buy or make bean flour with a grain mill. *Bob's Red Mill* is a brand that sells a variety of bean flours.
  ✦ See Page 155 for more information.

Bean Nutrition

- ❖ Protein: one-half cup of cooked beans has 7-9 grams protein
- ❖ Fat and cholesterol: naturally low in total fat, less than a half-gram of saturated fat per serving, and no cholesterol
- ❖ Fiber: one-half cup has 4-7 grams total fiber and 1/2-3 grams soluble fiber
- ❖ Carbohydrates: Low glycemic complex carbohydrates that are absorbed much more slowly than carbohydrates in sugars and flour
- ❖ Minerals: 1/2 cup provides
  - ✦ Iron: 20-35% DV (Daily Value)
  - ✦ Calcium: 3-11% DV
    - Navy, great northern and soybeans are highest
  - ✦ Copper: 7-14% DV
  - ✦ Magnesium: 10-28% DV
  - ✦ Potassium: 8-16% DV, may reduce your risk of stroke and high blood pressure
- ❖ B Vitamins:
  - ✦ Folate reduces the risk of heart disease
    - 3 ounces of soybeans provide 289 milligrams folate
    - 3 ounces of lentils provide 200 milligrams folate
  - ✦ Choline: a B vitamin that may reduce homocysteine levels
- ❖ Phytosterols: plant compounds that lower LDL cholesterol
- ❖ Anthocyanins which are antioxidants that fight inflammation
- ❖ Resistant starch which provides the benefits of both soluble and insoluble fiber. It resist digestion and acts as a form of fiber.

Nutritional information calculated using The Food Processor software by ESHA Research, Salem, Ore.

Don't Like Beans

Sometimes what people mean is they don't like the gassiness they experience from beans, but the suggestions mentioned on the next page may help.

If the tough skin or texture is bothersome, try varieties that have softer skins. For example, lentils (especially the red ones) or split peas (green or yellow) don't need to be soaked and become very soft. You may also blend or mash them into hummus or bean spreads. Check the recipe section, Page 443, for using beans in chocolate cake.

NUTRITION NOTE

When you start to add beans, add a few tablespoons a day to your meals.

It may be helpful to try several varieties of beans to see which ones you prefer. White beans such as great northern will blend into light-colored foods better than the dark-colored kidney beans. Red lentils seem to disappear in pasta sauce where the brown ones are more noticeable.

Beans freeze very well. When you start to add beans, add a few tablespoons a day to your meals. You may find that it is easier to store the extra beans in the freezer so that you can enjoy a variety of different beans throughout the week. When you open a can, drain, rinse, and then spread them out in a single layer on a cookie sheet that has been lined with aluminum foil. Place in the freezer and after about 30 minutes you can pull up the foil and pour the individually frozen beans into a zip-top plastic bag. Then, when you are ready to use them, you may easily remove a tablespoon or two instead of having a large clump of frozen beans.

What About Baked Beans?

Baked beans are not the best choice since the added sugars and salt make them less healthy. Also, they are not as versatile when adding to other dishes.

Ways To Decrease Gas

One concern you may have is that eating these nutritious foods will produce intestinal gas. Beans contain two natural sugars called oligosaccharides. When these sugars pass into the intestines, they allow the bacteria in our gut to feed on these sugars, thus producing gas. Some people have more gas producing bacteria than others. However, if you add beans slowly, your body will adjust. Try adding 1 tablespoon per day; after about three weeks, most people will adapt and find that they produce less gas. You can then increase the 1 tablespoon portion to 2 tablespoons.

If you prepare beans from their dried form, the gassiness may be reduced by soaking the beans before cooking. If you soak beans overnight, 75 percent to 90 percent of the gas problem is removed. You may try adding ingredients such as ginger; epazote; asafetida, an Indian spice (available at www.penzeys.com); kombu (a type of seaweed) when cooking to help reduce the gassiness further. Some recommend chewing on Fenugreek seeds (a spice found in Indian stores) when eating beans to reduce gas.

There is also a product called *Beano* that contains the enzyme alphagalactosidase, which may help break down the sugars before they reach the intestines. You need to add this product just before you eat the first bite of gas-producing foods. It will not help if you develop gas and then take it. For more information, visit their Web site (www.beanogas.com). Experiment with the amount needed since results vary.

Some beans, such as soybeans, produce more gas than others. Low gas producers are split peas, lentils, adzuki, anasazi beans, garbanzo and black-eyed peas.

NUTRITION NOTE

Low gas producers are split peas, lentils, adzuki, anasazi beans, garbanzo and black-eyed peas.

Bean Equivalents

1 lb. dry beans = 2 cups dry beans
1 cup dry beans = 3 cups cooked
1 lb. dry beans = 6 cups cooked
1 (15-ounce) can beans = 1-2/3 cups drained beans

Varieties Of Dry Beans and Peas (Legumes)

Some of the more common varieties are adzuki beans, anasazi beans, black beans (turtle beans), black-eyed peas, cannellini (white kidney), chickpeas (garbanzo beans), cranberry beans, dark- and light-red kidney beans (Mexican or small red beans), fava, great northern beans (white beans), soybeans (edamame), kidney beans, lentils (green, red, brown, chana dal), lima beans, navy beans (pea beans), pink beans, pinto beans, small red beans (Mexican red beans), and split peas (yellow and green). There are also a number of heirloom bean varieties.

Bean Flour

Bean flour is a great way to increase the use of beans or other legumes, and no one will know they are eating beans.

❖ Use bean flour instead of wheat flour to thicken gravies and sauces. Flour made from small white beans or lima beans is the mildest. Use pinto or kidney for darker-colored sauces.

❖ Make instant creamy bean soups. Bean flour combined with water cooks in about 3 minutes.

❖ Make quick bean dips or refried beans from pinto, black, kidney and garbanzo beans.

❖ Bean flour can be added to any recipe calling for wheat flour. Replace up to 1/4 of the total amount of all-purpose, wheat flour with bean flour.

Resources For Bean Flour

❖ www.beanflour.com
❖ www.bobsredmill.com
❖ *Country Beans* by Rita Bingham has information on how to use bean flour, along with 120 recipes that use bean flour. It will change the way you use beans.

Make Your Own Bean Flour

You will need a grain mill to grind the beans into flour. If making small amounts, a hand mill, such as *Back to Basics* grain mill, works well.

To grind beans, first sort them, checking and discarding dirty beans or rock pieces. Follow the directions of your mill.

Store flours in resealable plastic bags or other food storage containers and refrigerate or freeze if possible. Flours last about six months at room temperature. After that time, a bitter aftertaste may start to develop.

Beans & Legumes Quiz

1. One-half cup of beans per day may lower cholesterol by 8 percent.
   ❏ T   ❏ F

2. Beans are a good source of folate, a B vitamin that lowers homocysteine.
   ❏ T   ❏ F

3. Beans are high-carbohydrate foods that are high glycemic.
   ❏ T   ❏ F

4. Canned beans should not be used since they are high in sodium.
   ❏ T   ❏ F

5. A good way to include beans in your diet is vegetarian baked beans.
   ❏ T   ❏ F

6. Green peas are legumes.
   ❏ T   ❏ F

7. If beans cause intestinal gas, eating them in smaller amounts on a regular basis will allow your body to adjust.
   ❏ T   ❏ F

8. The commercial product *Beano* should be taken at the first signs of having gas after eating beans.
   ❏ T   ❏ F

9. One-half cup of beans has more potassium than half of a banana.
   ❏ T   ❏ F

10. Beans may be made into flour and used to thicken soups or added to other foods.
    ❏ T   ❏ F

ANSWERS
On Page 280.

28

Soy Foods

oybeans are legumes. The soybean is unique in that the protein in the soybean is a complete protein containing all the essential amino acids needed for adults and children over the age of four. There are many different soy foods made from soybeans, such as soy milk, roasted soy nuts and soy burgers.

Initial studies that used soybeans or soy foods made from the soybean found soy was good for heart health, leading to an FDA-approved health claim in 1999 for soy foods that contain at least 6.25 grams of soy protein per serving.

To allow the health claim, the FDA looked primarily at a meta-analysis (which combines previously done studies so their results can be analyzed together). This meta-analysis study found 25 grams of soy protein lowered LDL cholesterol about 13 percent.[71]

Soy lowers LDL cholesterol about 4 percent. However, two other meta-analyses since then found that the reduction was not as great as previously stated. It was only 4 percent in one and about 5 percent in another, even with large amounts of 50 grams of soy protein daily. Triglyceride reductions averaged about 8 percent, much lower than the initial meta-analysis indicated.

Soy lowers heart disease risk but not by lowering LDL. The benefits of soybeans are that they are a great source of protein that is low in saturated fat and contain fiber. The American Heart Association (AHA) issued a statement in January 2006 stating, *"use of isoflavone supplements in food or pills is not recommended."* However, the AHA remained optimistic that *"many **soy (food) products should be beneficial** for cardiovascular and overall health because of their high content of unsaturated fats, fiber, vitamins and minerals and low content of saturated fat."*[72]

This means that eating a high saturated fat diet and drinking a soy smoothie or taking a soy supplement will not provide the same benefits as replacing a large steak dinner with a tofu and vegetable stir-fry or replacing a high-fat burger with a veggie burger.

NUTRITION NOTE

Soy lowers LDL cholesterol about 4 percent.

Soy lowers heart disease risk but not by lowering LDL.

Once again, supplements of isoflavones are not recommended since they are highly processed. These refined products probably act differently than eating a food. We have seen the same problem when a beneficial component of vegetables such as beta-carotene or fiber is removed from foods and used as a supplement but fails to provide the expected results, and in some cases may cause harm.

Although the recent studies found that diets high in soy protein did not change LDL as much as previously thought, there may be other beneficial effects. In one study, soy decreased apolipoprotein B (Apo B) and LDL particle number. Therefore, even if LDL cholesterol does not decrease, if particle numbers decrease this would be heart protective.

Researchers at Iowa State University identified IP6 phytate as the substance in soy that reduced c-reactive protein, homocysteine and iron levels.

Whole Soy Foods

Choose whole soy foods: soy milk, tofu, tempeh, unsalted soy nuts, edamame (sometimes called green soybeans or sweet beans), soybean sprouts, and soy nut butter. Full-fat soy foods are also good sources of the omega-3 fatty acid, ALA. Beware that reduced-fat and low-fat soy foods have the good fats removed, along with some isoflavones, and may not be as beneficial.

Highly processed soy products such as snack foods, beverages and bars made from soy protein isolate and other highly refined sources of soy have the concerns found in all processed foods.

Fermented Soy

Some suggest that the only soy foods we should consume are fermented soy foods such as tempeh and miso. There is little evidence that fermented soy foods offer any advantage, and there is no research to prove that use of unfermented soy foods is dangerous. A study at Tufts University found that blood levels of active compounds were the same whether fermented or unfermented soy.

Organic Soy

In 2004, 85 percent of the U.S. soybean crop was genetically engineered. Genetic engineering is the manipulating of genes in a way that does not occur naturally. If you choose soy products that list organic soybeans in the ingredients, they are not genetically altered soybeans.

Soy Foods Smart 4 Your Heart

Adding Tofu To Your Diet

You may think you don't or won't like tofu even if you have never tried it. You may fear your family will reject soy foods. You know your family — if they are not open to new ideas, perhaps it is best to say nothing about tofu being an ingredient until after it has been tried and approved.

Start with silken tofu because it can be easily blended with other ingredients. If your family enjoys dessert, begin there since tofu may replace some of the high saturated fat items such as heavy cream. Pureed silken tofu is quick and easy as a creamy topping. It's tasty in chocolate mousse or in a smoothie (see recipe section). Odds are, people will like them because we tend to like desserts. Next, try some of the suggestions on the next page.

BOTTOM LINE: Eat Soy Or Not?

Whole soy foods have a place in your healthy diet. There may be other benefits even though cholesterol levels show only minor improvement. If you don't want to take cholesterol-lowering drugs or cannot tolerate them, every little bit that you may lower cholesterol is important because it adds up.

The greatest benefit of soy is probably when you substitute it for high saturated fat foods. Eating a soy burger instead of a beef hamburger, or soy crumbles instead of ground beef or ground poultry; or replacing a full-fat dairy product like cream or cheese with soy dairy products may help lower total saturated fat intake.

Forget the soy protein powders, bars, chips and pills created by manufacturers.

You may wish to consult your physician before consuming large amounts of soy foods if you are a breast cancer patient, have a history of oxalate kidney stones, or suspect an intolerance or allergy to soy.

NUTRITION NOTE
Choose organic soy to avoid genetically engineered varieties.

NUTRITION NOTE
You may wish to consult your physician before consuming large amounts of soy foods if you are a breast cancer patient, have a history of oxalate kidney stones, or suspect an intolerance or allergy to soy.

Allergies

Some individuals are allergic to soy, just as allergies to any food are possible. Obviously, if you are allergic to soy, you should not eat it.

Breast Cancer

It appears that eating soy foods from birth is protective. At least this has been the case in animal studies. A serving of soy foods daily is not harmful, but isoflavones supplements are not recommended. The best resource that I am aware of for anyone with breast cancer concerns is a dietitian who herself is a breast cancer survivor. Visit Diana Dyer's Web site at www.cancerrd.com.

Ways To Increase Whole Soy Foods In Your Diet

❖ Use soy milk on cereal. Check the label to be sure it has calcium and vitamin D added unless you are taking a supplement to meet those needs. Look for it in the refrigerated section or on shelves in aseptic, shelf-stable boxes. The plain, unsweetened variety is best.

❖ Combine each egg with 1/4 cup of mashed silken tofu, beat together and scramble like you usually do.

❖ Cube silken tofu and add to canned or homemade soup.

❖ Puree silken tofu and add for a cream-based soup.

❖ Add canned soybeans to any casserole, soup or side dish made with rice or barley.

❖ Mash soybeans into a bean spread or dip.

❖ Replace half of the ricotta cheese in dishes like lasagna or stuffed shells with silken tofu that has been mashed with a fork.

❖ Add pureed silken tofu to mashed potatoes.

❖ Try ready-to-eat baked tofu. Slice it onto a green salad or a pasta salad, use it in your sandwich, or heat and eat.

❖ Puree silken tofu, add a package of dry ranch salad dressing mix, and try it as a dip.

❖ Try a new vegetable, shelled edamame or green soybeans without the pods. They can be found in the freezer section in many grocery stores. Serve as a side vegetable or puree into a dip along with avocado.

❖ Snack on edamame in pods. Eat them right from the pod; eat the beans inside, discarding the pod.

❖ Cube regular (not silken as it tends to be too soft) tofu, brown in olive or canola oil, and toss into casseroles or stir-fries. Make extra to toss on your salad the next day.

❖ Use textured soy protein or textured vegetable protein wherever you use ground meat – chili, pasta sauce, lasagna, tacos or enchiladas. Substitute it for part or all of the ground meat in meatloaf, meatballs or anywhere else you use ground meat.

❖ Grill cubes of marinated tofu or tempeh along with the veggies and meat on your shish kebab.

❖ Add soy nuts to salads, and trail or snack mixes.

Soy Quiz

1. Soy foods may lower LDL cholesterol 4 to 5 percent and triglycerides about 8 percent.
   ❏ T ❏ F

2. Soy isoflavones supplements are an easy way to get heart protective benefits of soy foods.
   ❏ T ❏ F

3. Soy may decrease the number of LDL particles and Apo B, the primary carrier of cholesterol to tissues.
   ❏ T ❏ F

4. Soy must be fermented such as tempeh or miso to be beneficial.
   ❏ T ❏ F

5. Whole soy foods may improve heart health. Which of the following are considered whole soy foods?
   a) soy milk
   b) soy protein powder
   c) soy chips
   d) soy nuts
   e) ready-to-eat cereal with soy added
   f) tempeh

6. The healthiest way to add soy foods to your diet is:
   a) soy smoothie instead of bowl of oatmeal
   b) soy crumbles to replace ground beef
   c) soy bar instead of almonds

7. Soybeans are legumes.
   ❏ T ❏ F

8. Soy foods are most beneficial when they replace foods that high in saturated fat.
   ❏ T ❏ F

9. Silken tofu is a good substitute for high saturated fat dairy items such as sour cream and heavy cream.
   ❏ T ❏ F

10. Soybeans are a good source of plant omega-3 and soluble fiber.
    ❏ T ❏ F

ANSWERS
On Page 280.

TABLE 28.1
Where Do You Find Protein?

To determine how much protein you need each day, see Page 18.

PROTEIN	FOOD
7 grams	1 ounce fish
7 grams	1 ounce poultry, no skin
7 grams	1 ounce lean meat (beef, pork, lamb, veal)
7 grams	1/4 cup canned tuna or salmon
6 grams	1 ounce steamed shrimp
7 grams	2 egg whites
6 grams	1 egg
7 grams	1/4 cup egg substitute
8 grams	8 ounces milk
6 grams	1/2 cup plain yogurt
7 grams	1 ounce almond cheese
7 grams	1 ounce reduced-fat cheese
6.5 grams	1/4 cup cottage cheese or ricotta cheese
6-9 grams	1/2 cup legumes (black bean, kidney, garbanzo, etc.)
3-6 grams	1 ounce nuts
9 grams	1 ounce pumpkin seeds
8 grams	2 tablespoons nut butter (peanut, etc.)
9 grams	1-1/2 ounce *Bocca* vegetarian soy burger
8 grams	4 ounces tofu
10 grams	2 ounces tempeh
10 grams	1 cup (3 ounces) *Quorn Chik'n tenders*
20 grams	1/4 cup whey protein powder
8 grams	1/2 cup shelled edamame (green soybeans)
3 grams	1/2 cup cooked broccoli
7 grams	1/2 cup cooked quinoa

NOTE: Fruits and vegetables have small amounts of protein.

29

Carbohydrates –
Making Better Choices

arbohydrates are what we use for fuel. For a long time, carbohydrates were thought of as a "good" replacement for fat. Yet we continued to gain weight as a nation and the very low carbohydrate diets became popular. Do they cause you to get fat as the low-carbohydrate diets claim? One of the problems is there are a lot of carbohydrate food choices for quick and easy, low-cost eating that may not be the healthiest way to get carbohydrates. The truth is, large portions of any food, whether it is carbohydrate, fat or protein that provides too many calories, is what will cause you to gain weight.

About 35 percent to 50 percent of our total calories should come from carbohydrates. The leaner and more active you are, the higher your percent of carbohydrates can be. The type of carbohydrates is also important. The carbohydrates that you want are found in legumes, fruits and vegetables as well as whole, intact grains, rather than from highly refined foods made from flour such as cookies, breads, crackers, snack bars and white pasta.

A lower carbohydrate level (40 percent of calories) from whole unprocessed foods is recommended if you want to lose weight, need to lower triglycerides, need to raise HDL, or have insulin resistance or diabetes. If more than 60 percent of your calories come from carbohydrates, it may cause good HDL cholesterol to decrease and triglycerides and blood sugar levels to increase.

For some highly sensitive individuals with metabolic syndrome, insulin resistance or many small dense LDL particles, eating foods from whole-wheat flour, such a whole-wheat bread, whole-wheat crackers and whole-wheat cold cereals, may need to be limited or eliminated. When whole grains are finely ground into flour, the glycemic index is higher.

Many low-carbohydrate diets recommend levels of 10 percent to 20 percent of calories as carbohydrate. To follow a level that low discourages you from eating most fruits and some vegetables and legumes, all of which are healthy carbohydrates. Therefore, these extreme very low carbohydrate diets are not advised.

NUTRITION NOTE

See Page 180 for a sample menu plan with 38 to 39% of calories from carbohydrates

Carbohydrates

Better Carbohydrate Choices
Every day foods

Intact Grains	Fruit	Vegetable	Dairy	Other
Whole, intact kernels of grains: *(see Page 146 for complete list:)* • Amaranth • Brown rice • Barley • Oats, steel-cut • Quinoa • Wild rice • Sprouted wheat bread (flourless)	• Whole fruits with peel if edible	• Vegetables, *all except the ones listed in poor choice* • Green, leafy salad greens • Sweet potato • Green peas • Legumes • Dried beans • Lentils	• Milk (skim, soy, rice, almond) • Yogurt unsweetened preferred	• Cold cereal (first ingredient: rolled oats or barley and 5 grams or less of sugars)

Whole Grains Ground Into Flour (choose less often than whole, intact grains)

- Whole-wheat bread
- Whole-grain cereal
- Whole-grain crackers

Poor Carbohydrate Choices
(refined, processed, low in fiber, some high fat/or sugar)

Ground grains high glycemic (limit)	Fruit (limit)	Vegetable (starchy) (limit)	Dairy (limit)	Other (limit)
• White bread • Bagels • Sugary or low-fiber cereals • Crackers • White rice • Instant oatmeal • Pretzels	• Fruit juice • Fruit drinks	• White potatoes • Baked beans • French fries • Fried or battered vegetables • Corn	• 2% and whole milk • Full-fat or sweetened yogurt • Frozen custard • Premium ice cream	• Sherbet, ices • Desserts • Granola bars • Doughnuts • Cakes • Cookies • Candy • Sweetened beverages • Soda • Lemonade • Punch

Carbohydrates Smart 4 Your Heart

Glycemic Index (GI)

Not all carbohydrates act the same in regard to how quickly they are digested and absorbed. Those carbohydrates that break down and are digested quickly raise blood sugar (glucose) rapidly. The glycemic index (GI) is a system used to classify carbohydrates based on blood glucose response. High GI meals may lead to increased hunger and increased food intake, making weight loss difficult.[73] The more overweight and inactive someone is, the more harmful a high-glycemic diet will be. Studies suggest that diets that include large amounts of high GI foods may be associated, not only with the development of diabetes, but also with metabolic syndrome.[74]

In general, processed foods made from flour have a higher GI than eating the whole, intact grain. Cold cereals, crackers, breads, snack bars, pretzels, even when they are made from whole-wheat or whole-oat flour, have a high GI. Cold cereals made of mostly rolled oats or added fiber and breads that have coarse pieces of grain throughout have a lower GI. Carbohydrates from legumes have a low glycemic response.

You won't find many foods with their glycemic index displayed in the U.S. where it remains highly debated. In some countries such as Sweden and Australia, it is widely available on labels.

Glycemic Load (GL)

The glycemic load (GL) is actually a better measure since it takes two things into account – the amount of food normally eaten and how long it takes to get into the bloodstream.

The GI is based on a portion that contains 50 grams of carbohydrates, which is not necessarily the quantity of a normal portion size. For some foods, eating a portion that has 50 grams of carbohydrates may be much more than what is typically eaten at one time. For other foods, 50 grams is a smaller portion than most people typically eat. Adding the glycemic load takes into account the quantity of a food typically eaten in real life and is the better measure.

Some foods that have a high GI have a low glycemic load. An example is a fruit such a watermelon. A serving of watermelon has a GI of 72 (over 70 is high). However, watermelon, which is mostly water, requires a serving of almost 5 cups diced, for 50 grams of carbohydrates. Watermelon has a low GL of 4 (less than 10 is low) when the typical serving size is also considered.

Another example of a high GI but low GL food is carrots. Many diet books tell people to avoid eating carrots, as they are considered higher in carbohydrates, with a high GI of 92. However, to get 50 grams of carbohydrates from carrots, you would need to eat 1-3/4 pounds in one sitting, certainly more than most people would eat at one time. So when a typical serving size of approximately 3 ounces is considered, the glycemic load of carrots is low at 3.9, making them a good carbohydrate choice. Whether carrots are cooked or raw, they have a low glycemic load.

NUTRITION NOTE

A large intake of high glycemic carbohydrates increases your blood sugar and insulin levels.

High levels of insulin are associated not only with the development of diabetes but also metabolic syndrome – a risk factor for heart disease.

NUTRITION NOTE

The glycemic load of carrots is low, which means they do not raise blood sugar quickly.

GI Foods That Do Not Have Carbohydrates

Foods that do not contain carbohydrates cannot have a GI. Meats, fish, tofu, nuts, eggs, oils and butter cannot be assigned a GI because they do not have carbohydrates or are too low in carbohydrates to test. Often foods that are very low in carbohydrate are assigned a low GI, but that is incorrect. If they have not been tested they, cannot be classified.

During GI testing, it was discovered that some starchy carbohydrates, called complex carbohydrates, which were previously believed to raise blood glucose slowly, actually caused a rapid rise. For example, bread made from finely ground flour, whether it was white flour or whole wheat, raised blood glucose about the same amount. Some complex carbohydrates may raise blood glucose as much as sugars. Of course sugars are still empty-calorie foods but effect on blood sugars may be the same as the starchy complex carbohydrate foods. A meta-analysis of randomized, controlled trials, designed to determine if low-GI diets improved blood glucose control in diabetes, indicated that it did have a small, but useful, effect.

Used alone, the GI could lead you to eat foods that are too high in unhealthy fats since adding fat to a food, even unhealthy fats, may lower the GI. For example, high-fat, premium ice cream has a lower GI than a baked potato; however, the ice cream is loaded with saturated fat and is not recommended, even if it has a low GI.

The GI and GL may be useful as an additional tool. There is no single, perfect way of classifying food for good health. For example, if you classify foods based on fat content, you would incorrectly classify low-fat but high-sugar foods such as hard candy, sugary cereals or fat-free salad dressings as healthy foods. Similarly, if you select low-carbohydrate foods, then you could classify a food high in saturated fat, like prime rib, as a healthy food and place carrots as unhealthy. Using several classification systems together works best to select the healthiest foods. Using GI and GL when deciding between healthy carbohydrate foods within similar foods, such as which cereal or which bread to choose, may help to narrow the choices among those that are already whole grain, high fiber with healthy fats.

Most vegetables have a low GL and are also high in fiber, low in calories and full of nutrients. Vegetables are good for any condition, whether for weight loss, diabetes or heart disease.

In real-life situations, you do not eat a food alone but in combination with other foods. Therefore, your blood glucose response may vary by the combination of foods you eat together. The GI of foods at lunch or evening meals may be affected by foods you have eaten earlier in the day, unlike in testing where the foods are eaten after an overnight fast. Lower the GI of a meal by eating a salad with vinegar and oil dressing or squeezing lemon juice on your vegetables.

NUTRITION NOTE

Not all carbohydrates are equal.

Carbohydrates in some foods will cause a higher rise in blood sugar than an equal amount of carbohydrates in another food.

Glycemic Index Lowered By

❖ High amounts of fiber, fat and protein
❖ Adding lemon juice or vinegar (acids)

Glycemic Index Raised By

❖ Very ripe fruits (banana with brown flecks is higher than slightly green)
❖ Finely grinding grains into flour
❖ Cooking foods for a long time (soft pasta instead of al dente)

Glycemic Index and Heart Disease

As glycemic load increases, HDL decreases, and triglyceride and c-reactive protein increase. All of these issues are related to an increased risk for heart disease. Low glycemic load diets improve insulin sensitivity and blood cholesterol levels.[75, 76]

How To Use The Glycemic Index (GI) and Glycemic Load (GL)

❖ Replace a high GI food with a lower one at each meal or snack.
❖ Eat more vegetables, except for white potatoes which are better classified as a starch.
❖ Eat fruit as whole pieces and especially berries of all types. Limit juices to a single 4 oz. serving.
❖ Add whole, intact grains, such as cooked barley, brown rice or quinoa to soups, salad or side dishes, to lower the overall GI for the meal.
❖ Add legumes to your meals. They are low GI and low GL foods that are high in fiber.
❖ Sprinkle or stir in oat bran.
❖ Add protein or healthy fat to every meal or snack instead of eating carbohydrates alone.
❖ Snack on nuts and seeds, unsweetened yogurt and vegetables rather than refined-grain snacks like granola bars.
❖ Choose plain, unsweetened yogurt. Add your own safe sweetener (see Page 435).
❖ Aim for foods that are higher in fiber, contain good fats such as olive or canola oil, have less saturated fat and no trans fat.
❖ Choose breads that are grainy, coarse, contain sprouted grain, or have a measured GI rating (see Page 168).
❖ Avoid processed, low-fiber cereals. Choose cold cereals that list rolled oats or another rolled grain as the first ingredient, rather than those made from flour, rice, corn or wheat that are formed into a variety of shapes. Cereals that are high in fiber (bran listed first) are also a good choice. For a lower GI breakfast, see the recipe for muesli on Page 315.
❖ Watch portion size. Eating large amounts of low GL foods can still raise blood sugars.

To learn more about GI and GL, visit the Web site www.glycemicindex.com where you can search for foods from a database. Another Web resource is Rick Mendosa's Web site at www.mendosa.com. His Web page discusses a little known lentil, chana dal, which looks like a yellow split pea, but is different and has a very low GI.

If you prefer a book, try *The New Glucose Revolution*, by Dr. Jennie Brand-Miller and the latest editions of the annual *Shoppers' Guide to GI Values* by the same author, which lists GI and GL for more than 500 foods.

Breads With A Low Glycemic Index and A Low Glycemic Load

❖ Bread with at least 50% intact grainy kernels or 45% or more oat bran
❖ *Food for Life, Ezekiel Sprouted Grain* Bread
❖ *Alvarado Street Bakery* Diabetic Lifestyles bread (GI 5, GL 0.9)

Cereals With A Low To Moderate Glycemic Load and Low Glycemic Index

❖ Oat Bran
❖ *Nature's Path* Smart Bran with psyllium and oat bran
❖ *Whole Control* Golden barley cereal
❖ Oatmeal, rolled oats, (thick-cut)

Sources: product labels; product Web sites; and American Journal of Clinical Nutrition, Vol. 76, No. 1, 5-56, 2002; International table of glycemic index and glycemic load values: 2002 Kaye Foster-Powell, Susanna HA Holt and Janette C. Brand-Miller.

High Fructose Corn Syrup

NUTRITION NOTE

Fructose and high fructose corn syrup have been shown to raise cholesterol, VLDL, triglycerides and insulin resistance.

High fructose corn syrup (HFCS) is a sweetener made from corn. In 1967, we consumed less than a tenth of a pound of high fructose corn syrup per person annually, and by 2004, we were eating 59 pounds per person. Check the ingredient list of packaged foods, and you will find it in many foods, even healthy-sounding foods.

The concern is that fructose and HFCS may increase the risk of heart disease and high blood pressure. They have been shown to raise cholesterol (both VLDL and LDL), raise triglycerides and increase insulin resistance.[77]

Fructose is a sugar that is more easily converted into fat than glucose and may also cause weight gain. Excess fat is sent to the blood in the form of triglycerides. Fructose also increases uric acid levels. Uric acid interferes with nitric oxide availability. Insulin requires nitric oxide to use glucose. Increased uric acid levels may be a cause of metabolic syndrome.

A 2 percent increase in fructose raises LDL a little more than 1 percent. In one study, when fructose increased from 3 percent to 20 percent of total calories, triglycerides increased 9 percent and LDL increased 11 percent.[78, 79, 80]

It is not unusual for many individuals, especially children and adolescents, to consume 30 percent of their daily calories from sucrose (table sugar) and fructose.[81]

Besides the effect of HFCS on blood lipids, there is evidence that fructose may be linked to obesity and metabolic syndrome in animals.[82]

HFCS seems to trick your body into thinking it is hungry. Studies done at the University of California-Davis, found that hormones involved in body weight regulation act differently when we eat fructose than if we eat other types of sugars. Fructose does not increase production of the hormones insulin and leptin like other sugars would. Insulin needs to increase for cells to take in blood sugar and use it for energy. Leptin signals the brain to decrease appetite. As a result, you want to eat more and those calories are easily stored as fat. Eating fructose increased abdominal obesity, which is the most harmful type of obesity.[83, 84]

Foods that are most likely to use HFCS are sweetened beverages, soda, lemonade, punch, sweetened tea, cakes, cookies, pies, pastries, ice cream and pudding. Cutting back on HFCS is not as simple as avoiding obviously sweetened foods. You may find HFCS in many other packaged foods like instant oatmeal, low-fat fruit-flavored yogurt, soups, pasta sauce, jams, jellies, ketchup and fruit drinks. You may even find it in some brands of whole-wheat bread because it helps the bread stay softer. Take a look at the ingredient list of the foods in your cupboard, and you may be surprised where you find it.

To avoid HFCS, check the ingredient list of all packaged foods. You might try the natural foods sections if you are not having any luck avoiding HFCS with traditional brands. Ideally, choose foods without added sweeteners. If they do use a sweetener, choose ones with the least amount. It is less desirable if the sweetener used is HFCS. Don't believe the slick marketing that tries to persuade you that its safe to eat in moderation. It is not healthy and is not found in any food naturally. Avoid HFCS organic, natural or otherwise.

NUTRITION NOTE

Organic and natural do not necessarily mean healthy. Organic high fructose corn syrup is one example. If synthetic fixing agents are kept seperate during the manufacturing of this chemically derived sweetener it can be labeled as natural.

Is The Fructose I Get In Fruit Okay?

If you eat a piece of fruit, it contains the sugar fructose but won't cause the same problems as the corn-derived crystalline fructose or HFCS. Whole fruit contains pectin, a soluble fiber that causes these sugars to be absorbed slower, along with other nutrients which provide additional benefits to heart health. Those with diabetes, who follow a carbohydrate-controlled meal plan, may exchange fruit for other carbohydrate foods within their meal allowance.

Crystalline Fructose

Crystalline fructose is produced from a fructose-enriched corn syrup (www.sugar.org). It comes from highly refined corn, not fruit as the name implies. HFCS and crystalline fructose are very different than the fructose you get in a piece of fruit.

In one study, consumption of crystalline fructose also caused a rise in fasting bloods sugars and triglycerides.[85] Crystalline fructose was previously recommended for use in meal plans for those with diabetes, but in light of the harm it may do to cholesterol, it is no longer suggested.

The glycemic index (GI) of crystalline fructose is 32, lower than table sugar's GI of 92, but HFCS has a similar GI to sugar of 89. In spite of the low GI for crystalline fructose, it cannot be recommended.

Corn Syrup Or Glucose Syrup

Corn syrup sold in stores and glucose syrup found on food labels is mostly glucose, but most brands of corn syrup list high fructose corn syrup as one of the ingredients. A substitute for corn syrup is brown rice syrup.

Agave

Juice from agave plant is converted through enzymatic action into hydrolyzed inulin syrup, high in fructose. Low glycemic does not automatically make a sweetener healthy. In spite of its low glycemic index and claim to be a "natural" sweetener, high intake of fructose has serious negative health implications as previously discussed on page 168.

Fructose and Obesity

No single factor is responsible for the increased prevalence of obesity. Certainly, increased caloric intake and decreased physical activity are an important part of why we are getting heavier. There are those who argue that the problem is not HFCS but the fact that we eat so much of it. From 1967 to 2004, we decreased our cane and beet sugar intake, but increased our HFCS intake, resulting in a net increase of 22 pounds of sweetener.[86] However, that increase did not account for all of the increase in obesity; therefore, increased use of HFCS may be involved.

BOTTOM LINE

If you only consider calories, HFCS is no better or worse than table sugar and both are empty calories. But, HFCS is chemically different and appears to have additional harmful effects beyond calories such as raising triglycerides, LDL cholesterol and insulin resistance – making it a very poor choice.

Sugars

The new food pyramid does not provide guidelines on amounts of added sugars; instead, it has a *"discretionary calorie"* allowance that includes calories from added sugars, alcohol and added fats.

The World Health Organization (WHO) has a much stronger message on limiting sugars.[87] Their recommendation is that we not get more than 10 percent of our calories from added sugars. The sugar industry objects to that recommendation. For a person eating 1,800 calories a day, 10 percent would be 11 teaspoons a day, yet the average for all sweeteners consumed is more than four times that amount.

How Much Added Sugars Are Hidden In Your Food	
Soda (12 oz.)	9-12 tsp.
Yogurt, sweetened (8 oz.)	7 tsp.
Toaster pastry	6 tsp.
Sherbet (1/2 cup)	5 1/2 tsp.
Tomato soup (1 cup)	4 tsp.
Honey nut toasted oat cereal (1-1/2 cup)	4 tsp.
Vanilla ice cream (1/2 cup)	3-1/2 tsp.
Chocolate chip cookie (large)	3 tsp.
Jam (Tbsp.)	3 tsp.
Pasta sauce (1/2 cup)	3 tsp.
Barbecue sauce (1 Tbsp.)	2 tsp.
Fat-free dressing (2 Tbsp.)	1-2 tsp.

It is reasonable to assume that an occasional small amount of table sugar in a diet that consists of mostly healthy foods is of little concern. The problem is that nearly all processed foods add sugars. Table sugar contains 50 percent fructose, so eating large amounts of it could also increase LDL cholesterol. Overall, you want to decrease consumption of all sugars and sweeteners.

Organic, Natural Sugars

There are some organic, raw and less-processed sugars that claim to be healthier than table sugar or brown sugar. These "natural" sugars have some of the natural molasses, and some may cause a slower rise in blood sugars. Evaporated cane juice has up to 2 percent molasses. Sucanat and rapadura have about 13 percent natural molasses. These products are grainy, brown colored, have a distinct flavor, and do not dissolve as easily as table sugar. Small amounts of the minerals magnesium, calcium, iron and manganese remain in these less-refined sweeteners, and, though the small amounts would appear negligible, they may regulate how quickly food breaks down and can get into our bloodstream. This does not mean that you can eat unlimited amounts or small amounts daily. Trying to make traditional sweets with healthier, more natural ingredients so that we can consume them daily along with other simple carbohydrates is not possible. All sweeteners should be used only occasionally – no matter how unrefined and natural.

Honey, Molasses, Maple Syrup, Brown Rice and Barley Malt Syrup

Blackstrap molasses is high in iron, calcium and other minerals, and has a distinct, strong flavor. Honey and maple syrup have small amounts of vitamins, minerals and antioxidants and are less processed than table sugar. Brown rice and barley malt have enzymes and complex carbohydrates that are more slowly digested. Raw honey is not heat treated to prevent crystallization, so it still contains enzymes. Replacing granulated, refined white sugars with these is possible but requires experimenting if used in baking since the replacement cannot often be done in equal amounts. Since they are liquid, adjustment of another liquid is suggested when used in baking. Natural sweeteners also have their own distinctive flavors, unlike white granulated white sugar that is neutral in taste. The flavors need to be matched to what they are being used in, according to your personal preference.

Fruit Juice Concentrates

Fruit Sweet made by *Wax Orchards* is made from concentrated fruit juice. It is naturally sweeter than sugar, which allows you to use one-third less. A tablespoon has 10 grams of sugar(s), which would provide the same sweetness as 4 teaspoons of table sugar (16 grams). It works well in items that have a liquid that can be reduced or where adding additional liquid will not affect the item.

Sugar Alcohols

The structure of sugar alcohols resembles sugar and an alcohol, but it contains neither ethanol found in alcoholic beverages or sugar. Sugar alcohols are typically genetically modified from corn or wheat, although there are non-GMO organisms that may be used. On food labels, they are listed under the carbohydrates as "*sugar alcohols.*" In the ingredient list, you will see words that end in "ol" such as erythritol, lactitol, maltitol, mannitol, sorbitol and xylitol. Some of these may be purchased in health food stores and used to sweeten foods you prepare.

Sugar alcohols are not calorie-free but have about half the calories of other carbohydrates for the same taste of sweetness. They are assigned a calorie content of 2.4 calories per gram. Sugar has 4 calories per gram. They are often found in foods that are labeled "sugar-free" or "low-carb."

Since sugar alcohols are not completely absorbed by the intestine, some individuals are sensitive to the gastrointestinal effects that they may cause, such as bloating, rumbling in the intestines, and diarrhea. This varies with each type of sugar alcohol and with continued use you may find the effect decreases.

Erythritol (er-ĭth-ri-tol) is a sugar alcohol with the least effect on the GI tract because it is absorbed in the intestine and is excreted in the urine. There are organic versions that state they are GMO-free. *Wholesome Sweeteners* makes an organic erythritol product called *"Zero."*

BOTTOM LINE

Sugar alcohols appear to be safe in small amounts. Remember, sugars do not improve your heart health no matter how little it has been refined or how environmentally friendly it is, especially when large amounts are used. Moderation is still needed, no matter what the choice, since no sweetener is an everyday food. The best choice for sweetening foods is adding naturally sweet fruits and dried fruits.

What About Artificial Sugar Substitutes?

I don't recommend them. They may be as harmful as the sugar you want to avoid. A whole-food diet is one that focuses on naturally sweet food and avoids the extreme sweetness from artificial sweeteners.

Rather than give up or cut back on those foods that provide little in the way of nutrition, we look for a way to be able to consume them without any of the negative effects and guilt. There is no magic, safe alternative. Consider the foods you eat that contain sweeteners and ask yourself how much nutrition they provide and what benefits they have for your health. Are foods and beverages made with a sugar substitute okay in unlimited amounts? Not really! A piece of cake or a can of soda provides little in the way of nutrition, no matter what sweetener or artificial sweeteners were used. The goal is not to eliminate all sweets but to use more naturally sweet foods and to rethink how we can enjoy sweet-tasting foods in a healthy diet.

Many artificial sweeteners that are created from chemicals are surrounded by controversy. Even the newest one, *Splenda*, also known as sucralose, has two Web sites with opposing views. It is difficult to get totally unbiased information when these new sweeteners are introduced into the market because we don't have long-term experience of what effects they may have. The truth is, no one really knows for sure if these chemically created sweeteners, no matter how natural they are made to sound in advertising clips, are truly safe.

In a study where rats were fed artificial sweeteners, they ate three times more calories than rats given table sugar. The researchers suggested that the artificial sweeteners could be interfering with the rats' natural ability to regulate how much they ate. Another explanation suggested that the body

NUTRITION NOTE

Artificial sweeteners may be as harmful as the sugars you want to avoid.

There is no reason to put chemically created sweeteners into a healthy, whole foods diet.

doesn't know what to do when the brain registers sweet but there are no calories to process. Yet another study found that women who drank diet drinks instead of regular versions did not cut calories on a daily basis; instead, they ate more calories following meals that included diet drinks. These are small studies and more studies are needed before any definitive conclusions can be made; however, this should give pause to those who drink diet drinks or use sugar substitutes regularly.[88]

BOTTOM LINE

Forget the "fake-foods" and satisfy your sweet cravings with fruit, nature's way of providing sweets. If you want an occasional treat, eat a very small piece of the real thing rather than a larger portion that you have justified having daily because it contains a sugar substitute.

Drink water as your beverage of choice. Yes it may seem boring at first, but add a twist or squirt of lemon or lime instead of drinking soda or diet soda. Try 100-percent fruit juice, diluted 50:50 with water, gradually working in a higher proportion of water as your taste buds adapt. If you want to use a calorie-free sweetener, consider stevia.

Stevia

Stevia is a shrub in the chrysanthemum family with naturally sweet leaves. Those who want a natural sweetener with zero calories, zero carbohydrates, and no effect on blood sugar levels may use the herb as a natural sweetener. Stevia also has many phytonutrients, but the nutritional benefits, when used in the amounts needed as a sweetener, are very small.

The sale of stevia is allowed in the United States, as long as it is not called a sweetener. To date, the FDA has not approved stevia as a sweetener, although it did approve it in 1995 as a dietary supplement. The reason the FDA has not approved stevia is because of some concerns from animal studies. The World Health Organization reviewed studies in 2006 and found two of the sweet compounds in stevia are not genotoxic. In December 2008 FDA stated it did not object to the claim that rebaudiside A, one ingredient found in stevia, is generally recognized as safe (GRAS) sweetener. Stevia extracts are now entering the market as highly purified, refined and extracted forms of stevia. These are not the same as the dried leaves of the stevia plant and some question if it remains the same when you remove it from the original plant.

Stevia has been used in Asia, Canada, South America and Europe for years. Choosing an herb which has a history of being used safely in other countries seems a safer alternative than choosing a sweetener that is a chemist's creation, with no history of long-term use. However, this remains a personal choice.

NUTRITION NOTE

Stevia may be found in health food stores and some grocery stores with the dietary supplments. It is available in a liquid, powder and in packets.

Truvia and PureVia

Rebiana, the highly purified sweet extract from stevia leaves in combination with erythritol is available as a calorie free sweetener. The Coca-Cola Company has teamed up with Cargill and introduced a brand of sweetener called *Truvia*. Pepsi-Cola Company has plans for their version caled *PureVia*. The safety of these individual extacts and how the body reacts has not been assessed.

Homemade Jams With No Sugars

If you make your own jams, you are probably familiar with pectin, a product used to make jam set up, which requires a lot of sugar. If you cut back on the sugar, you end up with syrup instead of jam. However, there is a low methoxyl type pectin extracted from citrus peel. It is activated by calcium instead of sugar. Since it does not require sugar to jell, jams and jellies may be made with less or no sugar, as well as any other sweetener. *Pomona* is the brand. It may also be used to turn 100-percent juice into a gelatin. If you cannot find it in stores, it is available at their Web site, www.permaculture.com.

Tips To Use Less Sweetener

Try the following tips to help moderate or eliminate the amount of added sugars in your diet:

❖ Most instant hot cereals have added sweeteners; it is best to use the regular types (steel-cut oats and old fashioned oats) and sweeten with naturally sweet fruits.

❖ Sweeten your cereal with banana slices or dried fruit such as dates or raisins instead of artificial sweeteners or table sugar. If you have diabetes, count the fruit as part of your allowed carbohydrates.

❖ If you eat cereal, buy whole-grain, high-fiber, low-GI cold cereals (Page 168) with the least grams of sugars per serving. Also, see that there are no sugar substitutes in the ingredient list of "lower sugar" cereals. Check the ingredient list for sucralose or aspartame (sugar substitutes.)

❖ If you want fruit in your cereal, add your own and avoid the extra sugars and partially hydrogenated oils that manufacturers add to prevent dried fruit from getting hard when added to cereal boxes.

❖ Buy plain yogurt and sweeten with fruit. An 8-ounce container of plain yogurt with nothing added still has 12 grams of sugars that occur naturally from the milk sugars. For even less sugar, buy Greek-style yogurt, such as *Total 0%* by *Fage*.

❖ Drink water instead of sweetened beverages, such as juice drinks, punch, sweet tea or lemonade.

❖ Limit juice to one 4-ounce serving a day of "100%" fruit juice, then switch to water. Dilute your juices with water or sparkling water such as *LaCroix* to lower calories.

❖ Choose fresh fruit, canned or frozen without sugars, for dessert. Eat fresh peach slices (grilled if you like) instead of peach cobbler.

❖ Check food labels. There are 4 grams of sugars in a teaspoon of sugar. If you do the math, you can visualize the amount of sugars in a serving.

❖ Eat sweets less often. Make your own and reduce the amount of sugars in your favorite recipes. You may be surprised that some recipes taste the same even when you reduce the sugar content by one-fourth to one-third. If it calls for 1 cup of sugar, try 3/4 cup or 2/3 cup. If a half cup, try 5-6 tablespoons.

❖ Hidden sources of sweeteners may be in soups, mayonnaise, ketchup, salad dressings and other condiments. Check the ingredients.

❖ Use of artificial sweeteners reduces intake of other sugars, but the adverse effects of these chemicals reduces any benefit.

Carbohydrate & Sugars Quiz

1. Which foods have carbohydrates?
   a) olive oil   c) 100% whole-wheat bread   d) chicken breast
   b) apple   with 5 grams fiber per slice   e) broccoli

2. Foods that are quickly digested and raise blood sugars are high glycemic.
   ❑ T   ❑ F

3. Grinding kernels of wheat into flour to make 100 percent whole-wheat bread raises the glycemic index.
   ❑ T   ❑ F

4. Glycemic load is a better measure since it considers portion size.
   ❑ T   ❑ F

5. Fish and chicken are:
   a) low glycemic
   b) moderate glycemic
   c) cannot be assigned a value since they have no carbohydrates

6. Individuals with diabetes may eat low glycemic foods without concern about the carbohydrates in those foods.
   ❑ T   ❑ F

7. Fructose increases LDL cholesterol and is associated with abdominal obesity.
   ❑ T   ❑ F

8. Organic foods may have high fructose corn syrup.
   ❑ T   ❑ F

9. We are eating less sugar and more high fructose corn syrup, and the total sugars have been increasing over the years.
   ❑ T   ❑ F

10. The World Health Organization recommends that not more than 10 percent of our calories come from added sugars, yet we consume four times that amount on average.
    ❑ T   ❑ F

11. Natural sugars may be eaten without concern.
    ❑ T   ❑ F

12. Sugar alcohols are calorie-free.
    ❑ T   ❑ F

13. Instead of sugar, the use of artificial sugar substitutes are recommended.
    ❑ T   ❑ F

14. Stevia is an herb that is sweet and may be used as a no-calorie sweetener.
    ❑ T   ❑ F

ANSWERS
On Page 280.

Smart 4 Your Heart

Type 2 Diabetes

30

The risk of developing pre-diabetes or metabolic syndrome was discussed on Page 41. You may improve the odds that you won't get Type 2 diabetes or will postpone getting it by simple lifestyle changes. If you have metabolic syndrme you may reduce the risk of getting Type 2 diabetes by adding a small amount (30 to 45 minutes) of physical activity on most, if not all, days; losing a little weight (10 percent of your current weight); and eating a healthier diet.

If you have diabetes, your risk for heart disease increases. You are at the same risk of having a heart attack as someone who already has had a heart attack. This means that anyone who has diabetes should be following strategies to improve their heart health, along with keeping blood glucose in control.

When you eat food, it is broken down during digestion into several components. One of these components is glucose, a form of blood sugar your body uses for energy. Insulin is the key that allows glucose to enter cells where it can be used for fuel. Normally, as blood glucose rises after eating, your pancreas makes more insulin to cover the rising blood glucose. When you have diabetes, insulin is either not available or not working as it normally would.

Diabetes is a disease of carbohydrate metabolism. There are two types of diabetes. With Type 1, your body doesn't make any or enough insulin. With Type 2, your body's cells no longer recognize the insulin your body is making or does not efficiently use what is made, resulting in a buildup of glucose in the blood. If this condition is not treated, blood loaded with glucose will damage the blood vessels.

When blood glucose is not in good control, triglyceride levels may also increase in the blood, and your good cholesterol (HDL) decreases. HDL is intertwined with triglyceride metabolism so when triglycerides go up, HDL often goes down. A1C is a test that gives the average of your blood glucose (sugar) levels over the past three months. When the A1C blood test goes from being too high to a normal range, there is also a significant increase in desirable HDL cholesterol.

Individuals with diabetes and heart disease often ask, "If I can't have sugars and can't have fat, what can I eat?" The same principles that guide eating for heart health are also good for diabetes management. Choosing healthy fats and healthy carbohydrates from whole grain, fruits and vegetables, along with managing weight and increasing exercise, is good for heart health and regulating

NUTRITION NOTE

If you have diabetes, your chance of having a heart attack is the same as someone who already has had a heart attack.

NUTRITION NOTE

Carbohydrate is the nutrient in food that affects blood sugar (glucose) the most.

NUTRITION NOTE

Special diabetic
foods and the
use of artificial
sweeteners are
not necessary.

The curcumin in
turmeric and curry
lessens insulin
resistance.

NUTRITION NOTE

The portion of
food that contains
15 grams of
carbohydrates
equals one
*"serving or
choice"* of
carbohydrate.

blood glucose. Limiting intake of saturated fats and eliminating trans fats is important for those with diabetes as well as heart disease. Eating soluble fiber, which helps to remove cholesterol, also helps to regulate blood glucose. Fish, a good source of healthy omega-3 fat, is recommended for both.

By choosing a lower carbohydrate diet that includes more fish and poultry with small amounts of lean meats, along with healthy fats, you will have better blood glucose control that is also better for your heart. Since carbohydrates have the biggest effect on blood glucose, it may be tempting to follow a very low carbohydrate diet, with 20 percent or less calories from carbohydrates. However, when carbohydrates are very low, food choices are limited and the carbohydrates are often replaced with protein and fat. If this increases your intake of saturated fat and trans fats, it will be bad for heart health.

An area of confusion for those living with diabetes is food labeled "diabetic" or "no sugars added." Special diabetic foods and the use of artificial sweeteners are not necessary. These foods give the impression that you can eat as much of them as you want, but this is not true. Foods that have no added sugars or those that use a sugar substitute may still have a significant amount of calories and refined carbohydrates, which raises your blood glucose. It's better to think of sweets as occasional foods rather than everyday foods, no matter what sweetener is used. Substitute these foods for other carbohydrate choices rather than simply adding them. For example eat a smaller portion of bread, pasta or rice to allow for the carbohydrates in a small portion of dessert.

Learn to check the total carbohydrate content on food labels, not only the grams of sugar. The portion of food that contains 15 grams of carbohydrates equals one "serving or choice" of carbohydrate. If your goal is to lose weight, aim for two to three choices for women or three to four choices for men per meal. If your goal is to maintain your weight, then women may choose three to five choices and men four to six choices. If you snack between meals, decrease your meal choices to use for snacks.

CARBOHYDRATE SERVINGS OR CHOICES		
Carbohydrate choices include milk, fruit, starches (bread, cereal, etc.). A choice or serving is a portion that has 15 grams of carbohydrates.		
	Women	Men
Lose weight	2-3 per meal	3-4 per meal
Maintain weight	3-4 per meal	4-5 per meal

Adjust the food portions you eat to keep within the number of servings or choices set as your goal. Use the plate example described on Page 51 to help you eat a balanced diet.

You may find that spacing meals four to five hours apart will help with blood glucose control, whether you rely on your pancreas or medications to provide insulin.

Reduce as much as possible, processed, refined, high-glycemic foods such as sugars and white flour that have less nutrition. Choose whole, intact grains such as steel-cut oats instead of instant oats.

Choose carbohydrate foods that are more nutritious. Eating an apple is a better choice than a candy bar, yet they both have carbohydrates. A 15-gram serving of carbohydrates requires the same amount of insulin whether it is in the form of an apple or a candy bar. However, there are nutritional differences between them. Whole grain, fruits and vegetables are heart protective and full of nutrients; eat those more often instead of the ones that are lower in nutrients. Some carbohydrates have a higher glycemic load (Page 165), which may affect blood glucose response.

Exercise also affects blood sugar (glucose). If you will exercise within an hour of eating, you may need less insulin for that meal.

When insulin is required to manage your diabetes, it is necessary to balance the amount of carbohydrate with the insulin you take. Consult a certified diabetes educator or registered dietitian to learn carbohydrate counting for meal planning to give you more flexibility in food choices while keeping blood glucose at a safe level. If you need insulin, a diabetes health professional will help you determine your insulin to carb ratio so that you know how much insulin is needed to cover the carbohydrates in a particular meal. By keeping track of what you eat and testing blood glucose, you will learn how foods affect you and what you can do in these situations. For example, pizza, which is high in carbohydrates and fat, may not raise blood glucose as high as expected after a meal but can cause delayed high blood glucose that requires an adjustment to insulin dosing.

Controlling diabetes is not easy, but it is manageable. Seek help when you need it.

SAMPLE HEART HEALTHY DIABETIC MENU		
BREAKFAST	**1,500 Calories** Serving = g carbs	**2,000 Calories** Serving = g carbs
Fresh orange	1 = 15g	1 =15g
Steel-cut oatmeal or rolled barley	1/2 cup = 15g	1 cup = 30g
1/2 cup egg substitute, 2 egg whites or 1 egg	0g	0g
Natural peanut butter added to oatmeal	0g	1 Tbsp. = 0g
along with 1/4 tsp. cinnamon	Free	Free
Skim milk	1 cup = 12g	1 cup = 12g
Water, coffee, herbal or green tea	Free	Free
NOON MEAL		
Cooked shrimp added to:	2 oz. = 0g	3 oz. = 0g
Cold pasta salad	1/2 cup = 15g	1 cup = 30g
Carrot, celery, broccoli, bell pepper	1 cup = 5g	1 cup = 5g
Fresh apple sliced	1(6 oz.) = 22g	1(6 oz.) = 22g
Water, coffee, herbal or green tea	Free	Free
EVENING MEAL		
Grilled salmon or chicken	3 oz. = 0g	4 oz. = 0g
Baked sweet potato or 1/3 cup brown rice	3 oz. = 15g	3 oz. = 15g
Broccoli florets, steamed	1 cup = 10g	1 cup = 10g
Spinach salad with tomato	0g	0g
Vinegar and oil dressing	1 Tbsp. = 0g	2 Tbsp. = 0g
Slivered almonds	1 oz. = 0g	1 oz. = 0g
Olive oil	1 Tbsp. = 0g	1 Tbsp. = 0g
Chilled fresh fruit cup	3/4 cup = 22g	3/4 cup = 22 g
Water, coffee, herbal or green tea	Free	Free
EVENING SNACK (PROTEIN + CARBOHYDRATE)		
Lean Protein: tuna, salmon, chicken, turkey, shrimp, 1/2 cup beans	1 oz. = 0g	1 oz. = 0g
CARBOHYDRATE CHOICES	**CHOOSE ONE**	**CHOOSE 2 ITEMS**
Medium piece of fruit	1 piece = 15g	1 piece = 15g
Skim milk or yogurt	1 cup = 12g	1 cup = 12g
Popcorn, popped	3 cups = 15g	3 cups = 15g
Hummus with celery and carrots	1/4 cup = 11g	1/4 cup = 11g

2,000 calorie, 191 grams carbohydrate (38%), 115 grams protein, 82 grams fat, (17 g saturated) 32 grams fiber, 1,527 mg sodium

1,500 calories, 146 grams carbohydrate (39%), 98 grams protein, 59 grams fat, (12 g saturated) 26 grams fiber, 790 mg sodium

Type 2 Diabetes Smart 4 Your Heart

31

Sodium

Sodium is one of two ingredients found in salt. Sodium causes the body to retain extra water. The extra water creates more pressure in the blood vessels, resulting in higher blood pressure. Blood pressure is the force of blood against artery walls. High blood pressure causes arteries to stiffen and narrow. The heart has to work harder to pump the extra fluid, which puts a strain on your heart, potentially causing the heart muscle to thicken and enlarge.

But what if you don't have high blood pressure? Is restricting sodium necessary? Some studies have found that even if blood pressure is not high, an individual may be salt sensitive. The salt sensitivity increases stickiness of platelets and reduces the flexibility of blood vessels, which increases the risk for heart disease. There are no standard tests for salt sensitivity so moderation is advised for everyone.

Excess sodium causes a depletion of potassium, which may lead to a lack of energy, muscle cramps, stomach disturbances and an irregular heartbeat. Excess sodium may also cause stroke and kidney disease, as well as affect bone health and contribute to stomach cancer. It makes sense to reduce sodium to lower the risk of future health problems.

If you have received conflicting advice about sodium, it is because the debate about sodium can quickly divide health professionals. Some think it is important for everyone to reduce sodium intake, while others believe that unless you have high blood pressure, you don't need to be concerned about salt intake. The scientific evidence is mounting against sodium. Poorly done studies sponsored by the Salt Institute which found sodium is harmless, are being questioned. Well-designed studies, such as the ones used in the DASH diet, show that less sodium is better for your health as it reduces blood pressure.[89]

The U.S. Government guidelines recommend no more than 2,300 milligrams of sodium daily. According to the data collected from The Third National Health and Nutrition Survey (NHANES III), about 95 percent of men and 75 percent of women get more than that daily. The highest intakes are for adult males between the ages of 31 and 50 who average 4,300 milligrams.[90]

NUTRITION NOTE

The U.S. Government guidelines recommend no more than 2,300 milligrams of sodium daily.

Where We Get Sodium

Surprisingly, very little of the sodium we get comes from foods naturally; even less is added with a salt shaker at the table. About 10 percent of the sodium we eat comes from a salt shaker, and the remaining 15 percent is in foods naturally.[95] The majority of salt comes from the processing, as 75 percent of the sodium we eat is from processed packaged, boxed, canned, quick, easily prepared foods, and foods we get from delis and restaurants – whether it is fast food or fine dining. Packaged foods are required to list the amount of sodium per serving on the label so you can see how much they have. Sometimes the foods are not even the salty-tasting ones. Sometimes they are the low-fat, healthy-sounding items. Low-fat salad dressings are often higher in sodium. Pizza, processed cheese, frozen dinners and even bread may all contribute to the sodium we get. Cold cereals and breads – even the healthy versions – are often a major source since we eat so much of them.

Salt adds flavor to food and trying to change this habit overnight is not effective. You can decrease your preference for salt after two to three months by gradually eating less salt. At first, food will taste bland, but give your taste buds time to adjust to a lower level and you will soon discover that foods taste great even without all the added salt. Your old favorites will then taste too salty to you.

NUTRITION NOTE

1 teaspoon salt has 2,325 mg sodium.

SODIUM

Flaked cereal, ready-to-eat per cup . . . . 170-350 mg

Bread per slice . . . . 110-175 mg

Deli meat per ounce . . . . 175-350 mg

Pizza per slice . . . . 500-1,200 mg

Frozen dinners . . . . 460 to 1,600 mg

Soups . . . . 325 to 1,300 mg

Salad dressing per 2 Tbsp. . . . . 35 to 325 mg

Cottage cheese, low fat 1/2 cup . . . . 460 mg

Note: amount of salt can vary widely by brands.

Eating canned, *no-salt-added* soups and vegetables by themselves is a recipe for failure as the lack of taste is disappointing to most people. However, using canned *no-salt-added* tomatoes in cooking to make stews, casseroles, chili or spaghetti, which have other seasonings, will make the lack of salt less noticeable.

What About Iodized Salt?

Iodine is needed for a healthy thyroid and prevention of goiter. In the U.S., table salt is iodized to provide iodine. One third teaspoon of iodized salt meets the iodine needs in preventing goiter for an average adult. If you eat a low-salt diet or salt that is not iodized, there are good food sources for iodine. Fish from salt water is one of the best sources for iodine, as well as kelp or seaweed, asparagus, garlic, mushrooms, lima beans, spinach, soybeans and turnip greens. Another way is to take a daily vitamin/mineral supplement that contains iodine.

Sodium and Bone Health

High blood pressure is not the only health concern with salt and sodium; osteoporosis is another. The more sodium you consume, the greater the amount of calcium you lose in urine, which may increase the risk of developing osteoporosis.

Is Sea Salt A Better Choice?

The sodium content is the same. Much of the sea salt we find in stores and added to processed foods has been highly refined to remove all traces of minerals. There are a few brands such as *"Real"* and *"Celtic"* sea salt that still retains the minerals which appear as small, dark particles in the salt, making them flow less freely from the salt shaker.

There currently is little data on how refined and unrefined sea salt affects cardiac health. There are animal studies that suggest that refined salt causes more hypertension. We learned from the "DASH" diet that it is not only sodium but other minerals such as potassium, magnesium and calcium that affect blood pressure. However, since processed, packaged and restaurant foods supply 75 percent of the sodium in the form of highly refined salt in your diet, using sea salt at the table will have little impact on the overall sodium intake of the average diet. For most people eliminating the major source of sodium would require cooking without the use of any of the convenience items such as canned soups, canned tomatoes, *"tenderized"* meats and rotisserie chicken. It would also limit eating out, take out such as pizza or deli sandwiches.

NUTRITION NOTE

Eating a high-sodium diet reduces bone density.

NUTRITION NOTE

Coarse or kosher salt has less sodium per teaspoon because less "fits" in the spoon than finely ground table salt.

Weight of 1 teaspoon salt

Coarse/kosher: 4.8 grams

Table salt: 6 grams

Tips For Less Sodium

1. **Choose fewer processed packaged foods.**
   By eating more fresh, whole and minimally processed foods, you can easily reduce your intake of sodium. Frozen with no added salt is also a good choice.

2. **Choose more fresh fruits and vegetables.**
   Eating a diet that includes plenty of fruits and vegetables lowers blood pressure. Fresh fruits and veggies are ideal. They are naturally low in sodium, fat-free and packed with potassium which blunts some of the effect of sodium. Fruits and vegetables also have disease-fighting plant chemicals (phytonutrients).

3. **Check it before you eat it.**
   Packaged foods are required to list sodium per serving. This gives you the information you need to make smart sodium choices. For healthy adults, the goal is no more than 2,300 milligrams of sodium per day. If you have high blood pressure or heart failure, aim for 2,000 milligrams or even less.
   ❖ Consider mail order sources for hard to find items. *Healthy Heart Market* www.healthyheartmarket.com or 1-888-685-5988 is one source for mail order.

4. **Be aware when you eat out.**
   If several meals each week are prepared by restaurants or from a deli or take-out, you probably are getting more sodium than you think. Light, low-fat and heart healthy foods may be lower in fat or calories but are often higher in sodium to compensate for the loss in flavor.
   ❖ Skip the soups, even low calorie are high sodium. Get the sauces, gravies and dressings on the side, and dip your fork into the dressing or sauce and then into your food.
   ❖ Go easy on deli meats. Even the healthy sounding turkey and lean cuts are high sodium.
   ❖ Ask if nutrition information is available for any of the menu items. Check Web sites of chain and fast-food restaurants, as most have nutrition information available. See Page 249 for more tips.

5. **Select foods with no added salt for use in cooking.**
   At the grocery store, you may reduce your sodium intake by picking brands with "no added salt" that work well when used with other ingredients to add flavor. A tomato or pasta sauce recipe using regular canned, crushed tomatoes would yield a finished sauce with 591 milligrams of sodium per cup, before you add any salt to the recipe. If you add a teaspoon of salt, the amount jumps to 879 milligrams. If you substitute salt-free, crushed tomatoes for the regular canned tomatoes and add one half teaspoon of salt, each cup of sauce would contain only 174 milligrams of sodium. Adding salt to the sauce containing no-salt-added tomatoes when you are cooking it, makes a flavorful and lower in sodium sauce than if you used tomatoes canned with salt.
   ❖ Salt loses its flavor during long cooking times. Adding a small pinch of salt at the end of cooking helps you get more taste from smaller amounts of sodium.

6. **Rinse canned vegetables, tuna, salmon, chicken and beans.**
   The sodium is higher in canned versions than fresh or frozen with no salt added. The sodium content can be reduced 33 to 43 percent if you place food into a colander (or large sieve) and rinse under cold running water for 30 seconds. Soak olives for 10 to 15 minutes in cold water to reduce sodium.

7. **Cook with more herbs and spices.**
   ❖ Don't add salt to water when cooking pasta, rice, hot cereals, or when blanching vegetables. These are culinary techniques used by chefs who are more concerned with appearance than nutrition.
   ❖ To boost flavor, add wine to stews, casseroles, sauces and gravies, but don't use "cooking wine" which contains salt. Use only wine you would drink.
   ❖ Learning to cook with more seasonings is a delicious way to minimize sodium and maximize flavor. Use individual herbs and spices or try a salt-free seasoning blend.
   ❖ Try a variety of salt-free herbs and seasoning mixes until you find ones you like. The quality and tastes of different brands vary considerably, so don't give up. If you don't like the first one, try another one.

   Salt-free seasonings:
   - *Salt-Free Spike* and *Vegit* by Modern Products
   - Penzey's Spice House has a wide variety available. www.penzeys.com
   - Pleasoning www.pleasoning.com, or 1-800-279-1614. Low or no sodium and potassium-free seasonings.
     — *Mini-Mini Salt* (110 mg sodium per 1/4 teaspoon)
     — *Tasty 2 Pleasoning* (45 mg sodium per 1/4 teaspoon.)
     — *All-Purpose Pleasoning* (130 mg sodium per 1/4 teaspoon)
   - *Chef Seasoning* is a popular salt-free, potassium-free, pepper-free seasoning blend that is not sold in stores. www.dcdistributors.com or 1-800-827-6763

   ❖ Light-salt or 1/3-less-sodium salt have fillers added. These still contain sodium but taste less salty; therefore, if you salt to taste, beware that you may get just as much sodium if you continue to shake it on until you get the "salty" taste you prefer.
   ❖ Salt substitutes that contain potassium often have a bitter taste. One brand that has potassium but no sodium with less after-taste is *AlsoSalt* at www.alsosalt.com. Because of their high potassium content, salt substitutes should be avoided by people who take certain medications, such as ACE inhibitors (used to lower blood pressure). Always check with the doctor or pharmacist if in doubt.

8. **Go easy on condiments.**
   Many condiments like ketchup, mustard and pickles, may be high in sodium. Check out the the lower-sodium varieties like reduced-sodium soy sauce and no-salt-added ketchup.

9. **Check the sodium in your water supply.**
   ❖ If you drink bottled water, select those that do not have any sodium. The average amount of sodium for public water is 12 mg per 8 ounces. You can contact your local water company and ask for the sodium content. If you have a well, it may vary from 0 to 1,000 miligrams, so you might want to have it tested for sodium content.
   ❖ If you have hard water and use a water softener, the sodium added to soften the water will depend on the water hardness. The harder the water, the higher the sodium. To avoid adding sodium to drinking water and water you use for cooking, designate one faucet, usually the cold water faucet to the kitchen, plumbed to bypass the water softener. Another option is to use potassium salt. Those individuals who have been advised to limit potassium because of medications, such as ACE inhibitors, should not use these.

Cooking To Reduce Sodium

When cooking, use the following table to estimate how much sodium (in milligrams) per serving will be added from salt. (For example, a recipe that serves four and calls for 1 teaspoon of salt will have 575 milligrams of sodium per serving from salt.)

Amount of salt	Number of Servings in Recipe				
	1	2	4	6	8
1/8 tsp.	290	145	72	48	36
1/4 tsp.	581	290	145	97	73
1/2 tsp.	1,162	581	290	194	145
1 tsp.	2,325	1,162	581	387	291
1-1/2 tsp.	3,487	1,743	872	581	436
2 tsp.	4,650	2,325	1,162	775	581

How to modify a lasagna recipe to lower sodium by half.

ORIGINAL RECIPE 8 SERVINGS	ORIGINAL RECIPE SODIUM	CHANGE SUGGESTED	SODIUM IN SUGGESTED ITEM
9 Lasagna noodles, cooked in unsalted water	10	No change in sodium but healthier to use whole-wheat	10
2 jars pasta sauce	6,100	1 jar sauce + 28 oz. *no-salt-added* crushed tomatoes	3,147
1 cup cottage cheese	920	*No-salt-added* cottage cheese	30
1 egg	95	No change	95
1/4 cup Parmesan cheese	310	No change	310
2 packages (8 oz. each) Mozzarella shredded cheese	2,810	Use less 1 package cheese	1,405
1/2 pound ground turkey	130	No change	130
Total sodium for entire recipe	10,375	Total sodium with changes	5,127
Total sodium ÷ 8 servings =	**1,296**	**Total sodium ÷ 8 servings =**	**641**

Sodium Quiz

Select the choice with the most sodium.

1. (a) Grilled chicken breast sandwich
        or
    (b) 5 large black olives

2. (a) 1 cup canned vegetable soup
        or
    (b) Baby dill pickle

3. (a) Medium French fries
        or
    (b) Low-fat oat bran muffin

4. (a) 2 slices 100% whole-wheat bread
        or
    (b) 1/4 cup salted peanuts

5. (a) 1 cup macaroni and cheese
        or
    (b) 2 ounces deli ham

6. (a) 1 cup bran flakes
        or
    (b) 2 strips bacon

ANSWERS
On Page 281.

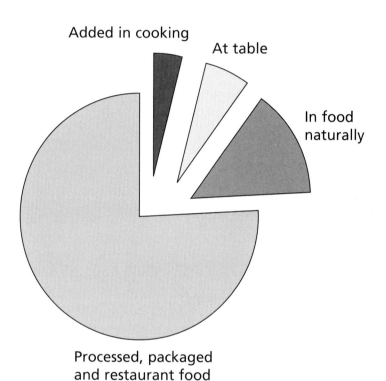

Added in cooking

At table

In food naturally

Processed, packaged and restaurant food

32

Blood Pressure

About 65 million people in the U.S. have high blood pressure. According to the National Heart, Lung and Blood Institute, individuals with normal blood pressure at age 55 have a 90 percent chance of developing high blood pressure during their lifetime. The higher the blood pressure is, the greater the chance of heart attack, heart failure, stroke and kidney disease. Blood pressure is measured in millimeters of mercury (mmHg) and is recorded as two numbers, systolic and diastolic. For every 10 points that systolic blood pressure increases, there is a 22 percent increase in your risk for cardiovascular disease. Systolic (which is the top number) measures the force of blood being pumped through the arteries. Systolic numbers over 140 mmHg, in those over age 50, are a more important risk factor than the diastolic blood pressure (the bottom number) recorded when the heart relaxes between beats.

High blood pressure may also affect your brain. It is the number one cause of strokes. Even if a stroke does not occur, high blood pressure reduces the amount of blood to some parts of the brain.

MEASURING BLOOD PRESSURE

When your blood pressure is measured at a screening or office visit, you should be seated quietly for at least five minutes in a chair, with both feet flat on the floor and your arm supported at your heart level by the individual taking your blood pressure, not resting on a table or arm of a chair which makes the pressure higher. Lying down or having your feet dangle off an exam table is not correct. The blood pressure cuff should be on bare skin, not over clothing. Plan to wear clothing that easily exposes your arm. If you roll up your sleeves, the clothing should not form a tourniquet around your upper arm.

Optimal Blood Pressure: Less than 120/80 mmHg

Blood Pressure* (mmHg)	**Desirable/Normal:** systolic less than 120 and diastolic less than 80
	Prehypertension: systolic 120-139, diastolic 80-89
	Hypertension Stage 1: systolic 140-159 and diastolic 90-99
	Hypertension Stage 2: systolic 160 or higher and diastolic 100 or higher

Source: The Seventh Report of the Joint National Committee on Prevention, Detection, Evaluation and Treatment of High Blood Pressure.

Changing your lifestyle according to the Joint National Committee on Prevention, Detection, Evaluation and Treatment of High Blood Pressure (JNC-7) may decrease blood pressure and lower risk for heart disease.

LIFESTYLE CHANGES THAT MAY LOWER YOUR BLOOD PRESSURE

❖ Losing weight if overweight

❖ Adding physical activity

❖ Lowering alcohol consumption

❖ Eating less sodium and more fruits and vegetables rich in potassium, magnesium and calcium

❖ Replacing 25 grams of protein with 1/2 cup of dry roasted, unsalted soy nuts

A DASH-type diet that limits sodium to 1,600 milligrams may lower blood pressure as much as taking a single blood pressure lowering drug. If other lifestyle changes listed below are added, there is an even greater benefit.

TABLE 32.1
EFFECT OF LIFESTYLE CHANGES ON BLOOD PRESSURE

Lifestyle Change	Recommendation	Systolic BP Reduction
Weight loss	Maintain a normal body weight, and a normal BMI of 18.5 to 24.9. (See BMI chart, Page 264.)	5 to 20 points per 22 lbs. or per 10 kg lost
An eating plan based on DASH diet	4 to 5 servings fruits, 4 to 5 servings vegetables, low-fat dairy, saturated and total fat reduced	8 to 14 points
Decrease salt	Limit sodium to 2,400 milligrams per day from all sources. Decrease to 1,600 mg if necessary.	2 to 8 points
Increase physical activity	30 minutes of aerobic physical activity most days of the week, such as brisk walking	4 to 9 points
Moderate alcohol	Limit alcohol to no more than 2 drinks per day for men and 1 for women	2 to 4 points

Source: JNC-7 "It's more than high blood pressure." Journal of the American Medical Association 289 (2003): 2573-2575.

Soy Nuts

In one study, women who substituted a half cup of unsalted soy nuts for protein from other foods lowered systolic blood pressure by 10 percent if they had high blood pressure and 5 percent if they had normal blood pressure. This diet also lowered LDL cholesterol 11 percent and Apo B levels 8 percent.[92]

Potassium

Blood pressure control is much more than not adding salt to your food. Increased potassium intake lowers your blood pressure.[93] While sodium is important, the ratio of sodium to potassium is also important. While sodium increases blood pressure, potassium blunts some of that effect. Getting 1-1/2 times as much potassium as sodium in one study lowered the systolic (top number) blood pressure by 2.4 points in four weeks.

The recommended amount of potassium is 4,700 milligrams each day from food, not supplements. Most Americans are not getting that amount. The average intake of potassium for men is only 2,900 to 3,200 milligrams. For women, the average is 2,100 to 2,300 milligrams.

Potassium comes from fruits and vegetables which are often lacking in our time-pressed, hectic lifestyles. Potassium is water soluble so boiling or soaking vegetables with large amounts of water will cause them to be lower in potassium. The DASH diet (2,000 calorie) suggests four to five servings of fruits plus four to five servings of vegetables daily, which can provide the potassium needed. When you eat a high-sodium meal, such as a restaurant meal, deli sandwich or canned soup, balance it by adding high-potassium foods such as a big green leafy salad, fresh fruits, vegetables and legumes.

Can You Get Too Much Potassium?

For most individuals with healthy kidney function, excess potassium is not a problem. Potassium from foods is not a concern but potassium supplements may be a concern. Those people with known kidney problems and on certain medications, such as digoxin or ACE inhibitors or beta-blockers, should not take potassium supplements or use salt substitutes with potassium. Follow the guidelines that were given with your medications or by your physician.

Magnesium

MAGNESIUM IS OFTEN LOW IN:

- Type 2 diabetes
- Heart failure
- High blood pressure
- High cholesterol
- Gum disease
- PMS
- IBS

Foods that contain magnesium, such as nuts and seeds, dark green vegetables, soybeans, whole grains, wheat bran, and seafood, are beneficial in lowering blood pressure, decreasing risk of heart disease, and stroke and Type 2 diabetes.[94] For food sources of magnesium see Table 32.3 on Page 193. Processing and refining foods removes much of the magnesium.

The amount of magnesium required daily for a woman is 310 to 320 milligrams; for men 400 to 420 milligrams. If you are like 75 percent of the U.S. population, you don't get enough magnesium.

Fish Oil Lowers Blood Pressure

Studies using 3 to 7 grams of fish oil daily found that it lowered blood pressure from 1.6 to 2.9 mmHg. It appears that it is the DHA, not EPA, that lowered blood pressure.[96, 97]

Blood Pressure Smart 4 Your Heart

TABLE 32.2 FOODS RICH IN POTASSIUM
(most to least by group)

Fruits	POTASSIUM	Calories
Banana, (7-8 inches long)	422 mg	105
Cantaloupe, 5oz	368 mg	47
Apricot, dried, 7 halves	346 mg	71
Kiwifruit, 1 medium	240 mg	50
Orange, navel, 5 oz.	232 mg	68
Avocado, 1 oz. (1/5)	170 mg	55
Fig, dried (1)	114 mg	53
Nuts		
Soy nuts, 1/4 cup	308 mg	95
Pistachio, 1 oz.	290 mg	158
Peanut butter, 2 Tbsp.	238 mg	188
Almonds, 1 oz.	206 mg	163
Legumes & Soy Foods		
Adzuki, 1/2 cup cooked	612 mg	147
Green soybean, edamame, 1/2 cup cooked	485 mg	127
Textured vegetable protein (TVP), 1/4 cup dry	462 mg	51
Pink beans, 1/2 cup cooked	429 mg	126
Lentils, 1/2 cup cooked	365 mg	115
Black beans, 1/2 cup cooked	305 mg	113
Kidney beans, 1/2 cup cooked	358 mg	112
Northern beans, 1/2 cup cooked	346 mg	104
Garbanzo, 1/2 cup cooked	239 mg	134
Vegetables		
Potato sweet, 1/2 cup mashed, (5 oz.)	674 mg	128
Tomato paste, 1/4 cup	664 mg	54
Potato (white), with skin, baked, 5-1/2 oz.	610 mg	145
Tomato juice (choose low sodium), 6 oz.	448 mg	40
Spinach, 1/2 cup cooked, or 2 cups raw	419 mg	21
Acorn squash, 1/2 cup	322 mg	40
Butternut squash, 1/2 cup cooked	284 mg	40
Fish and seafood		
Halibut, 3 oz. baked	490 mg	120
Clams, about 12	470 mg	110
Cod, 3 oz.	460 mg	90
Salmon, wild, 3 oz. baked	430 mg	118
Scallops, 6 large, 14 small	430 mg	140
Rainbow trout, 3 oz.	375 mg	144
Sardine, 3.75 oz.	365 mg	191
Tuna, canned, light, in water, 3 oz.	201 mg	98
Dairy		
Yogurt, plain, nonfat, 8 oz.	579 mg	127
Soy milk, unsweetened, 8 oz.	300 mg	80

TABLE 32.3 FOODS RICH IN MAGNESIUM
(most to least by group)

Nuts & Seeds (1 oz.)	MAGNESIUM	Calories
Pumpkin seed	152 mg	153
Flaxseed, ground nuts	111 mg	151
Brazil nuts	107 mg	186
Sunflower seed	100 mg	162
Sesame seeds	99 mg	162
Cashews	83 mg	157
Almonds	78 mg	165
Peanuts	50 mg	166
Legumes		
Soybeans, 1/2 cup cooked	74 mg	149
Navy beans, 1/2 cup cooked	62 mg	148
Black beans, 1/2 cup cooked	60 mg	114
Northern, 1/2 cup cooked	44 mg	104
Pinto, 1/2 cup cooked	43 mg	122
Kidney, 1/2 cup cooked	42 mg	110
Garbanzo, 1/2 cup cooked	39 mg	134
Dark Green Vegetables		
Spinach, 1/2 cup cooked	78 mg	21
Swiss chard, 1/2 cup cooked	75 mg	17
Edamame, 1/2 cup cooked	54 mg	127
Broccoli, 3.5 oz. cooked	21 mg	35
Dark green leafy (romaine, green, leafy), 2 cups	16 mg	19
Asparagus, 3.5 oz. cooked	14 mg	22
Seafood, (3.5 oz.)		
Shrimp	34 mg	98
Tilapia, cooked	34 mg	127
Salmon, cooked	33 mg	138
Tuna, canned	33 mg	127
Whole Grains		
Amaranth, 1/2 cup cooked	86 mg	121
Quinoa, 1/2 cup cooked	59 mg	105
Steel-cut oats, 1/2 cup cooked	48 mg	67
Wheat bran, 2 Tbsp.	44 mg	16
Brown rice, 1/2 cup cooked	42 mg	108
Oats, old fashioned 1/3 cup dry (1 cup cooked)	40 mg	103
Millet, 1/2 cup cooked	38 mg	103
Oat bran, 2 Tbsp.	28 mg	29
Whole-wheat flour, 2 Tbsp.	21 mg	51
Barley, pearled, 1/2 cup cooked	17 mg	96
White rice, 1/2 cup cooked	9 mg	103
OTHER		
Chocolate, unsweet, 1 oz.	93 mg	142
Molasses, 1 Tbsp.	49 mg	59
Chocolate, semi-sweet, 1 oz.	33 mg	136
Banana, medium	31 mg	105
Avocado, 1/2	29 mg	161
Cocoa powder, 2 Tbsp.	24 mg	53
Fig, dried (1)	12 mg	47

DASH Diet: Dietary Approaches To Stop Hypertension

In research by the National Heart, Lung and Blood Institute, the DASH diet was very effective in lowering blood pressure. For more information, see the Web site: www.nhlbi.nih.gov/health/public/hbp/dash.

While the DASH diet works, there are many changes that might improve the DASH diet that were not studied. One such variation on the DASH diet occurred in a later study, the OmniHeart Study, which used the DASH diet but replaced some of the carbohydrates with protein or monounsaturated fat. When protein was increased, half of the protein came from plant sources, which helped to keep saturated fat low, since an increase in saturated fat is not heart healthy. Blood pressure was lowered even more when lean protein or healthy fat replaced carbohydrates (sweets).[35]

The DASH Eating Plan For Two Calorie Levels			
Number of Daily Servings			
1,600 calorie	2,000 calorie	Serving size	Foods
6	7-8	1-ounce or 1/2 cup	Grains and grain products (these can include whole-grain breakfast cereal, whole-grain bread, brown rice, whole-wheat pasta
3-4	4-5	1/2 cup cooked, 1 cup raw	Vegetables
4	4-5	1/2 cup or medium piece	Fruit
2-3	2-3	8 oz. milk or yogurt, 1-1/2 oz. cheese	Low-fat or nonfat dairy foods or calcium-rich foods (see Page 221)
1-2	2	3 oz.	Fish, poultry, lean meat
3-4 per week	4-5 per week	1/4 cup nuts, 1/2 cup beans	Nuts, seeds and legumes/beans
2	2-3	1 teaspoon of oil, 1 Tbsp. of regular salad dressing or mayonnaise	Fats and oils
0	5 per week		Sweets (1 Tbsp. jam, or 1/2 cup low-fat ice cream or 1 cup sweetened beverage) **See Nutrition Note in side bar**

NUTRITION NOTE

Blood pressure was lowered even more when lean protein or healthy fat replaced carbohydrates from grains and sweets.

Blood Pressure DASH Smart 4 Your Heart

BOTTOM LINE

To control your blood pressure:

❖ Eat lots of fruits and vegetables rich in potassium, magnesium and calcium.
❖ Snack on a small handful of unsalted nuts, especially soy nuts daily.
❖ Eat primarily whole grains.
❖ Eat more fish, rich in omega-3 fatty acids and take fish oil supplements.
❖ Limit packaged, processed and restaurant foods, which are high in sodium.
❖ Limit alcohol and caffeine.
❖ Exercise daily.
❖ Lose weight if you are overweight.
❖ Check vitamin D levels (Page 217) and correct if needed.

Blood Pressure Quiz

1. High blood pressure increases risk of heart attack and stroke.
   ❏ T ❏ F

2. Systolic (top number) is more important than diastolic (bottom number) for increased risk of heart disease.
   ❏ T ❏ F

3. It is important to be seated for five minutes before taking a blood pressure reading.
   ❏ T ❏ F

4. The desirable range of blood pressure is:
   a) less than 100 systolic and less than 70 diastolic
   b) less than 120 systolic and less than 80 diastolic
   c) less than 140 systolic and less than 90 diastolic

5. Fish oil supplements should not be taken if you have high blood pressure.
   ❏ T ❏ F

6. Fruits and vegetables rich in magnesium and potassium may lower blood pressure.
   ❏ T ❏ F

7. The DASH diet recommends that for a 2,000 calorie diet, you have:
   a) 4-5 servings of vegetables and
      4-5 servings of fruits daily
   b) 2 fruits and 3 vegetables daily
   c) 4 vegetables and 4 fruits daily

8. Potassium is best taken as a supplement.
   ❏ T ❏ F

9. Unsalted soy nuts may lower systolic blood pressure.
   ❏ T ❏ F

10. Which foods are good sources of magnesium?
    a) pumpkin seeds
    b) sunflower seeds
    c) salmon
    d) cocoa powder

ANSWERS
On Page 281.

Beverages
(Water, Coffee, Tea,
Cocoa and Alcohol)

33

There are entire aisles at the grocery store devoted to beverages. Check the ingredient list and the majority will have added sweeteners which contain calories; others have no calories but use artificial sweeteners. A good rule of thumb is to skip beverages if they have added sweeteners or artificial sugar substitutes. The best beverage is plain water.

Plain water may take some getting used to because your taste buds have become accustomed to being stimulated with those other beverages. If you need something added as you make the adjustment, try squeezing a section of lemon, lime or orange into the water for a bit of flavor, or use bottled lemon or lime juice. You can even buy a lemon – or lime – flavored dry packaged, crystallized powder which comes in packets or shaker bottles called *True Lemon* and *True Lime* that is 100 percent natural and does not contain any sweetener, sodium or preservatives. Check if your store carries it, or order it online at www.truelemon.com.

Water is important to every cell in your body. Your body weight is 55 to 75 percent water. The amount you need varies with the weather, altitude, amount of fiber intake, how much water you lose, and how much you exercise. As you get older, thirst is not a good indicator of when you need fluids since thirst becomes less accurate with age.

The standard guideline of eight (8-ounce) glasses each day works well for most people since we lose about 2 quarts of fluids daily from normal body functions.

Get in the habit of drinking a glass of water with each meal and a glass between each meal. Take a water bottle with you when you are out, and keep a glass on your desk or near your work area to help meet your fluid needs. If you are not allowed to have water where you work, then drinking water at every break is important. Some of your fluid requirement can be met with other beverages, such as milk, 100% juice (limit to a single 4-ounce serving a day) and decaffeinated beverages, as well as fruits and vegetables, which contain a fair amount of water.

Is Bottled Water Better?

Bottled water is the fastest growing segment of the beverage industry and you may find it sold as mineral, spring, carbonated, oxygenated, flavored and

and vitamin-enhanced. Water that comes from a bottle does not automatically mean it is cleaner, safer or lower in sodium than the tap. The safety and quality varies by the regulations of the state in which it is bottled in, or by the FDA if it is sold outside of the state in which it is bottled. The goal is to make bottled water equal to tap water, not better.

If plastic bottles are exposed to high heat, some of the components from plastic bottles may leach into the water. Chemicals such as phthalate may be added to plastic to keep it flexible. This chemical may exhibit hormone-like behavior and act as an endocrine disrupter. Safe plastics are those coded with 1, 2, 4 and 5. Avoid plastics with the codes 3, 6 and 7.

BOTTOM LINE

Bottled water is not necessary since reasonably reliable, safe water is available from the nation's public drinking water. Our daily needs can be met with tap water. If using bottled water means that you drink more water, by all means buy it bottled. If you prefer carrying your own water, then use an unlined stainless steel or a glass bottle if possible. Be sure to let the container dry out between uses.

Softened Water

If your water is softened, it will add a significant amount of sodium to your water, depending upon how hard your water is. Softened water is better for machines, not humans, who benefit from the minerals in hard water. The minerals in hard water, primarily calcium and magnesium, are exchanged for sodium during the softening process. There are potassium pellets that may be used to soften water for those who wish to avoid the added sodium, but they are harder to find and cost more. The best way to avoid excessive sodium used in drinking and cooking is to have the faucet in the kitchen bypass the water softener. If you cannot change the existing system, you can remove sodium from softened water with the use of a distillation system, though many people feel distilled water tastes bland and flat. You can buy bottled water for cooking and drinking, but check the sodium levels.

Sports Drinks

Sports drinks are not necessary unless you exercise vigorously enough to produce significant sweating for more than an hour or are training for an athletic event or competition. It is likely that your electrolyte needs can be met with water and food. Check the ingredients as some of these are sweetened with high fructose corn syrup or artificial sweeteners.

Coffee

Nearly half of all Americans drink coffee to start their day. Studies continue to be done on the benefits and risks of coffee with conflicting results. On the one hand, you are warned of the risks of caffeine's effects, while others promote the benefits of the phytochemicals found in all plants, including coffee beans.

For some individuals, caffeine acts as a stimulant that may increase anxiety and causes problems with sleep. If you are caffeine sensitive, headaches and reflux may also occur.

Caffeine may affect your blood pressure, raise homocysteine levels, increase inflammation, and raise the stress hormones such as cortisol. It causes you to lose more magnesium, an important mineral for maintaining proper heart functioning. These side effects may play a role in increasing risk for heart disease; however, studies have been conflicting.

Paper Filters

Coffee contains two plant chemicals called diterpene compounds (cafestol and kahweol). These chemicals may raise LDL cholesterol and triglyceride levels. The diterpines are extracted from the coffee when exposed to hot water, but are removed with paper filters. One study showed that five cups a day of unfiltered coffee caused cholesterol to rise by 5 to 10 percent.[98] Therefore, drink coffee that has been brewed using a paper filter. Percolators, espresso machines, French presses, or cafetiere machines, as well as boiled coffee (common in some Scandinavian countries), use brewing methods that do not use paper filters. Gold mesh or metal filters are also not recommended as there is no paper filter used.

Coffee filtered through paper is low in these chemicals. Espresso has moderate amounts, and boiled or percolated coffee is highest.

NUTRITION NOTE

Drink coffee that has been brewed using a paper filter.

Benefits Of Coffee

Coffee is a source of antioxidants because it is a plant, and all plants have antioxidants. Coffee is consumed by so many Americans in such large amounts – more so than other antioxidant-rich fruits and vegetables. Because of this, it appears that coffee is one of the richest sources of phytochemicals in the American diet. This is misleading because coffee is not a better source of antioxidants than vegetables and fruits, but we drink more coffee than we eat vegetables. If we increased vegetable and fruit intakes, they would quickly surpass coffee.

A few observational studies have found coffee decreased the risk of developing Type 2 diabetes and possibly lowered the risk of Parkinson's and Alzheimer's. Remember that these observations are not the same as a clinical trial, and more studies will be needed before we may determine if coffee is beneficial. Based on what we currently know, there is no reason to begin drinking coffee or to drink more to obtain phytochemicals. However, expect more research to be done looking for the beneficial effects of coffee, along with studies that discover the negative effects.

NUTRITION NOTE

Coffee is not a better source of antioxidants than vegetables and fruits. But because more coffee is consumed than vegetables in the U.S. it seems to be a better source.

Teeccino

For those who want to find a substitute for coffee that is caffeine free and still enjoy a beverage that tastes and brews like coffee, the product *Teeccino*, which is made from herbs, grains, fruits and nuts, is a good choice. It is a no-caffeine beverage, unlike decaf, which still contains some caffeine and is high in acidity. Look for *Teeccino* in your grocery store or at www.teeccino.com.

Coffee Whiteners

If you don't drink your coffee black, there is little to recommend in the way of coffee whiteners from an optimal health viewpoint. The majority of coffee whitener choices are combinations of chemicals and ingredients such as high fructose corn syrup, artificial sweeteners, or partially hydrogenated oils. Check the ingredient list even if they are fat free, sugar free or carbohydrate free.

The best choice is to add a whitener with no sweeteners, such as liquid milk, evaporated skim milk, dry milk powder, soy milk or dry soy milk powder. Another option from the refrigerated section is a coffee creamer made by *White Wave* called *"SILK Creamer,"* which contains canola oil and uses evaporated cane juice for a sweetener.

If you find those choices unacceptable or unavailable, then the use of half–and-half in moderation would be a better choice than the products that imitate cream, with all of their bad fats, additives and chemicals. Half-and-half contains 1 gram of saturated fat per tablespoon. A moderate amount of a tablespoon or less is advised to stay within your daily saturated fat limits.

Tea

The scientific evidence that tea may reduce the risk of cardiovascular disease continues to grow. If you are choosing between tea and coffee, tea is the healthier choice for heart health based on what we presently know. A high intake of flavanoids decreases the risk of heart disease. Antioxidants in tea may reduce the oxidation of LDL cholesterol and may block platelets from sticking to artery walls. In one clinical trial, drinking five cups of black tea a day reduced total cholesterol by 6.5 percent and LDL by 11 percent.[14]

If you drink tea, it is best to brew it from loose leaves or tea bags rather than using bottled or instant, which contain less catechins. Tea, freshly brewed from tea leaves, has a higher antioxidant level than that found in powdered, instant and bottled tea. Bottled, sweetened teas often have none of the antioxidant benefits found in freshly brewed tea. Try to drink three to four cups per day.

There are several different catechins found in tea. Catechins are natural plant chemicals that belong to a group of antioxidants called polyphenols. The most important catechin for heart health may be (epigallocatechin gallate) EGCG, which acts as an antioxidant.

Decaffeinated Tea

Green tea contains about 20 milligrams of caffeine in a 6-ounce cup. For comparison, 6 ounces of coffee has 68 milligrams. There are decaffeinated teas but they are lower in antioxidants. Try rooibos tea which has no caffeine.

NUTRITION NOTE

If you drink tea, it is best to brew it from loose leaves or tea bags rather than using bottled or instant, which contains less catechins.

NUTRITION NOTE

EGCG in 3.5 oz. brewed tea
- Green tea, brewed, 78 mg
- Green tea, decaffeinated, brewed, 26 mg
- Green tea, bottled, 3.96 mg
- Green tea, instant, 0.49 mg
- Green tea, instant, decaffeinated, 0.45 mg

What About Green Tea Extract Supplements?

While it is thought that EGCG is the active compound responsible for the benefit to heart health, it is not certain. It may turn out that this compound, along with many other ingredients in the tea, has a synergistic effect that a supplement where the isolated, single compound exists, cannot offer. Drink 3 to 4 cups of tea daily – forget the pills.

Rooibos Tea

Rooibos, pronounced "roy-boss," comes from a South African flowering shrub. It may be marketed as red tea. Rooibos contains numerous polyphenol antioxidants and trace amounts of the minerals copper, iron, potassium, calcium, zinc, and magnesium. This tea is caffeine-free and low-tannin. It contains almost no oxalic acid, making it a good beverage for people prone to kidney stones.

Cocoa

Cocoa has nearly twice the antioxidants as red wine and up to three times that found in green tea. The phenolic phytochemicals or flavanoids that are found in the cocoa bean are what provides health benefits in chocolate. However, roasting and alkali treatment such as dutching may reduce the flavanoids by as much as 90 percent.

The best idea is to purchase cocoa that is natural, not dutched, and make your own cocoa mix for hot chocolate. See Page 303 for a recipe. Popular brands of natural cocoa are made by *Hershey, Ghirardelli* and *Scharffen Berger.*

Alcohol and Red Wine

While all alcohol may raise the good cholesterol, additional benefits from red wine come from resveratrol and flavanoids called anthocyanins and other polyphenols found in the wine. Anthocyanins are also found in purple fruits and vegetables.

Moderate alcohol consumption, considered to be one serving per day for women and two per day for men, may lower overall mortality risk by 30 percent. In the *Health Professionals Follow-Up Study,* those who had one to two drinks per day, not daily, but three to four times per week, decreased their risk of a heart attack as much as 32 percent.[99] In the *Copenhagen City Heart Study,* those who drank wine had half the risk of dying from coronary heart disease or stroke as those who never drank wine.[100]

Not all studies have found benefits for red wine. Alcohol may also increase the blood fats called triglycerides. Excessive alcohol use may lead to liver damage, pancreatitis, motor vehicle accidents and addiction.

Increasing alcohol or wine consumption for cardio-protective benefits is not recommended by the American Heart Association.

NUTRITION NOTE

Purchase cocoa that is natural, not dutched.

NUTRITION NOTE

Moderate alcohol
- 1 drink per day for women
- 2 drinks per day for men

What is a "Drink"
Serving size:
- 12 ounces regular beer
- 5 ounces wine
- 1.5 ounces 80-proof distilled spirits

NUTRITION NOTE

If you don't drink alcohol, don't start. If you do drink, do so in moderation.

If you have high triglycerides, avoid alcohol, as it may raise triglycerides.

Beverage Quiz

1. As you get older, thirst is a good indicator of when you need to drink more.
   ❏ T   ❏ F

2. Bottled water is better than tap water because the FDA regulates bottled water.
   ❏ T   ❏ F

3. Softened water is higher in sodium.
   ❏ T   ❏ F

4. Caffeine does not affect blood pressure.
   ❏ T   ❏ F

5. Coffee that is brewed without the use of a paper filters can raise LDL cholesterol.
   ❏ T   ❏ F

6. Antioxidants in tea may prevent oxidation of LDL cholesterol.
   ❏ T   ❏ F

7. Drinking bottled tea is a good way to obtain antioxidants.
   ❏ T   ❏ F

8. Cocoa is a richer source of antioxidants than green tea and red wine.
   ❏ T   ❏ F

9. A serving of alcohol is:
   a) 12 ounces regular beer
   b) 5 ounces wine
   c) 1.5 ounces 80-proof spirits
   d) all of the above

10. Moderate alcohol intake is two servings per day for men and women.
    ❏ T   ❏ F

11. Alcohol raises HDL and lowers triglycerides.
    ❏ T   ❏ F

ANSWERS
On Page 281.

Smart 4 Your Heart

34

Vitamin K and Warfarin

I f your doctor is concerned that your body may form blood clots that block blood circulation or move to another part of your body such as to your brain and cause a stroke, then you may be prescribed a blood-thinning medication. This medication reduces the ability of your blood to form clots but does not dissolve a clot if it already exists.

Warfarin, a drug better known by its brand name *Coumadin*, is the drug most commonly used in the United States to prevent blood clots. In this chapter, we will refer to the two names interchangeably. There are other coumarins used in other countries that require the same precautions. While taking *Coumadin*, you will have blood testing called prothrombin time (Protime), which measures your International Normalized Ratio (INR) and warfarin's effect on the blood. Testing will also help to establish the correct dose and then monitor it in case it needs to be changed.

There are several factors that can affect your INR test results. Any over-the-counter medication or vitamin, mineral or herbal supplement that you take or stop taking should be reported to your doctor. Your doctor can then monitor your INR levels closely.

Vitamin K not to be confused with potassium, for which the element symbol "K" is used. For example, bananas contain a lot of potassium but not a significant amount of vitamin K.

Vitamin K_1 (phylloquinone) is found in plants and is used to make clotting factors. Vitamin K_2 is made by bacteria in your intestines. *Coumadin* lowers both types of vitamin K, increases your INR and thins the blood. Vitamin K, taken in excess amounts, will work against *Coumadin*, decrease your INR, and reduce protection against blood clotting.

Vitamin K is found in green vegetables. A common misunderstanding is that you should avoid eating green vegetables when you are taking warfarin.

The vitamin K content of green vegetables varies widely. It is most important that you keep your diet consistent in vitamin K content (or intake). If you avoid all foods with vitamin K, you will have very low vitamin K in your body, making you more sensitive to small amounts of vitamin K. This will make regulating your dose of *Coumadin* more difficult. Some doctors do not restrict your food and vegetable intake. Check to see what your doctor recommends.

NUTRITION NOTE

A common myth is that vitamin K increases blood clotting. Too much vitamin K works against *Coumadin* and its protection against blood clotting.

NUTRITION NOTE

It is a myth that you should avoid all green vegetables when taking *Coumadin*.

NUTRITION NOTE

The vitamin K
daily requirement

for men is 140
micrograms (mcg)

for women is
90 mcg daily.

Vitamin K plays a role in maintaining healthy bones. Your bones are constantly breaking down and reforming, and vitamin K helps to reform bones. Use of *Coumadin* for more than a year increases the risk for osteoporosis, which is linked to bone fractures, especially in men. Exercise and adequate intake of calcium and vitamin D are important for maintaining bone health, as well as getting a consistent daily amount of vegetables containing vitamin K.

Eating vegetables consistently will allow the benefits of eating healthy and getting enough vitamin K for bone health, without increasing your risk of blood clots.

Amounts Of Vitamin K Per Meal

A small minority of individuals with low vitamin K status are highly sensitive to foods or supplements containing even small amounts of vitamin K. But for most individuals, a single meal or a vitamin/mineral supplement containing less than 100 mcg of vitamin K that is taken daily would not interfere with blood thinning medication in most cases.

A single, occasional meal containing 250 mcg vitamin K will usually not be a problem either, but consuming 250 mcg vitamin K for several days reduces the effect of *Coumadin* and requires a dose adjustment. Single meals with 700 to 1,500 mcg vitamin K may measurably change the INR.

Not all green vegetables are high in vitamin K. Foods highest in vitamin K are the darkest green leafy vegetables, especially cooked greens such as spinach, collards and kale. Lighter greens have less vitamin K, and outer leaves that are darker green have more than lighter leaves. Iceberg lettuce is very low. Romaine, Bibb and Boston lettuce have much lower vitamin K content than spinach. Most fruits are low, with the exception of kiwifruit, which is moderate in vitamin K. Most nuts, with the exception of pine nuts and cashews, are not a significant source of vitamin K. See Page 207 for specific foods.

Snack and Processed Foods

Foods that are fried in vegetable oils such as soybean oil, high-fat processed foods, and fried restaurant foods may be a source of vitamin K. Potato and tortilla chips made with the artificial fat substitute *Olestra* contain added vitamin K.

Juices and *Coumadin*

There have been reports from the United Kingdom of cranberry juice associated with increased risk of bleeding while taking *Coumadin*. Nothing has been reported to date in Canada or the United States. In some cases, the amounts consumed were excessive — two quarts or more daily. If you have difficulty with INRs and drink cranberry juice, you may want to stop drinking it to see if that resolves the problem.

In some cases, other juices such as grapefruit, berry juices and herbal teas have been reported by individuals to affect INRs.

Green Tea

Drinking tea in the amounts most individuals drink is not a concern. It is not recommended that you eat the leaves, as has been promoted by some for health benefits. Drinking the tea made from tea leaves is of little concern since a tea bag contains a small amount of tea leaves by weight. Some charts indicate that green tea is high in vitamin K when they compare foods by 100-gram servings. This would be about 50 tea bags since each bag is only about 2 grams. In one case reported, drinking one-half to 1 gallon of green tea daily decreased the effect of *Coumadin*.

Alcohol and *Coumadin*

Social drinking of alcohol with food does not appear to be a concern. Moderation is considered to be consuming one to two drinks a day. An occasional large amount of alcohol will increase INR (thin the blood more). But excessive alcohol intake that occurs regularly can lead to the opposite and decrease the INR.

Low-Carb Diets May Require More *Coumadin*

High-protein, low-carbohydrate diets may decrease INR and require a larger dose of medication. If the diet is stopped, then the amount of medication may need to be reduced. These diet changes will require that your INR is monitored since everyone does not respond in the same way.

Fish Oil and *Coumadin*

There are many benefits of fish oil, such as decreased inflammation and lowered triglycerides. Fish oil may have a weak antiplatelet effect, somewhat similar to taking aspirin. Some have raised concerns that fish oil in large doses containing more than 4 grams of omega-3 fatty acids, which is the dose required to lower triglycerides, may increase bleeding when combined with *Coumadin*. There is no strong evidence to prove this in the published literature. This perception of increased risk does not mean that patients on *Coumadin* cannot take fish oil. Most patients who take fish oil do not see any change in INR. Monitoring INR more closely initially when fish oil is added is recommended, similiar to the monitoring suggested with the addition of any other supplement or change in diet. Determining the individualized response to each new combination is important.

NUTRITION NOTE

Caution should be taken when consuming certain supplements that add green tea extract.

More frequent blood testing should be considered to find out the affect on INR.

Others That May Affect Anticoagulation

Smokeless tobacco may interfere with warfarin, as it is high in vitamin K. Tobacco products in any form should be avoided for many other reasons as well.

Natto, a fermented soybean product that contains bacteria that produces large amounts of vitamin K in the intestines, may decrease INR.

Other herbals such as garlic, vitamin E, green tea extracts, CoQ10, ginger, aspirin, wheat grass, flax oil, and over-the-counter weight-loss products to name a few, may also thin the blood and should only be taken under supervision of your doctor who can closely monitor your INR to determine their effects. St. John's wort, ginseng and soy isoflavones, as well as soy milk, have decreased INR. These have been reported in a few cases, but true risk is unknown, so frequent testing and monitoring of the INR is the best way to know how you respond.

The use of acetaminophen may raise INR. Other over-the-counter pain medications; changes in prescription drugs; and changes in your environment, amount of exercise, general health, sleep amount and travel schedule may also have an effect.

Tips For Taking Warfarin (*Coumadin*)

❖ Take your dose every day.

❖ Do not stop taking your dose before talking to your doctor.

❖ You may take it with or without food.

❖ Take it at the same time of the day.

❖ If you forget and remember within eight hours, take the dose.

❖ Do not take a double dose.

❖ If you forget your dose more than one day in a row, call your doctor.

❖ Before taking over-the-counter supplements or herbals such as garlic, gingko biloba, fish oil, vitamin E or C, etc., check with your doctor who can monitor your INR more closely to see how you respond.

❖ Store medicine at room temperature, but not in the bathroom, which tends to be too damp.

❖ Wear or carry identification that states you are taking warfarin.

TABLE 34.1　Vitamin K Content of Foods

	Serving Size	Vitamin K (mcg)
Leafy Salad Greens, Raw		
Arugula	1-1/2 cups (30g) (1 oz.)	33
Escarole	1-1/2 cups (75g) (2.5 oz.)	173
Curly endive/chicory/frisee	1-1/2 cups (75g) (2.6 oz.)	173
Boston	1-1/2 cups (82g) (3 oz.)	84
Bibb	1-1/2 cups (82g) (3 oz.)	84
Iceberg lettuce	1-1/2 cups (85g) (3 oz.)	20
Looseleaf, green leaf	1-1/2 cups (84g) (3 oz.)	147
Red leafy lettuce	1-1/2 cups (84g) (3 oz.)	119
Radicchio	1-1/2 cups (60g) (2 oz.)	153
Romaine	1-1/2 cups (84g) (3 oz.)	86
Spinach, raw	1-1/2 cups (84 g) (3 oz.)	405
Watercress	1-1/2 cups (51g) (1.8 oz.)	127
Leafy Greens, Cooked Unless Indicated		
Beet greens	1/2 cup (72g) (2.5 oz.)	348
Collard	1/2 cup (95g) (3.4 oz.)	623
Kale	1/2 cup (65g) (2.3 oz.)	531
Mustard greens	1/2 cup (70g) (2.5 oz.)	209
Rabe, rapini, raw	1/2 cup (75g) (2.5 oz.)	192
Spinach, cooked	1/2 cup (90g) (3 oz.)	444
Swiss chard	1/2 cup (87g) (3 oz.)	122
Turnip greens	1/2 cup (72g) (2.5 oz.)	264
Fresh Vegetables		
Artichoke, boiled	1 medium (113g) (4 oz.)	17
Asparagus, cooked	5 spears (75g) (2.6 oz.)	38
Avocado	1/2 medium (100g) (3.5 oz.)	21
Bamboo shoots, canned, drained	1/2 cup (75g) (2.6 oz.)	ND
Basil (fresh)	2 Tbsp. chopped (5.3g) (0.2 oz.)	22
Bean sprouts, raw	1/2 cup (113g) (4 oz.)	37
Beans, green, cooked	1/2 cup (62g) (2.2 oz.)	10
Beets, cooked	1/2 cup (81g) (2.8 oz.)	0.16
Bell pepper, green, chopped	1/2 cup (74g) (2.6 oz.)	5
Bell pepper, red, chopped	1/2 cup. (74g) (2.6 oz.)	4
Bok choy, cooked	1/2 cup (85g) (3 oz.)	29
Broccoli, raw	1 cup (88g) (3 oz.)	90
Broccoli, cooked	1/2 cup (92g) (3.25 oz.)	91
Broccoflower, cooked	1/2 cup (78g) (2.75 oz.)	ND
Brussel sprouts, cooked	1/2 cup (77g) (2.75 oz.)	150
Cabbage, green, raw	1 cup shred (70g) (2.4 oz.)	42
Cabbage, green, cooked	1/2 cup (75g) (2.6 oz.)	37
Cabbage, nappa, cooked	1/2 cup (54g) (2 oz.)	ND
Cabbage, red, raw	1 cup shred (70g) (2.4 oz.)	27
Cabbage, red, cooked	1/2 cup (75g) (2.6 oz.)	36
Cabbage, savoy, raw	1 cup shred(70g) (2.5 oz.)	48
Carrot, baby, raw	3/4 cup (85g) (3 oz.)	8
Carrot, cooked	1/2 cup (73g) (2.5 oz.)	7
Carrot juice	4 oz.	18
Cauliflower, raw	1 cup (85g) (3 oz.)	14
Cauliflower, cooked	1/2 cup (90g) (3.17 oz.)	11
Celery, raw, stalks	2 medium (80g) (2.82 oz.)	13
Celery, cooked	1/2 cup diced (75g) (2.6 oz.)	28
Celery root, raw	1/2 cup (78g) (2.7 oz.)	32
Chives	2 Tbsp. (6g) (0.2 oz.)	13

ND –
no data
available

	Serving Size	Vitamin K (mcg)
Coleslaw	1/2 cup (66g) (2.3 oz.)	38
Cilantro/coriander, raw	2 Tbsp. (2g) (0.07 oz.)	6
Corn, sweet, cooked	1 medium ear (85g) (3 oz.)	0.5
Corn, cooked	1/2 cup (77g) (2.7 oz.)	0.02
Cucumber, raw	1/3 medium with peel (99g) (3.5 oz.)	116
Cucumber, raw	1/3 medium peeled	9
Eggplant, cooked	1/2 cup (48g) (1.7 oz.)	1.4
Edamame (green soybeans)	1/2 cup (90g) (3 oz.)	28
Fennel, raw	1 cup (87g) (3 oz.)	ND
Garlic	1 clove (3g) (0.1 oz.)	0.04
Jicama, raw	1/2 cup (60g) (2 oz.)	0.2
Kohlrabi, cooked	1/2 cup (82g) (2.9 oz.)	0.08
Leeks, raw	1/2 cup chopped (44g) (1.5 oz.)	21
Mixed vegetables, cooked	1/2 cup (82g) (3 oz.)	10
Mushroom, portobello, raw	1/2 cup (85g) (3 oz.)	0.02
Mushrooms, raw	5 medium, 1-1/4 cup sliced (87g) (3 oz.)	0.02
Mushroom, canned	1/2 cup (85g) (3 oz.)	0.09
Okra, cooked	1/2 cup (85g) (3 oz.)	42
Onion, yellow or red	1 medium (150g) (5.3 oz.)	0.6
Onion, green, chopped	1/2 cup (25g) (0.88 oz.)	52
Onion, green	1 bulb + top (15g) (0.5 oz.)	31
Parsley	2 Tbsp. (7.5g) (0.25 oz.)	123
Parsnips, cooked	1/2 cup boiled (78g) (2.75 oz.)	1
Pea pods, cooked	1/2 cup (82g) (2.9 oz.)	20
Pea pods, raw	1/2 cup (85g) (3 oz.)	21
Peas, cooked	1/2 cup (80g) (2.8 oz.)	18
Pickle, dill, spear	4" (30g) (1 oz.)	5
Pickle relish	2 Tbsp. (30g) (1 oz.)	6
Potato, baked, w/skin	1 medium (170g) (6 oz.)	3
Potato, no skin	1 medium (70g) (6 oz.)	0.5
Pumpkin, canned	1/2 cup (122g) (4.3 oz.)	20
Radishes	1 medium (2g) (0.07 oz.)	0.03
Rapini (broccoli-rabe), cooked	1/2 cup (85 g)	217
Rutabaga, cooked	1/2 cup mashed (120g) (4 oz.)	0.4
Sauerkraut	1/2 cup (71g) (2.5 oz.)	41
Sweet potato	1 medium (155g) (5.5 oz.)	4
Squash, butternut, cooked	1/2 cup (120g) (4.2 oz.)	1.3
Squash, spaghetti, cooked	1/2 cup (77g) (2.7 oz.)	0.6
Squash, winter, cooked	1/2 cup (102g) (3.6 oz.)	4
Squash, zucchini	1/2 medium (98g) (3.5 oz.)	4
Tomatillo, raw	1 (34g) (1.2 oz.)	33
Tomato	1/2 medium (90g) (3 oz.)	7
Tomatoes, canned	1/2 cup (113g) (4 oz.)	3
Turnip, cooked	1/2 cup (78g) (2.75 oz.)	0.1
Fresh Fruit - Berries		
Blackberries	1 cup (144g) (5 oz.)	28
Blueberries	1 cup raw (145g) (5 oz.)	28
Cherries, sweet	21 or 1 cup (140g) (5 oz.)	3
Cranberries	1 cup (95g) (3.3 oz.)	4.8
Raspberries	1 cup (123g) (4.3 oz.)	9.6
Strawberries, sliced	1 cup (166g) (5.8 oz.)	3.6
Fresh Fruit - Melons		
Cantaloupe, cubes	1 cup (160g) (5.6 oz.)	4
Honeydew, balls	1 cup (177g) (6.2 oz.)	5
Watermelon, diced	1 cup (152g) (5.3 oz.)	0.1

ND –
no data
available

Fruit	Serving Size	Vitamin K(mcg)
Fruit cocktail, canned	1/2 cup (118g) (4 oz.)	3
Peaches, drained	1/2 cup (111g) (3.9 oz.)	2.9
Pears, drained	1/2 cup (100g) (3.5 oz.)	4.5
Pineapple, crushed, drained	1/2 cup (97g) (3.4 oz.)	0.6
Fresh Fruits - Other		
Apple, w/peel	1 medium (138g) (4.8 oz.)	3
Apple, peeled	1 medium (138g) (4.8 oz.)	0.8
Apricot, fresh	1 (35g) (1.2 oz.)	1.1
Banana	1 medium (118g) (4 oz.)	0.5
Fig, fresh	1 (50g) (1.7 oz.)	2.3
Guava	1 (82g) (3 oz.)	2.1
Grapes, Thompson or red grapes	1/2 cup (80g) (2.8 oz.)	11.6
Grapefruit	1/2 medium (91g) (3.2 oz.)	0
Kiwifruit	1 large (74g) (2.6 oz.)	30
Lemon	1 medium (58g) (2 oz.)	0.1
Lime	1 medium (67g) (2.4 oz.)	0.4
Mango, slices	1/2 cup (82g) (3 oz.)	3.5
Nectarine	1 medium (136g) (4.8 oz.)	3
Orange	1 medium (131g) (4.6 oz.)	0.1
Papaya	1/2 cup (70g) (2.4 oz.)	1.8
Passion fruit	1 (18g) (0.6 oz.)	0.13
Peach	1 medium (98g) (3.5 oz.)	2.5
Pear, all varieties	1 medium (139g) (4.9 oz.)	6.2
Pineapple, diced	1/2 cup (77g) (2.7 oz.)	0.5
Plantain	1/2 cup (77g) (2.7 oz.)	0.5
Plum	1 medium (66g) (2.3 oz.)	4.2
Pomegranate, 3-3/8"diameter	1 each (154g) (5.4 oz.)	7
Rhubarb, chopped	1/2 cup (61g) (2 oz.)	25
Starfruit	1 (91g) (3.2 oz.)	0
Tangerine	1 medium (109g) (3.8 oz.)	0
Dried Fruits		
Apricots	2 pieces (1/4 oz.)	0.02
Dates	2 each (1/4 oz.)	0.4
Fig	1 each (0.6 oz.)	2.9
Prunes	1 each (0.3 oz.)	5
Raisins, not packed	1/4 cup (1 oz.)	1
Dried cranberries	1/4 cup (1 oz.)	1.1
Nuts		
Almonds	1 oz.	0
Brazil nuts	1 oz.	0
Cashews	1 oz.	9.84
Hazelnuts	1 oz.	4.03
Macadamia nuts	1 oz.	0
Peanuts	1 oz.	0
Pecans	1 oz.	0.99
Pine nuts	1 oz.	15.28
Pistachios	1 oz.	3.71
Soy nuts	1 oz.	10.49
Walnuts	1 oz.	0.77

Nutritional information calculated using The Food Processor software by ESHA Research, Salem, Ore.

VITAMIN K

ND –
no data
available

Vitamin K Quiz

1. Vitamin K works against *Coumadin* (warfarin), a drug which protects against blood clots.
   ❏ T ❏ F

2. Vitamin K is found in green vegetables, so avoiding all green vegetables is a good idea.
   ❏ T ❏ F

3. Foods highest in vitamin K are:
   a) cooked leafy greens
   b) iceberg lettuce
   c) green beans

4. Over-the-counter herbal supplements may interfere with *Coumadin*.
   ❏ T ❏ F

5. Eating consistent amounts of vitamin K makes it easier to regulate your *Coumadin* dose than trying to eat very low amounts of vitamin K.
   ❏ T ❏ F

6. A single meal of 100 mcg of vitamin K or less is acceptable for most individuals.
   ❏ T ❏ F

7. A single meal of 3 cups of raw spinach or 1 cup of cooked provides more than 700 mcg of vitamin K and would affect INR.
   ❏ T ❏ F

8. Vitamin K is important to maintain healthy bones.
   ❏ T ❏ F

9. Fish oil cannot be taken when using *Coumadin*.
   ❏ T ❏ F

ANSWERS
On Page 281.

Multivitamin/Mineral Supplements

35

Two-thirds of Americans describe themselves as "healthy eaters." A survey of dietary habits finds that only 5 percent of American adults actually consumed a diet with the recommended amounts of vegetables and fruits, so we are not eating as healthy as we seem to think.

We know vitamins and minerals are micronutrients essential to a healthy heart, and the supplement industry offers them to us in the form of pills. The *Journal of the American Medical Association* recommends that all adults take a multivitamin daily, unless you are undergoing medical treatment and have been advised otherwise by your doctor.[102] Inadequate intake of several vitamins has been linked to chronic disease, including coronary heart disease, cancer and osteoporosis. But does that mean that you can forget the platefuls of broccoli and have a pill with your brownies and get the same effect? No pill or supplement can substitute for a healthy diet.

The USDA report of *"What We Eat in America"* found that 93 percent of Americans don't get enough vitamin E, a little over half did not get enough magnesium, one-third need more vitamin C, and 44 percent need more vitamin A in the form of carotenoids such as beta-carotene.[103] At the same time, we get too much added salt, sugars, saturated fat and trans fat, as well as too many calories. That makes us overweight but undernourished. Taking a multivitamin does not, in any way, mean that you can make up for a poor diet by taking a pill. It cannot replace eating well. There is a reason they are called supplements instead of replacements!

NUTRITION NOTE

Simply adding a vitamin/mineral supplement won't correct the problem of getting too many calories, the wrong fats or too much salt.

NUTRITION NOTE

We get too much:
- Salt
- Sugar
- Saturated fat
- Trans fat
- Calories

WE NEED MORE	WHERE YOU GET IT
Vitamin E	Nuts (hazelnuts, almonds), sunflower seeds, almond butter, salad dressing made with oil (Page 218)
Magnesium	Nuts, pumpkin seeds, flax seeds, dark green vegetables, soybeans, whole grains, seafood (Page 193)
Vitamin C	Strawberries, red bell pepper, kiwi, oranges, broccoli (Page 215)
Beta-Carotene	Green leafy vegetables, (collard, spinach, kale, Swiss chard, romaine) red pepper, sweet potato, pumpkin, carrots, broccoli, okra, brussels sprouts, winter squash

There are thousands of health-promoting things in foods besides vitamins and minerals – many that we are only beginning to know what they do. Things such as phytochemicals, some that have not yet been discovered, are seldom found in supplements. If they are, they act very differently than when found in foods. The synergy of whole food is more beneficial than when we isolate a specific component that is thought to be beneficial and put it in a pill.

If you choose to take a vitamin, knowing what to take is confusing because the science of what is needed constantly changes, and what you need will depend upon what you typically eat and your individual needs. Seek the help of a registered dietitian who can analyze your food intake to determine what you need and suggest ways to improve you diet or supplement wisely. As new trials using supplements are completed, the advice on what is helpful or harmful is likely to change. But the recommendation to eat plenty of healthy foods will not change as it is the safest way to get vitamins and minerals naturally.

Is Your Vitamin Absorbed?

Unless the pill you take breaks apart, your body will not get any of the benefits it contains. If you see "USP" (United States Pharmacopeia) on the label, it has passed the standard test that attempts to create what happens in your body. Some products carry the USP, but many good products do not. The most common pills that may not break apart are tablets or caplets which, if packed or coated, stay intact. There is less of a problem with chewable forms, if you do chew them, and with gelatin capsules which dissolve easily. Enteric-coated and timed-release pills should not break down as they are meant to release the contents differently.

You can attempt to duplicate the test using vinegar, which is about equal to the acidity found in the stomach. Heat the vinegar to body temperature (98.6°F). Add the pill and agitate occasionally, but do not hit the pill. Keep the temperature constant. In 30 to 45 minutes, the pill should fall apart.

What To Look For In A Multivitamin

There are many different choices of "multi's" and a wide variety of brands. The following guidelines will meet your basic needs in a reasonably safe manner.

❖ Visit www.consumerlab.com, an independent Web site for lists of supplements they have tested to determine if they contain what is stated on the label.

❖ For vitamin A, choose those with not more than "100%" of daily value, with some or all in the form of beta-carotene.

❖ Pick a supplement that fits your age and gender. For example, no iron if male or postmenopausal female, but most premenopausal women need iron.

❖ Do not take more than 400 mcg of folic acid (100% daily value).

How To Take A Multivitamin/Mineral

Take the supplement with food to avoid an upset stomach and with a meal that contains some fat for better absorption of fat-soluble vitamins. For example, taking them with applesauce or crackers would not provide any fat, but adding a few almonds would provide some healthy fat.

Take caffeine-containing beverages such as tea, coffee and colas several hours before or after taking supplements. If you have an iron deficiency, it is better to take calcium between meals or before bed to prevent it from binding with iron in foods.

What About Vitamin/Minerals With Added Herbs?

There are no government-established guidelines for daily intake of herbs. Multivitamin and mineral supplements will often add very small amounts. Even if these herbs are beneficial, the amounts are often not enough to make a difference. For example, lutein, according to studies, is effective at 6 milligrams a day for reduction of the risk of macular degeneration.[104] Some vitamin/mineral supplements provide small amounts in micrograms, not milligrams (250 mcg = 0.25 mg). It is better to eat a half cup of cooked kale, Swiss chard or spinach which provides the 6 milligrams of lutein needed.

Vitamin A/Retinol and Carotenes

Be careful to not take more than "100% daily value" of vitamin A. Too much of this fat-soluble vitamin is not good. High intakes of preformed vitamin A, or retinol, may increase risk for bone fractures and may build up in the liver. In pregnant women, too much may cause birth defects.

It is preferred to get it in the form of beta-carotene (15,000 IU or less), which is converted to vitamin A as the body needs it, rather than palmitate, retinol or acetate which could cause an overdose. Some multivitamins will include a combination of beta-carotene and vitamin A.

While beta-carotene is a safer form, you don't want too much. Supplementation of high doses of beta-carotene is now discouraged for smokers and former smokers. The amount of beta-carotene found in your multiple one-a-day supplements is usually not a concern as the amounts tend to be small. This risk was seen when taking 20 to 30 mg (33,000 to 50,000 IU) of beta-carotene as a separate supplement. There was an increased risk of cancer in smokers and ex-smokers but not in nonsmokers. Risk was also higher in those who drank above-average amounts of alcohol.

When you eat foods, you get a mixture of carotenoids. Some recommend mixed carotenoids rather than only beta-carotene when taking a supplement.

Foods with added vitamins, such as skim milk, yogurt, cold cereals and breakfast bars, protein and energy bars, and shakes and beverages may add vitamin A as retinol/palmitate or beta-carotene. Check the ingredient list. If retinol or palmitate is listed and the daily value for vitamin A is more than 10 percent, avoid or limit those foods.

NUTRITION NOTE

Limit vitamin A that is listed as palmitate, retinyl or acetate to 2,310 IU for women and 3,000 IU for men.

Limit beta-carotene from supplements to 15,000 IU.

B Vitamins: Folic Acid, B$_6$ and B$_{12}$

The B vitamins affect the body's production and use of homocysteine (ho-mo-SIS-teen). Homocysteine is an amino acid found in your blood that forms when you eat animal proteins such as eggs, cheese, beef and chicken. When homocysteine levels are too high, they contribute to the buildup of plaque. There is a correlation between high levels of homocysteine and an increased risk for heart disease and stroke. High homocysteine may also increase risk for Alzheimer's disease.

Taking B vitamins lowers homocysteine levels, although it is uncertain if lowering them with B vitamins protects against heart disease. If you are taking a multivitamin, it can easily supply the 400 mcg folic acid and other B vitamins. You may also get B vitamins in a vitamin B complex supplement if you are not taking a multivitamin. White flour that is "enriched" adds folic acid; and some cereals, energy bars and other "heart healthy" foods are also adding it.

Food Sources Of B Vitamins

❖ **Folic Acid:** Beans (legumes), vegetables (especially spinach), asparagus, romaine, brussels sprouts, beets and avocado. Fruits don't contain much, but banana, oranges and cantaloupe are best. Not much is found in animal and dairy foods. High levels of folic acid could delay the diagnosis of a vitamin B$_{12}$ deficiency if you have atrophic gastritis. Some studies have found that taking folic acid as a supplement in large amounts might increase growth of cancers in animals, and now some data suggests that is also the case in humans.

❖ **B$_6$ (pyridoxine):** Animal foods such as fish, chicken, pork, beef, eggs and dairy. For plant foods, banana, mango and whole-grain foods are best.

❖ **B$_{12}$:** Found only in animal foods – not plants. This vitamin protects the nervous system, and a deficiency may result in blindness, deafness and dementia. Most multiple vitamins contain B$_{12}$. If you are over 50, the IOM (Institute of Medicine) recommends taking B$_{12}$ as a supplement or from foods fortified with B$_{12}$. Up to 30 percent of adults over 50 have increased growth of intestinal bacteria that makes it difficult to absorb vitamin B$_{12}$ from foods or supplements even when they are receiving enough in their diet or supplements. They will develop anemia and cognitive impairment. A B$_{12}$ tablet is available that dissolves under the tongue (sublinqual), allowing it to get into the bloodstream instead of going through the stomach. The recommended daily allowance (RDA) for B$_{12}$ is 2.4 mcg for adults. B$_{12}$ is safe and has a low risk for being toxic.

Vitamin C

It is recommended that men get 90 milligrams and women get 75 milligrams of vitamin C. The upper limit is 2,000 milligrams per day. Some studies demonstrate a relationship between vitamin C intake and a lower risk for heart disease. It is not recommend that you take vitamin C as a supplement to prevent heart disease – instead eat foods rich in vitamin C.

See Table on next page for foods that are good sources of vitamin C.

NUTRITION NOTE

How much Folic Acid?
Not more than 400 mcg from supplements or fortified foods.

FOOD SOURCES
B$_{12}$:
• Rainbow trout
• Sockeye salmon
• Yogurt
• Clams
• Eggs

NUTRITION NOTE

How much vitamin C?
Men: 90 mg
Women: 75 mg

TABLE 35.1	Food Sources Of Vitamin C
FOOD	**VITAMIN C (mg)**
Guava, 1 whole	205
Papaya, 1/2 whole	94
Red bell pepper, 1/2 cup sliced, raw	87
Strawberries, 1 cup	82
Kiwi, 1 medium	72
Orange, 1	70
Green bell pepper, 1 small	66
Broccoli, 1/2 cup cooked	58
Mango, 1	57
Brussels sprouts, 1/2 cup cooked	48
Honeydew, 1 cup	42
Mandarin orange, canned, drained 1/2 cup	32
Cantaloupe, 1 medium wedge	29
Black berries, 1 cup	30
Sweet potato, 1 medium	28
Kale, 1/2 cup cooked	27
Cauliflower, 1/2 cup	27
Watermelon, 1 cup	27
Tomatoes, 1 medium	25
Collard, 1/2 cup cooked	22
Limes, 1	19
Mustard greens, 1/2 cup cooked	18
Cabbage, 1/2 cup cooked	15
Parsley, 2 Tbsp. chopped	10
Asparagus, 1/2 cup, 4 spears	10
Spinach, 1 cup raw	8
Orange peel, 1 Tbsp. fresh	8
Fennel, 1/2 cup sliced	5
Lemons, 1	4

Source: The Food Processor software by ESHA Research, Salem, Ore.

Vitamin D

When it was believed that vitamin D was a fat soluble vitamin there was concern that we could get too much. It is really a secosteroid. Studies are finding that people over age 50, or with dark skin, and anyone who does not get enough sunlight exposure, may be deficient. If you wear sunscreen when exposed to sun, you decrease vitamin D production to almost none.

A growing number of scientists who have reviewed studies from the past 25 years think that 1,000 IU (25 mcg) or more may be needed to prevent certain types of cancers, such as colon, breast, prostate and ovarian.[107] In the past, there was concern of potential toxicity, but the safety of vitamin D_3 at this level has been assessed and confirmed by the Council for Responsible Nutrition (CNR). The upper limit, which currently is set at 2,000 IU per day, may be safely raised to as high as 10,000 IU (250 mg). For more information

NUTRITION NOTE

How much vitamin D?

2,000 units for most people – will vary based on weight, age, sun exposure and where you live.

NUTRITION NOTE

For the latest
informaton on
vitamin D visit
the vitamin D
council Web site

as it becomes known visit www.vitamindcouncil.org.

Vitamin D in the form of D_3 (cholecalciferol) is better absorbed. If you are taking calcium as a supplement, you may be getting vitamin D in it. Most multivitamins have 400 IU. Vitamin D in the prescription form is D_2 (ergocalciferol), which is not absorbed as well and much more expensive. It is better to choose an over-the-counter, oil-based gel-cap of vitamin D_3 (cholecalciferol), as a separate supplement.

Most foods have little to no vitamin D. The best source is fatty fish such as salmon and sardines. While all cows' milk has added vitamin D, not all dairy will have vitamin D added. Yogurt and cheese typically do not.

TABLE 35.2   Food Sources Of Vitamin D

FISH (3 OUNCES)	VITAMIN D IU
Herring, pickled	582
Salmon, sockeye	505
Salmon, pink, canned	468
Mackerel, canned Jack	383
Salmon, coho/silver	373
Sardine, in oil	232
Salmon, sockeye, canned, drained	190
Tuna, light, oil packed	190
Halibut	170
Tuna, steak, bluefin	169
Tuna, white, oil packed	165
Tuna, white, water packed	137
Tuna, light, water packed	124
Shrimp	119
Salmon, smoked	90
Trout, rainbow	75
Sole	60
Cod	51
Haddock	34
Perch	34
Walleye	34
Scallops	4

OTHER FOODS	
Cod liver oil, 1 teaspoon.	433
Milk, all types (fortified), 8 oz.	100
Egg yolk, 1 large	107

Source: The Food Processor software by ESHA Research, Salem, Ore.

Vitamin D and Heart Disease

Vitamin D plays a role in heart health and development of high blood pressure. Having a low blood level of vitamin D is strongly related to the risk of developing heart disease and heart failure. Vitamin D acts as an anti-inflammatory and improves muscle function and blood pressure. Vitamin D has been shown to improve the body's ability to use insulin. Those with low HDL and vitamin D often see an increase in HDL when their vitamin D blood levels improve.

Testing Vitamin D Blood Levels

The only way to know if you have an adequate vitamin D level in your blood is to have your doctor order a blood test. Testing will allow you to know if you have a low level and need to correct a deficiency by taking a vitamin D supplement. Your vitamin D status is determined with a blood test called 25(OH)D or 25-hydroxy vitamin D. It should not be confused with another, more expensive vitamin D test, 1,25-Hydroxy (Calcitriol), which is used when calcium is high or there is a disease that might produce excess amounts of calcitriol. The 1,25-Hydroxy test could be normal even when 25(OH)D is low.

The lab that does your test will provide a set of reference numbers that are within the range of normal. Ideally your 25(OH)D is a minimum of 50 ng/ml (125 nmol/L). It is the level at which vitamin D begins to be stored for future use. Toxicity has not been documented at 25(OH)D levels less than 200 ng/ml.

Vitamin E

At one time, cardiologists routinely recommended vitamin E to their cardiac patients. After the GISSI and HOPE studies, researchers indicated that there was no benefit, and doctors became less likely to recommend vitamin E.[56, 119]

At this time, the frustrating truth is that there are not enough good clinical trials that can state conclusively that we should or should not be taking supplemental vitamin E.

Vitamin E contains many different active ingredients including four tocopherols and four tocotrienols. This is how vitamin E is found in foods. The RDA is 22 IU, taking 200 IU or less vitamin E as a mixture of mixed tocopherols and tocotrienols, rather than d-alpha alone, is ideal.

The best sources are foods rich in vitamin E, such as nuts, seeds, whole-grain foods, and leafy greens with salad dressing that includes oil rather than fat-free dressing. Most vitamin E is found in foods with healthy fats. If your diet is too low in fat, you will have cut out many good sources of vitamin E.

See Table 35.3 on the next two pages for foods that are good sources of vitamin E.

TABLE 35.3   Natural Food Sources Of Vitamin E

FOOD	VITAMIN E IU
OILS, 1 TABLESPOON	
Wheat germ oil	20.2
Hazelnut oil	9.5
Rice bran oil	5.8
Grapeseed	5.8
Sunflower oil	5.7
Almond oil	5.5
Safflower oil	4.8
Flaxseed	3.5
Olive oil	2.6
Canola oil	2.4
Palm oil	2.2
Peanut oil	2.2
Soybean oil	1.3
Mayonnaise soybean, regular	1.0
Palm kernel oil	0.8
Mayonnaise, fat free	0.7
Walnut oil	0.08
NUTS and SEEDS	
Almond butter, 2 Tbsp.	11.3
Sunflower seeds, 2 Tbsp.	9.3
Almonds, 2 Tbsp.	6.9
Almond paste, 2 Tbsp.	5.7
Peanut butter, natural, 2 Tbsp.	3.9
Hazelnuts, 2 Tbsp.	3.2
Pine nuts, 2 Tbsp.	2.4
Brazil nuts, 4 each	1.6
Peanuts, 2 Tbsp.	1.5
Sesame seeds, 2 Tbsp.	0.73
Pecans, 2 Tbsp.	0.71
Soy nuts, 2 Tbsp.	0.41
Pistachios, 2 Tbsp.	0.40
Walnuts, English, 2 Tbsp.	0.27
Cashews, 2 Tbsp.	0.19
Macadamia nuts, 2 Tbsp.	0.12
Flax ground, 2 Tbsp.	0.08
Pumpkin seeds, 2 Tbsp.	0.06
GRAINS*	
Quinoa, 1/4 cup dry	3.0
Wheat germ, 1 Tbsp.	1.5
Rice brown, 1/4 cup dry	0.8
Barley, 1/4 cup dry	0.4
Oats, Steel-cut, 1/4 cup dry	0.4
Oats, rolled, 1/4 cup dry	0.2
Rice, white, 1/4 cup dry	0.02

FOOD	VITAMIN E IU
FLOUR 1/4 cup	
Brown rice flour	1.41
Rye, flour, dark	1.34
Rye, flour. medium	0.60
Whole-wheat flour	0.40
Barley flour	0.31
Wheat flour, all purpose	0.03
GREEN, LEAFY VEGETABLES, COOKED	
Broccoli rabe, 1/2 cup	3.7
Spinach, 1/2 cup	2.8
Dandelion greens, 1/2 cup	2.7
Chard, 1/2 cup	2.5
Beet greens, 1/2 cup	1.9
Turnip greens, 1/2 cup	1.4
Mustard greens, 1/2 cup	1.3
Collards, 1/2 cup	1.0
Kale, 1/2 cup	0.8
Cabbage, 1/2 cup	0.1
OTHER VEGETABLES	
Taro, 1/2 cup raw slices	2.1
Tomato paste, 2 Tbsp.	2.1
Red bell pepper, 1/2 cup raw	1.1
Squash, butternut, 1/2 cup cooked, mashed	0.24
FRUIT	
Avocado, 1/2 medium	2.5
Mango, 1/2 cup slices	1.4
Kiwi, 1 medium	1.3
Blackberries, 1/2 cup	1.2
Raspberries, 1/2 cup	0.8
Cranberries, 1/2 cup raw	0.8
Pomegranate, 1/2 whole	0.7
Apricots, dried, 4 each	0.6
Blueberries, 1/2 cup	0.6
Strawberries, 1/2 cup	0.4
Olives, 4 small	0.3
MEAT AND FISH	
Salmon, coho, wild, broiled, (3 oz.)	1.03
Egg, large	0.64
Pork tenderloin, broiled, (3 oz.)	0.61
Beef tenderloin, 0" fat, broiled, (3 oz.)	0.49
Chicken breast baked, (3 oz.)	0.34
Cheese, cheddar, (1 oz.)	0.12

*Note: whole grains are good sources, refining and bleaching removes vitamin E.
Source: The Food Processor software by ESHA Research, Salem, Ore.

VITAMIN E

NUTRITION NOTE
**How much
Calcium?**
• Age 19-50:
   1,000 mg
• Age 51+:
   1,200 mg

NUTRITION NOTE
**How much
Magnesium?**
• Women:
   310-320 mg
• Men:
   400-420 mg

NUTRITION NOTE
**How much
Iron?**
• None if male or
postmenopausal
female

NUTRITION NOTE
It is possible to
meet all your
nutritional needs
with foods, but
that leaves very
little room in your
diet for alcohol,
sweets, and added
oils and fats.

Everyone has
different needs.

Consult a
registered dietitian
for a nutrient
analysis to meet
your unique needs.

Minerals

Choose chelated minerals that are bound to an amino acid because they are better absorbed. These are citrate, glycinate, arginate, orotate, malate, fumate and succinate rather than elemental or oxide forms. Take with a small amount of fat such as a handful of nuts which also increase absorption.

Calcium

Calcium is bulky so there won't be much in your vitamin/mineral supplement. Instead, take it as a separate supplement. Take it with vitamin D, which helps you absorb calcium. If you consume three servings of dairy or foods that have been fortified with calcium, you will meet your calcium requirements. Choose nonfat dairy to avoid saturated fat. If you need additional calcium, take it in a separate supplement since most multivitamins won't have enough. Calcium citrate is a better form of calcium than calcium carbonate because stomach acids decrease with age and it does not need acid to be absorbed.

Magnesium

Discussed on Page 192. Recommend taking along with calcium.

Iron

Only menstruating women or those who are diagnosed with an iron-deficiency anemia need iron in a supplement. Men and postmenopausal women should take a supplement without iron. Excessive iron may increase the risk for heart disease.

Selenium

Selenium is important to the immune system and the cell walls. It is an antioxidant that limits the oxidation of LDL cholesterol. Only after LDL is oxidized does it become harmful. Selenium is found in the soil. Selenium levels in grains, nuts and vegetables are determined by the amount of selenium in the soil in which it was grown. It is also found in fish. Selenium protects the body from mercury, which it binds and excretes. If you enjoy Brazil nuts, you could meet your selenium needs by eating one daily.

TABLE 35.4 Food Sources Of Selenium	
FOOD	**micrograms (μg)**
Brazil nuts, dried, 1 (5-gram) nut	90
Tilapia, cooked, (3 oz.)	46
Sardine, canned, drained, (3 oz.)	45
Salmon, wild, broiled, (3 oz.)	40
Shrimp, cooked, (3 oz.)	34
Tuna, light, canned in water, drained, 1/4 cup	31
Beef, sirloin cooked, fat trimmed, (3 oz.)	27
Chicken Breast, meat only, roasted, (3 oz.)	24
Barley, whole, cooked, 1/4 cup	18
Egg, whole, 1 large	16
Oat bran, dry, 1/4 cup	11

Source: The Food Processor software by ESHA Research, Salem, Ore.

TABLE 35.5 Calcium in Foods milligrams per serving size listed

Food	mg	Food	mg	Food	mg
Calcium-fortified orange juice, 8 oz.	300	Thyme, 1 Tbsp. dry	80	Blue corn tortilla chips, 1 oz.	20
Calcium-fortified soy or rice milk, 8 oz.	300	Tofu, *White Wave*, firm, 3.5 oz.	80	Cabbage, napa or green, 1/2 cup cooked	20
Milk, 8 oz.	300	Almonds, 1 oz.	70	Celery stalk, 11"	20
Yogurt, plain, 6 oz.	300	*Amy* light in sodium chili, 1 cup	60	Collard greens, 1/2 cup cooked	20
Yogurt, flavored, 8 oz.	300	Basil, 1 Tbsp. dry	60	Garbanzo beans, 1/2 cup cooked	20
Alpine Lace Swiss, reduced-fat, 1 oz.	280	Chili beans, 1/2 cup	60	Green beans, 1/2 cup cooked	20
Almond cheese, 1 oz.	250	Dill weed, 1 Tbsp. dry	60	Kidney beans, 1/2 cup cooked	20
Cabot 50% light cheese, 1 oz.	200	Dried figs, 1/4 cup	60	Kiwi, 1	20
Calcium-fortified apple juice, 8 oz.	200	Great northern beans, 1/2 cup cooked	60	Lentils, 1/2 cup cooked	20
Cheese, regular or reduced-fat, 1 oz.	200	Mustard greens, 1/2 cup cooked	60	Mint, 1 Tbsp. dry	20
Cream cheese, fat free, 1 oz.	200	Orange, 1 medium	60	*Mori Nu* tofu, silken, 3 oz.	20
Ricotta cheese, 1/4 cup	150	Rhubarb, diced raw, 1/2 cup	60	Onion, 1 medium	20
Smart Beat cheese, fat-free, 2/3 oz.	150	Sardines, no bones, 1 oz.	60	Parsley, dry, 1 Tbsp.	20
Poppy seeds, 1 Tbsp.	121	Swiss chard, 1/2 cup cooked	60	Pea pods, 1/2 cup fresh	20
Molasses, dark, 1 Tbsp.	100	Tarragon, 1 Tbsp. dry	60	Peanut butter, 2 Tbsp.	20
Almond butter, 2 Tbsp.	100	Tempeh, 3 oz.	60	Quinoa, 1/4 cup dry	20
Cottage cheese, nonfat, 1/2 cup	100	Meatless soy burger, 1	60	Romaine or green/red leafy, 1-1/2 cups	20
Salmon, canned with bones, 1.5 ounces	100	Brazil nuts, 1 oz.	50	Butternut squash, 1/2 cup cooked, mashed	20
Sardine, with bones, 1 oz.	100	Flaxseed, ground, 2 Tbsp.	42	Turmeric, ground, 1 Tbsp.	20
Sweet green soybeans, edamame, 1/2 cup	100	Broccoli, 1/2 cup cooked	40	*Veggie Slice* soy cheese, 1 slice	20
Turnip greens, 1/2 cup cooked	100	Chili powder, 1 Tbsp.	40	Wild blueberries, 1/2 cup	20
Sesame seeds, unhulled, 1 Tbsp.	87	Corn tortilla, 2 (6-inch)	40	Hummus, 2 Tbsp.	15
Amaranth grain, 1/4 cup dry	80	Cumin, ground, 1 Tbsp.	40	Salmon, no bones 1.5 ounce	12
Beet greens, 1/2 cup cooked	80	Kale, 1/2 cup cooked	40	Couscous, whole-wheat, 1/2 cup cooked	10
Cinnamon, 1 Tbsp.	80	Navy beans, 1/2 cup cooked	40	Portabello, raw, 3 oz.	10
Oregano, 1 Tbsp. dry	80	Sage dry, 1 Tbsp.	40	Barley, pearled, 1/4 cup cooked	8
Sour cream, fat-free, 2 Tbsp.	80	Squash, acorn, 1/2 cup cooked, mashed	40	Wheat germ, 2 Tbsp.	5
Soy flour, 1/2 cup	80	Tomatoes, stewed, 1/2 cup	40	Nori seaweed, 2 sheets	4
Soybeans, 1/2 cup cooked	80	*Veggie Ground Round*, meatless, 1/3 cup	40	Millet, 1/4 cup dry	4
Teff grain, 1/4 cup dry	80	Soy nuts, 1 oz.	37	Millet, 1/2 cup cooked	3
Textured vegetable protein, 1/4 cup dry	80	Maple syrup, 2 Tbsp.	30		
		Pistachios, 1 oz.	30		
		Walnuts, 1 oz.	28		
		Tahini (unhulled), 2 Tbsp.	20		
		Amy light in sodium split pea soup, 1 cup	20		
		Apricot, dried, 1/4 cup	20		
		Barley, 1/4 cup dry	20		
		Black beans, 1/2 cup cooked	20		
		Blackberries, 1/2 cup	20		

Source: Nutritional information calculated using The Food Processor software by ESHA Research, Salem, Ore.

Vitamin/Mineral Quiz

1. Americans get enough vitamin E, magnesium, vitamin D and beta-carotene.
   ❏ T   ❏ F

2. Americans get too much:
   a) salt
   b) sugar
   c) saturated fat
   d) trans fat
   e) calories
   f) all of above

3. Choosing a multivitamin that includes herbals such as lutein is a good way to get the added benefits.
   ❏ T   ❏ F

4. Vitamin A should be greater than 100 percent of the daily value since we need more.
   ❏ T   ❏ F

5. High intakes of vitamin A are good for bone health.
   ❏ T   ❏ F

6. Adults over age 50 need additional B_{12}.
   ❏ T   ❏ F

7. Most adults need more vitamin D than previously thought. About 1,000 IU is recommended for most.
   ❏ T   ❏ F

8. We have good evidence that taking vitamin E is beneficial for heart health.
   ❏ T   ❏ F

9. Calcium citrate is a poorly absorbed form of calcium.
   ❏ T   ❏ F

10. Men and postmenopausal women should choose a multivitamin/mineral that includes iron.
    ❏ T   ❏ F

ANSWERS
On Page 281.

Smart 4 Your Heart

TABLE 35.6 VITAMINS

NUTRIENT	Function	Upper Level (UL) for adults (Effects if too much)	RDA or AI (For adults)	Food Source
Vitamin A (retinol, retinyl palmitate, acetate or other forms retinol)	Healthy eyes, fight off virus and infections, strong bones, build new cells	UL 3,000 mcg or 10,000 IU from retinol can cause irreversible liver damage and birth defects. More than 4,333 IU increases the risk of hip fracture	Women: 700 mcg or 2,310 IU Men: 900 mcg or 3,000 IU (3.44 mcg retinyl acetate = 1 IU)	Animal foods. (Liver, cod liver oils, butter, eggs, milk, ice cream, cheese) Vitamin A added to foods such as cereals, energy bars, protein bars and others
Beta-Carotene	Body can make vitamin A only as needed from beta-carotene. Acts as an antioxidant.	Smokers who took 33,000-55,000 IU have a higher risk of lung cancer. High levels not advised for those on statin drugs or niacin, as may lower HDL.	IOM 3-6mg equivalent to 833-1667 IU Limit to 15,000 IU or less	Plant foods. Dark green, leafy vegetables or yellow/orange vegetables and fruits. (apricot, cantaloupe, carrot, beet greens, collards, kale, sweet potato, spinach, mango, broccoli)

All of the eight B vitamins are important to help release energy from the food you eat and to help in cell growth and division. The average diet usually provides enough. Alcohol, tobacco and digestive problems can decease how much you absorb. Most vitamin supplements have plenty of B vitamins added. Your body makes as much choline, inositol and PABA as it needs, so they are not technically B vitamins.

NUTRIENT	Function	Upper Level (UL) for adults (Effects if too much)	RDA or AI (For adults)	Food Source
B₁ Thiamin	Healthy nerve cell growth. Important for healthy nervous system.	None determined	Women: 1.1 mg Men: 1.2 mg	Wheat germ, brown rice, whole grains, legumes, soybeans, pine nuts, peanuts, peanut butter, sunflower seeds, pork, brewer's yeast, fish
B₂ Riboflavin	Healthy eyes and skin	None determined. Children and elderly may need supplement.	Women: 1.1 mg Men: 1.3 mg	Almonds, wheat germ, wild rice, mushrooms, soy flour, wheat bran, dairy, whole grains, green vegetables, meat, beans/legumes
B₃ Niacin (nicotinamide) This form does not work to lower cholesterol	Makes hormones, Needed in many different body processes.	**UL 35 mg synthetic** from fortified food & supplements. No limit when in foods naturally. Nicotinic acid lowers triglycerides in high doses.	Women: 14 mg Men: 16 mg	Whole grains; brown rice; peanuts; mushrooms; potatoes; protein foods such as milk, legumes, avocado, eggs, fish, chicken, meat
B₅ Panothenic Acid	Makes hormones. Helps cells produce energy.	**None**	5 mg safe and adequate for adults	Found in large number of foods, including milk, fish and poultry. Whole grains, brewer's yeast
B₆ Pyridoxine	Maintains immune and nervous system. Helps produce serotonin, insulin.	**UL 100 mg** Reversible nerve damage (tingling, numbness) Doses of 30 mg used in PMS, asthma	Women (age 19-50): 1.3 mg Women (age 50+): 1.5 mg Men 1.7 mg	Meats, whole grains, legumes (soybeans and peanuts), dried fruit, avocado, banana, seeds, nuts, brussel sprouts, walnuts

TABLE 35.6 VITAMINS (continued)

NUTRIENT	Function	Upper Level (UL) for adults (Effects if too much)	RDA or AI (For adults)	Food Source
Biotin (B$_7$ or Vitamin H)	Fat and amino acid utilization	None – made in intestine by gut bacteria when needed	30 mcg	Oatmeal, salmon, banana, cheese, eggs, soybeans, brewer's yeast, peanuts, whole wheat. No side effects reported from supplements.
Folic acid (folate, folacin or B$_9$)	Reduces risk of certain birth defects and may lower homocysteine levels	UL1,000 mcg applies only to synthetic or "added to," fortified foods. Masks B$_{12}$ deficiency if you get too much.	400 mcg, (0.4 mg)	Dark green, leafy vegetables; fortified cereals; lentils; oatmeal; pinto beans; spinach; navy beans; orange juice; asparagus; beets; sunflower seeds; soybeans
B$_{12}$ (cyanocobalamin)	As we get older, this is hard to absorb from food. Deficiency can cause memory loss and irreversible nerve damage.	None	2.4 mcg People over age 50 often need a supplement or fortified foods	Exclusively in animal foods, including clams, milk, yogurt, eggs, fish, chicken and meat. It's not in plants, but can be added to plant foods. Fortified foods: nutritional yeast, some cold cereals.
Vitamin C (ascorbic acid)	Antioxidant. Makes collagen for blood vessel walls, gums and bones. Important in healing wounds and fighting infections	UL 2,000 mg Loose stools and diarrhea if you take too much.	Women: 75 mg Men: 90 mg Smokers: add 35 mg	Citrus fruits, kale, collards, broccoli, brussel sprouts, cauliflower, vine-ripened tomatoes, red & green bell peppers, strawberries, cantaloupe, kiwi, mangoes, Swiss chard. Canned fruits have much less. See Table 35.1, Page 215.
Vitamin D Cholecalciferol D$_3$	Helps you absorb calcium for strong bones and teeth. Body can make from exposure to sun	UL current level probably too low Expect to increase to 10,000 IU	Current levels probably too low Expect recommendations to increase to 1-2,000 IU or more	Cold water, fatty fish and cod liver oil. Vegetables are low; best sources are dark green, leafy vegetables and shitake mushrooms. Fortified foods like cereal, milk, soy milk. See Table 35.2, Page 216.
Vitamin E (tocopherol) 4 tocopherols + 4 tocotrienols	Antioxidant, improves immune system	UL 1,000 mg or 1,100 IU synthetic 1,500 IU natural	15 mg or 22 IU natural, 33 IU synthetic if d – natural if dl – synthetic	Nuts and seeds; whole grains; wheat germ; egg yolk; green, leafy vegetables; asparagus; avocado; berries. See Table 35.3, Page 218.
Vitamin K (phylloquone)	Makes proteins for blood clotting. Improves bone health.	None Caution with *Coumadin*	Women: 90 mcg Men: 120 mcg	Green, leafy vegetables; brussels sprouts. See Table 34.1, Page 207.

TABLE 35.7   MINERALS

NUTRIENT	Function	Upper Level (UL) for adults (Effects if too much)	RDA or AI (For adults)	Food Source
Boron	Bone health, major role in calcium and magnesium use	UL 20 mg	None. 1.5-3 mg safe.	Fruits and vegetables, nuts, bean/legumes. Level depends on soil content of boron.
Calcium	Strong bones and teeth. Because it's bulky, most multis cannot fit enough into a pill	UL 2,500 mg High blood calcium may cause kidney damage	Age: 19-50 1,000 mg Age 51+: 1,200 mg	Many fortified foods, dairy and fortified soy milk, collards, kale, broccoli, bok choy, almonds, Brazil nuts, hazelnuts, amaranth. See Table 35.5, Page 221.
Chromium	Regulate blood sugar by working with insulin	None	Age 51+ Women: 20 mcg Men: 30 mcg	Whole-grain cereals, seafood, potatoes, mushrooms, prunes, nuts, asparagus, foods cooked in stainless-steel cookware
Copper	Antioxidant enzymes. Copper is needed to absorb iron and for healthy blood vessels.	UL 10 mg (10,000 mcg) Cupric oxide not well absorbed. Nausea, liver damage	0.9 mg (900 mcg) Works with iron	Legumes, lima beans, seafood, clams, whole grains, sunflower seeds, kiwi. Food cooked in copper pots. Too much zinc causes copper deficiency.
Iodine	Thyroid hormones; deficiency may cause mental retardation, goiter, dwarfism	UL 1,100 mcg	150 mcg	Iodized salt, some seafood. If following a low-sodium diet, take your multi with iodine. If consuming soy foods, make sure you have adequate iodine in your diet.
Iron	Iron deficiency is the leading cause of anemia. In some, iron overload may cause hemochomatosis.	UL 45 mg GI distress, constipation 0-10 mg in multi for men and postmenopausal women	Women 19-50: 18 mg (32 mg if vegetarian) 50+ Women and Men: 8 mg (20 mg if vegetarian)	Red meat, dark poultry, whole grains, raisins, legumes, wheat germ, blackstrap molasses, pumpkin. Vegetarians need to have about 1.8 times more iron. Vitamin C helps absorption, tannin in tea decreases iron absorption. Cook in uncoated, cast-iron pots to increase iron available in foods.
Magnesium	Helps to utilize calcium. Important for heart health, relaxes muscles, helps control blood sugar and blood pressure.	UL 350 mg synthetic Nausea, vomiting, low blood pressure, diarrhea	Women: 310-320 mg Men: 400-420 mg	Whole, not processed grains; figs; dark; leafy green vegetables; nuts and seeds; legumes; dark chocolate; banana. See Table 32.3, Page 193.
Manganese	Bone formation and protein metabolism	UL 11 mg Iron absorption lowered, neurological side effects	Women:1.8 mg Men: 2.3 mg	Nuts, legumes, tea, raisins, blueberries, spinach and whole grains

TABLE 35.7 MINERALS (continued)

NUTRIENT	Function	Upper Level (UL) for adults (Effects if too much)	RDA or AI (For adults)	Food Source
Molybdenum	Enhance enzymes, growth and development	**UL 2,000 mcg** Gout-like symptoms	45 mcg	Legumes, grain products and nuts, dependent upon amounts in soil where food is grown.
Potassium	Fluid balance, heart function. Regulate blood pressure.		4,700 mg	Tomatoes, spinach, bananas, oranges, avocado, legumes, broccoli, sweet potato, cantaloupe. See Table 32.2, Page 193.
Selenium	Antioxidant, may prevent cancers and heart damage.	**UL 400 mcg** Some suggest 200 mcg organic form. Excess nail or hair loss/ brittleness.	55 mcg	Seafood, whole grains, Brazil nuts. See Table 35.4, Page 220. *SelenoExcel* brand used in studies
Zinc	Immune system. Brain function, wound healing and sperm production. Vegetarians, alcohol drinkers and older individuals may need more.	**UL 40 mg** **Too much can lower copper levels, lower HDL.** **High dose can suppress immune response.**	Women: 8 mg Men: 11 mg	Oysters; wheat germ; yogurt; nuts; tempeh; barley; lentils; oatmeal; legumes; yeast leavened, whole-wheat products; lean red meats; egg; seafood; blackberries; kiwi To fight a cold, use zinc lozenges not pills you swallow.

Mineral supplements in the form of succinates, gluconates, citrates, picolinates and fumarates may be more soluble and easily absorbed by the body than inorganic salts such as sulfates.

Source: *Dietary Reference Intakes: Recommended Intakes for Individuals, Vitamins. Food and Nutrition Board, The Institute of Medicine National Academies.*

UL highest level of intake that poses no risk based on what we currently know. Limit for foods plus supplements unless it says "synthetic" (magnesium, niacin and folic acid), which means the amounts from fortified foods and supplements but not including what is found in your food naturally. (UL for other minerals that were set but are not listed in above chart: Nickel 1 mg and Vanadium 1.8 mg). Supplements are not required to provide UL information on labels.

RDAs (Recommended Dietary Allowances) are designed so that there is a 97-98% probability that you will exceed the minimum needed. It varies by age and gender. It is too much information to include on a label, so the FDA sets daily values to use on labels based on someone eating 2,000 calories daily.

DV or Daily Value: The FDA set the Daily Values you find on labels in 1968 based on the RDAs. Several RDAs have been changed by the Institute of Medicine of the National Academies. However, the FDA has not changed the label guidelines to reflect the changes.

Multivitamin/Mineral Smart 4 Your Heart

36

Other Supplements

D ietary supplements for heart health that have been approved to carry an FDA health claim are:

❖ Omega-3 fish oil supplements
❖ Soluble fiber

Both are covered in separate chapters in this book.

Plant (Phyto) Sterols

Plants such as legumes, soybeans, rice, nuts and seeds, naturally contain small amounts of noncholesterol plant sterols. The highest concentration of phytosterols occurs in vegetable oils. Plants do not contain cholesterol. Cholesterol is found only in animal foods. Plants contain close cousins called phytosterols. Though similar, they are not exactly the same, which makes them act very differently from cholesterol in the body. Phytosterols may lower blood cholesterol. They may also protect against cancer and have beneficial effects on the prostate. Phytosterols compete with cholesterol for absorption, which reduces the amount of cholesterol that may be absorbed. Think of it as a game of musical chairs. If the phytosterols get there first, the cholesterol doesn't have a chair, and without a place, it is eliminated from your body. Phytosterols occur in plants mostly as sterols and less often as stanols, their saturated counterpart.

For cholesterol-lowering benefits, the National Cholesterol Education Program, Adult Treatment III, recommends 2,000 milligrams (2 grams) a day. Consuming more than 2 to 3 grams offers no additional lowering of cholesterol.

A typical American diet provides 150 to 350 milligrams of plant sterols and 20 to 50 mg of plant stanols per day. Vegetarians eat more plants, but still take in only about 600 to 800 milligrams of phytosterols daily.

AUTHOR NOTE

The Adult Treatment Panel III of the National Cholesterol Education Program issues evidence-based guidelines on how to manage cholesterol.

Do They Work?

Phytosterols lower total cholesterol by about 6 to 10 percent and decreased LDL cholesterol by 6 to 20 percent.[108] They do not have any effect on the good HDL cholesterol or triglycerides. They have not been shown to affect morbidity or mortality.

Evidence that phytosterols lower LDL was strong enough that the FDA approved a health claim. The amounts needed to carry a health claim are based on whether they are esterified or nonesterified forms.

Numerous phytosterol products are available. Adding phytosterols to a food does not make it a healthy choice. If a food is highly refined or highly sweetened, contains high fructose corn syrup, or has unhealthy fats such as partially hydrogenated fat, then it remains a poor choice – even with the added phytosterols.

Plant sterols, but not stanols, decrease in their LDL cholesterol-lowering effect over time. Plant sterols decrease production of bile acids and this, over time, makes them less effective. After several months, the initial reduction is about half of the initial 15 percent reduction. Stanols, which do not have this levelling off effect, would be preferred for long-term management of cholesterol lowering.

Are They Safe? If They Are Absorbed, Can They Cause Harm?

Plant stanols' absorption is so low that it is considered insignificant. However, plant sterol absorption is about 10 times more efficiently absorbed. There are a few individuals who have a rare, inherited metabolic disorder called phytosterolemia, in which plant sterols but not stanols are absorbed at very high rates. These individuals develop multiple xanthomas or noncancerous deposits of fat that develop beneath the skin. They develop early, premature heart disease.[109, 110]

The question is do even the small amounts of sterols absorbed, which are then found in the blood and plaque of the arteries, increase the risk of heart disease? Does accumulating sterols instead of cholesterol have any effect on health? These are important questions investigators have raised to which we don't know the answers. In mice plant sterols increased plaque. If sterols accumulate in the artery walls, there may be increased potential that they promote plaque development. Sterols, unlike stanols, can also become oxidized, which may increase the possibility of contributing to atherosclerosis. At this time, there is no clear answer if this is necessarily bad.

Stanol Products

In the United States, stanols are currently available as *Benecol* spreads and chews. The margarine spreads require 2 tablespoons daily and contain partially hydrogenated oils. The chews require consuming four a day for a total of 12 grams of sugars. *Benecol* drinks are available in Europe and other countries but not in the United States at this time.

BOTTOM LINE

Stanols appear to be safe for nearly all individuals, including adults and children, who need to lower cholesterol. Stanols are saturated sterols that are not absorbed. Stanols can be used safely to reduce cholesterol absorption.

It is not recommended that sterol ester products be used until more is known. Some individuals may overabsorb sterols. Individuals with a strong family history of heart disease, as well as those taking cholesterol-lowering statin drugs and postmenopausal women, should be cautious about the use of products with added sterols, but not stanols, for cholesterol lowering.

Supplements That Are Not FDA Approved But Appear To Have Benefit

❖ Cinnamon
❖ Garlic
❖ Coenzyme Q10

Cinnamon

Adding 1 gram of cinnamon to your diet (slightly less than one-half teaspoon of ground cinnamon) seems to help lower blood sugars in some individuals. In people with Type 2 diabetes, 1 to 6 grams of cassia cinnamon lowered triglycerides by 23 to 30 percent and lowered the LDL cholesterol by 10 to 24 percent.[111] One study compared cassia cinnamon from several sources, Indonesia, China and Vietnam, and found them to be equal in effect. Adding cinnamon to your cereal or to a glass of milk or hot cocoa as a spice doesn't add calories and may help you reduce sweeteners since it adds a slight taste of sweetness. Getting your cinnamon from pastries or presweetened packaged cereals is not recommended. The effects of eating cinnamon continued three weeks after consumption had stopped, which indicates that you may not have to take it daily to get the benefit. It should also be noted that cassia cinnamon contains coumarin which could be toxic to the liver, however ceylon cinnamon has much smaller amounts of coumarin.

There are water-soluble extracts of cinnamon available in supplement form with the potential toxins removed if you don't enjoy the taste of cinnamon or prefer a pill form.

NUTRITION NOTE

Types of cinnamon
• Ceylon (true)
• Cassia

Garlic

NUTRITION NOTE

Chop your garlic, allow it to stand for 10 minutes, then eat it within 20 minutes after chopping for the most health benefits.

Some short-term trials lasting less than six months of garlic showed a small benefit, but other trials that were longer than six months showed no significant reductions in cholesterol because the lowering that happened in the beginning disappeared after it was used for a longer period. The conclusion for most people is that garlic does little for cholesterol reduction.[112] However, most garlic supplement companies have chosen to ignore the more recent studies and continue to promote their products based on those early studies. In Germany, where garlic's cholesterol benefits originated, the government no longer allows companies to claim that garlic may lower cholesterol.

Some feel that garlic studies have resulted in conflicting outcomes because there are so many different preparations of garlic and standardization is lacking. If you try garlic to see if you get any benefit, at best you might see a 5 percent decrease, too little to treat high cholesterol levels, but perhaps useful for someone who cannot tolerate drugs or needs only a small reduction.

If you enjoy garlic, include it in your diet as often as you wish since it is the most reliable way to obtain the health benefits. Be sure to chop your garlic and allow it to stand 10 minutes. However, eat it within 20 minutes after chopping for the most health benefits. When garlic is chopped or crushed, the enzyme allinase is activated and acts on the allin in garlic to produce allicin, which is thought to be the beneficial compound. Garlic that is cooked loses most if not all of the active ingredients as heat inactivates them.

A clove of fresh garlic that weighs 4 grams will yield 4,000 to 12,000 mcg of allicin. The studies where benefit was seen suggest a daily amount of 3,600 to 5,400 mcg of allicin per day. Eat a clove of fresh garlic daily to get this amount. Monitor lipids for three months to see if eating raw, chopped garlic is effective.

> ### BOTTOM LINE
> **Studies of garlic as a supplement have found that it does not consistently lower cholesterol. If you enjoy garlic, eat it daily as a food. Mince, let stand, then mix with extra-virgin olive oil and use on salad or to season vegetables after they are cooked.**

Coenzyme Q10

NUTRITION NOTE

How much CoQ10?
100-300 mg (choose one that lists oil in the ingredients)

The chemical name for coenzyme Q10 is "ubiquinone." It is also referred to as coenzyme Q10 or CoQ10. Your body makes this antioxidant. CoQ10 is found in all cells, including the heart muscle cells and is important for the production of energy.

Statin drugs lower cholesterol by inhibiting the production of cholesterol in the liver. This same part of the liver that is now blocked by statins also produces CoQ10, so it is also inhibited. Other drugs such as beta-blockers, fibrates and diuretics may also deplete CoQ10. Muscle-related aches and weakness while taking a statin could be the result of this decrease in CoQ10. The longer you take statins and the higher the dose, the more likely you may notice this. Many patients will stop taking their drugs because they feel so poorly. If you take statins, taking a supplement of CoQ10 (which is safe), may help with the symptoms of muscle aches for some, although not all find it beneficial.

If you are taking a statin and experience muscle aches, discuss it with your doctor, who will check to be sure it is not a serious side effect such as the extremely rare condition called rhabdomyolysis. In clinical trials, this serious muscle damage from statins occurred in only 1 to 2 percent of patients.

Studies on heart failure provide the strongest evidence of benefit for taking CoQ10. Those taking CoQ10 significantly improved heart muscle function while producing no adverse effects or drug interactions.[113, 114]

Can You Get It In Food?

Yes, but not enough. We probably can obtain up to 20 or 30 milligrams from foods. Many foods have not been analyzed for CoQ10 content. The best animal sources are fresh sardines and mackerel, the heart and liver of animals, and eggs. Vegetable sources include spinach, broccoli, peanuts and the germ portion of a whole grain.

How Much CoQ10?

The type and amount taken may determine whether it will work or not. You may want to try 100 milligrams a day of oil-based CoQ10 capsules. Within a week, if it is going to help, you will have noticed a difference, although it may take a month for the full effect. If you don't see relief, increase to a higher amount in two equally divided doses.

If you are on the drug *Coumadin* (warfarin), a blood thinner, your physician will want to check INR to see if there is any interaction. If you have diabetes, your physician may need to decrease your insulin requirements.

NUTRITION NOTE

CoQ10: oil-based capsule is better absorbed.

What Does "Maintain Normal Cholesterol Levels" Mean?

Often claims are misleading and confusing. All supplements are regulated as foods not drugs. A structure and function claim can be made with no research necessary before being sold. A disclaimer must be included that the supplement is not intended to treat, cure or prevent disease.

Be cautious where you get your advice regarding supplements. If the source that is providing it is also selling the item, the advice may be biased. Do your homework and get as much information as you can before making a decision. You should know the amount needed daily, and which compounds are necessary to get the intended benefit that may have been seen in studies.

Useful Website For Information

A Web site to help you find more information on supplements is www.consumerlab.com. The organization obtains funding by charging users an annual subscription fee, allowing them to provide unbiased analysis of a variety of brands as to whether they contain the amounts stated on their packaging. Some free information is also available on the site.

Supplements That Are Not Recommended

❖ Guggulipid
❖ Policosanol
❖ Red yeast rice extract sold in the U.S. cannot legally contain the active ingredient (lovastatin) and varies tremendously.
❖ No-flush niacin (Chapter 37, Page 237)

Guggulipid, Guggul, Guggulsterone

This is extracted from a tree and was shown to lower cholesterol in studies done in India. However, a randomized, controlled trial conducted in Britain resulted in increased LDL in the group taking guggulipids compared to the placebo group who did not take it. Additionally, one in 10 individuals developed a rash, suggesting an allergic reaction. The authors concluded that there was no benefit. It may also interfere with the effectiveness of statins, therefore, it is not recommended when taking a statin drug.[120]

Policosanol

The majority of data on policosanol's effectiveness has been from questionable studies done by the same researchers in Cuba. Those results have not been seen in other studies.

A German study that was well-designed, did not receive any drug company funding, and used the policosanol derived from sugar cane identical to what had been used in the Cuban studies, finally confirmed what was suspected by other researchers.[121] It doesn't work! The results showed no effect on total cholesterol, no LDL reduction, and no change in HDL or triglycerides.

> **BOTTOM LINE**
> While policosanol is not harmful,
> it is clear that there are no benefits either.

Red Yeast Rice Extract

Early studies showed over-the-counter red yeast was effective at lowering cholesterol because it naturally contained lovastatin. The red yeast rice that is currently available in the United States can no longer legally contain lovastatin since the FDA considers any supplement containing lovastatin an unapproved drug, following a lawsuit brought about by the original patent holder. The FDA has taken action against some red yeast rice products and warns consumers not to purchase them if it determines they contain the active ingredient.

Original forms of red yeast rice contained monacolin K, which is a natural form of lovastatin, the prescription cholesterol-lowering statin drug. The previous version of the brand *Cholestin*, which had been the most effective supplement from Chinese red yeast rice, has been reformulated and no longer has monacolin K or lovastatin. The original formula of *Cholestin* is reported to be available in some countries other than the U.S.

Red yeast rice is the result of fermentation of rice with various yeast strains. While some supplements state that they contain monacolins, they can no longer report levels, so there is no way to know what you are getting or how much to take. A study of nine different red yeast supplements available over-the-counter found that only one actually contained the standard quantity of monacolins to effectively lower cholesterol. Seven of the nine preparations contained citrinin, an unwanted byproduct of fermentation that is a suspected liver and kidney toxin.[122] Consumer labs has also evaluated red yeast products with the results available on their website at www.consumerlab.com.

Because there is no way to know for sure what is in a red yeast supplement bottle sold in the United States, results are not predictable. The only way to know if the product you buy is working is to monitor your cholesterol levels. Once you find a brand that works, they may reformulate it or be forced to remove it, if determined to violate FDA policy.

Red yeast rice that contains adequate levels to effectively lower cholesterol requires checking your liver enzymes, since side effects may develop just as they do when taking statin drugs.

NUTRITION NOTE

Red yeast rice supplements may contain the potential toxin citrinin.

BOTTOM LINE

The use of supplements and the results that you get will depend upon how a supplement was formulated and how it was manufactured. Check to see if enough of the active ingredient was used, as well as the quality of the ingredients. Supplements are not standardized and studies done on an ingredient in a supplement will not guarantee the same results. Doses that produced results in clinical trials may not be the same as what is recommended on the bottles.

Try one supplement at a time. Determine if it is effective before adding another. Measure your lipids before starting and after a month or two of taking the supplement to determine if it is beneficial. Remember, if you are also losing weight and changing the way you eat, those changes may be what gave you results, rather than a supplement. That is why it is recommended that you fix diet and lifestyle first, and then, if necessary, add a supplement or a drug for additional lowering.

Don't attempt to use a supplement to avoid seeing your doctor or to treat serious conditions, such as heart failure, and never stop taking your prescribed medications unless you have received approval to do so from your physician.

Supplements Quiz

1. Supplements that state "may reduce risk for heart disease" must have FDA approval.
   ❏ T ❏ F

2. Which phytosterols are absorbed?
   a) stanols
   b) sterols

3. Cinnamon may lower blood sugar levels.
   ❏ T ❏ F

4. Garlic is best used as a food rather than as a pill.
   ❏ T ❏ F

5. CoQ10 in an oil base is useful for some individuals who experience mild muscle aches while taking a statin.
   ❏ T ❏ F

6. No-flush niacin is recommended since it effectively raises HDL.
   ❏ T ❏ F

7. Guggulipid is an effective supplement discovered in India to lower cholesterol.
   ❏ T ❏ F

8. Policosanol, when obtained from sugar cane, is effective for naturally lowering cholesterol.
   ❏ T ❏ F

9. Red yeast rice sold in the United States contains a natural form of lovastatin that is less toxic to the liver than prescription statins so testing liver enzymes is not necessary.
   ❏ T ❏ F

ANSWERS
On Page 281.

37

Niacin

Niacin is one of the oldest effective agents used to lower cholesterol. It was used before statin drugs were available. It is no longer widely used even though it is relatively low in cost and is the best HDL cholesterol-raising drug currently available. The biggest challenge are the side effects that occur when niacin therapy is started. Niacin dilates blood vessels, creating a sensation of warmth often called a "niacin flush," and in some cases an itchy sensation. For niacin to be helpful, you need a doctor experienced in using it effectively to help you develop a tolerance to the effects of flushing. Flushing will, in most cases, go away within a couple of weeks of starting niacin. You need directions on how to start niacin at a low dose to develop a tolerance and slowly increase dosage over time.

Niacin is vitamin B_3, also called "nicotinic acid." Taken in high doses niacin acts like a drug providing health benefits not seen when taken in the recommended doses for a vitamin. Niacin is especially good for those who have low HDL and high triglycerides. Niacin is also effective to lower elevated Lp(a) and small dense LDL particles. Niacin is more effective than statins for raising HDL. Statins increase HDL 5 to 10 percent, but niacin will raise HDL from 15 to 35 percent, depending upon the dose.

Niacin is available as a prescription (*Niaspan*) as an extended or "intermediate-release" discussed in more detail later in this chapter. Niacin is also available over-the-counter without a prescription, as:

1. *Immediate-release* niacin or "crystalline," which causes the most flushing, is inexpensive but must be taken several times a day.
2. *Slow-release* niacin exposes the liver to small amounts of niacin for an extended time, so it is toxic to the liver and not recommended.
3. *Controlled-release*. The brand *Slo-Niacin* (Upsher Smith Pharmaceuticals), sold over-the-counter as was used in the HDL-Atherosclerosis Treatment Study (HATS) and has published data that proved it works and is safe with low risk to the liver.[123]
4. *"No-flush"* niacin, which does not work in humans like it worked in animal studies.

NUTRITION NOTE

Niacin lowers:
  Lp(a)
  Triglycerides
  LDL-P

Raises:
  HDL

Flushing

If you experience the side effect of flushing, you might fear that something very bad is happening. Actually, the opposite is true. The flushing in most cases is unpleasant but not harmful, and flushing means that the niacin is working. Individuals' responses vary from very little to intense. It may help you tolerate the side effects if you understand for many people, flushing shortens as they adjust to the niacin. If you continue to take niacin, don't miss a dose. The flushing diminishes after several weeks, and some patients report that it goes away. Flushing can temporarily occur again whenever you increase the dose. Flushing lasts 20 minutes on average for most, but can vary from 10 to 60 minutes.

Niaspan Prescription Niacin

Niacin is available in prescription form as *Niaspan*, an extended-release, FDA-approved prescription drug that is regulated and standardized like any other drug. It is effective and has less flushing than the over-the-counter, immediate-release types. It also has a low risk of causing damage to the liver. In clinical trials, it raised HDL more than the over-the-counter, sustained release types.[135]

If taking the prescription *Niaspan*, your doctor will determine the dose based on your response. Remember, you should be under a doctor's supervision if taking niacin at doses greater than 1,000 milligrams.

If you cannot afford the cost or your insurance won't cover it, the following information on over-the-counter niacin may be helpful.

Slo-Niacin, Over-The-Counter

Discuss this with your doctor who will want to monitor your liver function. If you have history of gout, gastritis, peptic ulcer or liver disease, niacin should be used only with caution and your doctor's approval. You can purchase it over-the-counter in pharmacies or via the Internet.

Take once a day at the evening meal. Starting dose is 250 milligrams once a day for 4 weeks. It is then increased to 500 milligrams. Increase by 500 mg every 4 weeks until the desired effect on cholesterol is reached. If taking more than 1,000 mg, have your liver blood tests done to monitor levels.

SLO-NIACIN DAILY DOSE	
Week	Total Per Day
1-4	250 mg
5-8	500 mg
9-12	1,000 mg

Immediate-Release "Crystalline" Niacin, Over-The-Counter

Immediate-release niacin has a high rate of flushing as it is immediately absorbed and must be taken three times a day. This means you may get flushing three times a day instead of once until tolerance is built up. The ingredients will state *nicotinic acid*.

Start with 250 milligrams at dinner for the first week. If flushing is more than you can tolerate, you may want to find 100 milligrams tablets to start with. Follow the schedule below for immediate-release crystalline niacin. Note that crystalline niacin requires two and three times a day doses.

IMMEDIATE-RELEASE NICOTINIC ACID DAILY DOSE*				
Week	Total per day	Breakfast	Lunch	Dinner
1	250 mg	None	None	250 mg
2	500 mg	250 mg	None	250 mg
3	750 mg	250 mg	250 mg	250 mg
4	1,000 mg	250 mg	250 mg	500 mg
5	1,500 mg	500 mg	250 mg	500 mg

* Consult your physician or health care provider before using and always follow the schedule prescribed. Continue to add in the same way if you need to increase dose.

Two Forms Of Niacin That Won't Improve Cholesterol Levels

No-Flush Niacin

It does not work! It contains inositol hexaniacinate but no nicotinic acid. While there were a few initial small animal studies that showed it did work in rabbits, further larger studies found that it does not work in humans because it takes as long as 48 hours to break down.

Nicotinamide

Another form of niacin is nicotinamide, also known as niacinamide. It does not contain nicotinic acid, so it is ineffective for cholesterol lowering though it has other applications, such as prevention of pellagra, a disease caused by a niacin deficiency. It is the form of niacin often used in multivitamin preparations as a water-soluble B vitamin. Stick to forms of niacin that have published studies on safety and effectiveness for cholesterol lowering.

NUTRITION NOTE

"No-flush" niacin, in the form of inositol hexaniacinate, in spite of the intense marketing, is not effective in improving cholesterol levels in humans.

Tips To Reduce Flushing From Niacin

❖ Flushing and itching are expected side effects that decrease with time. This does not mean you are allergic or cannot take niacin.

❖ Take a full-dose, adult (325 milligrams), regular aspirin, not the enteric-coated kind, about 30 minutes prior to taking niacin, if your doctor approves. Once the flushing has decreased, you may be able to decrease to an 81-milligrams dose aspirin.

❖ If you cannot take aspirin due to an allergy, try ibuprofen 200 to 400 mg. It is not as effective but may give some relief.

❖ Take niacin on a full stomach, at the end of your biggest meal. If taking niacin before bed, you will have less food in your stomach and may have more flushing. Take the aspirin, eat your meal, then take niacin.

❖ If you do take niacin before bed, try one-fourth cup of nuts such as almonds, or low-fat yogurt, which is more helpful than a snack of crackers or fruit.

❖ Drink a full 8-ounce or more glass of very cold water. If you do get a flush, at the first sign, quickly drink one or two more glasses of cold water.

❖ Avoid hot beverages or spicy foods until you have adjusted to taking the niacin.

❖ Limit alcoholic beverages in the evening until you no longer experience flushing.

❖ Avoid vigorous aerobic exercise or a hot bath or shower for several hours before taking niacin until you have adjusted to niacin.

BOTTOM LINE

Take prescription *Niaspan* if possible. Otherwise, take *Slo-Niacin* over-the-counter niacin. Both have clinical data to backup safety and effectiveness.

You may see a continued small rise in HDL, with the same dose of niacin, for up to a year before the full benefit occurs.

If you can tolerate the flushing and are willing to take it three times a day, the immediate-release niacin, also called crystalline niacin or nicotinic acid, is safe to take. It is available as over-the-counter niacin B_3.

No-flush varieties and nicotinamide have no effect for cholesterol management since they have no free nicotinic acid.

Niacin Quiz

1. Which is the most effective in raising your good HDL cholesterol?
   a) fish oil
   b) niacin
   c) statin drugs

2. Which is most effective to lower Lp(a), the independent genetic marker that correlates with increased risk for heart disease?
   a) fish oil
   b) niacin
   c) statin drugs

3. Immediate-release crystalline niacin causes the most flushing and must be taken more than once a day.
   ❑ T   ❑ F

4. *Slo-Niacin* is an over-the-counter brand of niacin that has published data from the HATS trial showing it is safe and effective.
   ❑ T   ❑ F

5. The prescription form of niacin, *Niaspan*, causes less flushing than immediate-release niacin.
   ❑ T   ❑ F

6. If you experience flushing when taking niacin, it means you cannot take it and should stop immediately.
   ❑ T   ❑ F

7. An effective way to minimize flushing is:
   a) taking it with a full meal
   b) drinking a large glass of cold water
   c) not missing a dose
   d) all of the above

ANSWERS
On Page 281.

38

Healthy Dining Out

I t is probably no surprise to hear that Americans are eating out more often. What used to be a special occasion is now a regular part of the week for many of us. Generally speaking, Americans spend nearly half of their food budget on dining out. For those who want to eat healthy, restaurant foods present a challenge as they rarely come with a food label. Only if a restaurant makes a health claim for a menu item are they required to provide nutrition information. Some of the large chain restaurants voluntarily provide information for some items. Fast-food restaurants generally provide the most information; their Web sites offer detailed nutrition information along with ingredients for nearly every item. Because their food is standardized, it is much easier to provide complete information. However, having that information at the time you order would be more helpful, since not everyone will have checked in advance. In restaurants where the menu often changes, and recipes are not standardized but left to the creativity of the chefs, it is much more difficult to provide that information, and most often it is not available. Learning a few strategies will help you keep your healthy eating habits even when dining out.

In most American restaurants, portions are getting larger, but many diners are unaware, as the plate diameters have also increased. Food, when served in separate courses such as appetizers, a bread basket and dessert, quickly adds up without you being aware of just how much it is. Large servings of meat, poultry and fish or carbohydrates, such as mountains of pasta, fill the platters. Vegetables and fruits are in smaller amounts, often served as a garnish unless ordered as a side dish. If you leave feeling "full," you have consumed too many calories. If you are feeling stuffed, you probably have consumed an extra couple thousand calories. Your goal should be to leave feeling satisfied but not full.

The good news is that all restaurants have healthy options if you look for them and make reasonable requests to modify what is typically served. Most restaurants and chefs are willing to make changes at your request. While they may not appear on the menu, if you ask, your requests will often be accommodated.

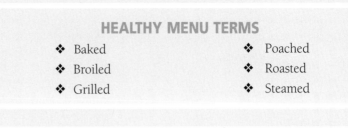

How To Avoid Trans Fats When Dining Out

Under a current FDA ruling on trans fats, restaurants are not required to disclose the amount of trans fats in their items or to provide any other nutrition information. Some chain restaurants have voluntarily provided that information. Assume that anything that is fried, breaded or battered contains trans fats, unless the menu states otherwise. What the server says is not legally binding, but what is stated in writing is. Restaurants often purchase foods prebreaded or "par-fried" as in the case of French fries. Trans fats may still be in the foods from this preparation, regardless of the oils used for the final frying.

Unless customers demand foods without trans fats and are willing to pay more for foods made with these healthier oils, most restaurants will not be willing to make the switch.

Menu Reading

As you browse the menu, think of it as a suggestion of all the possible options. For example, if you see a healthier sauce or side dish served with a different entrée, ask if you can have that instead of the French fries or chips listed by an item you are ordering. By picking and choosing, you can create a healthier meal from the items offered.

When reading the menu, look for terms that indicate a healthy cooking method, such as steamed; in its own juice (au jus); garden fresh; broiled; baked; roasted; poached; or stir-fried in broth, wine or lemon juice.

Terms that indicate less healthy options are terms such as, fried, crispy, creamed or creamy, in cream, butter or cheese sauce, au gratin, au fromage, escalloped, hollandaise, béarnaise, stewed, basted, sautéed, lightly sautéed, breaded, casserole, angus, prime, pot pie or pastry crust.

Smaller Portions

Don't mistake large for good. Much of the cost of a restaurant meal involves nonrelated food expenses, such as labor, so a restaurant can serve you a large amount of food for a relatively small additional cost. Restaurants know that Americans love getting a good deal and often those mountains of food will keep customers coming back to their establishments.

Most of us have great intentions of making up for those meals we ate that lacked vegetables and contained high amounts of sodium and unhealthy fats.

However, the next restaurant meal or occasion to splurge is probably just around the corner, with more leftovers to take home, and too often we don't balance them.

The exception to restaurants that serve monster-sized portions are upscale restaurants, where presentation and taste are more important than large, value-priced portions. If you think those places serve too little food, it may surprise you that those seemingly skimpy portions are closer to recommended serving sizes. However, sauces tend to be rich and used generously, which may increase calories in spite of small entrée portions. Even at an upscale restaurant, vegetables tend to be skimpy and are used mostly as a garnish with the main entree. However, a variety of side vegetables are readily available for you to order a la carte.

Split A Dish

Control serving sizes by splitting a dish with a companion or ask if you may order a half portion. If you split an entrée and they do it in the kitchen, most restaurants will fill the plate with the starchy side dish, and you may still end up with large amounts of food since sending out skimpy-looking portions makes an unfavorable impression to other diners.

Decide How Much To Eat

Unless you are employed in a job that requires heavy physical labor all day, you may need to cut back on how much of the food served you will eat.

When your plate arrives, if you are having a meat, fish or poultry entrée, cut off what you judge to be a 3-ounce portion. Think of a deck of cards or review portions from Page 272. Do the same with the starchy side dish, estimating how much is one or two servings. When you have eaten those portions, stop and leave the rest. If you absolutely can't bear to leave it, take it home. You might justify large, cheap portions by taking it home for the next day, but you will now have two meals of less healthy options instead of one.

If you feel that you are wasting food and throwing away money, think again. Remember, you can choose to waste it by leaving it or "waist" it by wearing it! Add up the cost of diets, books, special foods and all the other ways you will try to lose the excess pounds. That does not even take into consideration the cost to your health, self-image and emotions, which go along with being overweight. Eventually you waste money to fix a problem that came from not wanting to waste food.

Increase The Fruits and Vegetables

Lack of fresh fruit and colorful vegetables means you need to order them, if available, from the menu as an appetizer or side order. If they are not available, make up for them by eating fruits and vegetables at your next meal and choose them for snacks.

Ask For Whole Grain

Lack of whole-grain foods is often a problem. Even when breads sound healthy, such as rye bread, wheat bread, multigrain bagel or bran muffins, they are more often than not made with mostly white flour with only a handful of whole grain tossed in. Therefore, cutting back on refined grains when eating out is probably a good idea. If having a potato, rice or pasta with dinner, skip the bread or chip basket.

**Ask the server about ingredients or how foods were prepared.
Never assume anything.**

Tips For Eating Heart Healthy When Eating Out

Avoid Buffets

As you try to sample all the foods or are tempted to eat all you can since it is a good value, you will find it difficult to stick to the guidelines for heart health. Even healthy choices provide too many calories when eaten in large amounts.

Ask For What You Want

Get it your way. Restaurants are more willing to let you make requests because they have discovered that if they do, you will come back. Ask for dry broiled or poached fish, no butter on your vegetables, or to use only olive oil. Ask for herbs to be used instead of salt. Be specific. If you say just a little oil, to the chef, it may mean a quarter cup of extra-virgin olive oil, which contains 56 grams of fat and 504 unwanted calories.

Get Extras On The Side

To control fat and sodium, get gravy, sauces and salad dressings on the side. This allows you to decide how much to add, not the person in the kitchen. Dip your fork in the sauce or dressing and then your food for just a "taste."

Ask About Ingredients and Preparations

If your server can't tell you, have him check with the kitchen. See if an item can be baked, broiled, grilled, poached or steamed instead of fried. Unless items have been pre-prepared, you can probably get it your way.

Request Nutrition Information

Ask to see nutrition information for any item with a health claim such as "low fat" or "heart healthy." Federal law now requires that when restaurants make health claims, they must provide nutrition information upon request. When eating out, focus on taste and nutrition. By checking nutrition information, it is possible to have tasty and healthy food.

Substitute Where Possible

Most restaurants will allow reasonable substitutions, such as a small tossed salad instead of French fries or a larger serving of vegetable instead of fries or coleslaw. Some restaurants may have a small charge to make the change. If no substitutions are allowed, ask to have the item left off to avoid the temptation if it comes on your plate.

Aim For Balance

It may be okay to splurge on a steak if you choose a side salad and side order of steamed vegetables. The salad and vegetables are nutrient-dense, low-fat, low-calorie choices that balance out the higher fat steak. Only fried food are off limits. For other foods it depends upon what else you eat, how often you choose a food, and what size the portion is.

SPECIFIC TIPS FOR HEALTHY CHOICES

Fast Food

❖ Choose salads, the darker the greens the better. Choose a regular dressing since fat-free dressings are high in sugar and sodium. If it comes in a packet, dip your fork into the dressing to get just a "taste" with each bite rather than using the whole packet. It also slows you down as you have to keep dipping with each bite.

❖ Order a grilled chicken sandwich and ask for a dry, not buttered, bun with extra lettuce, tomato or other vegetables.

❖ Select small or regular-sized hamburgers or the plain roast beef sandwich.

❖ Ask for just a little sauce or mayonnaise or scrape off the excess before eating.

❖ Skip anything fried: fried fish, fried chicken strips, fried vegetables and french fries.

Breakfast

❖ Have fresh fruit or a small glass of citrus juice. Tomato and V-8 are high in sodium unless low-sodium varieties are available.

❖ Order whole-grain varieties of bread, half a bagel or English muffin with peanut butter. Spread thinly if watching calories.

❖ Choose whole-grain cereal with low-fat (1%) or nonfat milk.

❖ Have hot oatmeal with nonfat milk and top it with fruit. Ask them not to add any butter to your oatmeal before serving.

❖ If eating eggs or omelets made with eggs, balance the cholesterol later in the day, or choose egg whites or egg substitute. Ask for one egg plus several egg whites. Choose sautéed veggies without cheese if having an omelet.

❖ Ask for plain low-fat yogurt, then add high-fiber cereal such as oat bran flakes or muesli and fresh berries or other fruit. A little brown sugar, honey or stevia can be added if you need a touch more sweetness.

Beverages

Don't drink your calories. This may add up quickly for juice, wine, lemonade, soft drinks and sweetened tea. Limit calorie beverages to one and then drink lots of water. Choose:

- Water with lemon or lime.
- Flavored sparkling water (noncaloric).
- Milk, nonfat skim or 1%.
- Juice spritzer (half or less 100% fruit juice and half or more sparkling water).
- Tomato or vegetable juice (reduced-sodium).
- Iced or hot tea (unsweetened).
- Coffee drinks with skim milk or soy milk.

Bread

- If you plan to have potato, pasta or rice with your meal, skip the bread.
- If you want to have bread, eat one small piece with the meal to prevent taking in more calories than you need.
- A small loaf of bread and small dish with 1/4 cup of olive oil may add up to more than 1,000 calories.
- Ask to have the chips, fried wontons or bread served with the meal or move them to the far end of the table until your meal arrives.

Appetizers

Do you really need an appetizer considering the amount of food typically served? A large glass of water with a lemon twist may be the best bet. Even with careful choices, a multicourse meal will mean more food than you need. If you must have something to munch on, check out the other sections of the menu besides appetizers, such as salads or vegetables.

- Shrimp cocktail (red cocktail sauce – go easy, sauce is high in sodium). No need to concern yourself with cholesterol in shrimp.
- Melons or fresh fruit with a lime wedge.
- Fresh fruit cup, ask if you don't see it on the menu.
- Small side salad with dressing on the side (or add a bit of olive oil and vinegar).
- A la carte order of grilled vegetables.
- Raw vegetables with salsa.
- Vegetables with hummus or low-fat black bean dip.

Soups

- Broth-based soups are low in fat and calories, but all soups are high in sodium. Broth-based or cream-based soups will set you back at least 900 to 1,200 milligrams sodium per cup. Bowls contain even more.
- Choose soup that has vegetables, barley or legumes such as lentil, northern beans, split peas, etc.
- Seafood chowders may sound like a good way to get the healthy omega-3 fats, but very little fish are in these and if heavy cream is used as a base, they are also loaded with saturated fats.

Entrées/Main Course

❖ **Grilled, broiled or poached fish**, is best, especially fish such as wild salmon, which is higher in omega-3. Ask them not to melt butter on it after they cook it. If it comes with a sauce, ask for it on the side and then use just a bit for flavor by dipping your fork into it. Avoid deep-fried fish, which cancels out the benefit of eating fish. If you don't see poached on the menu, ask as it is an easy thing for them to do.

❖ **Poultry** is best broiled or baked, with the skin removed before eating. If it comes in a sauce or with added cheese, ask to have it served on the side or left off. Chicken is not automatically a heart healthy choice. Chicken Alfredo, deep-fried or breaded chicken, or chicken pot pie, even if it is made with all white meat, will be less healthy than a petite beef tenderloin steak.

❖ **Beef:** A small steak, such as a beef tenderloin or filet mignon, is your best choice. Portion control, the amount of marbling and how often you choose it, is key when choosing beef. If they have bison or grass-fed beef, they will be lean choices.

❖ **Vegetarian** does not automatically mean healthier or lower in calories or lower in saturated fat. Sometimes a heavy dose of full-fat cheese or high-fat dairy, as in vegetarian lasagna, will make a meatless choice even higher in saturated fat. Vegetables wrapped in a pastry crust with a white sauce and cheese is high in calories and saturated fats. Ask what is in the dish. Vegan dishes do not use cheese or dairy foods; the major source of saturated fats in vegetarian choices.

❖ **Pasta:** Red sauce is lower in fat than creamy sauces, but the addition of meat or sausage may make them just as high in fat. The average amount of pasta served is four cups which is eight servings! It may be low in fat but not low in calories when a large portion is served as a main course.

❖ **Sandwiches**
  • **Ask for a dry bun or bread.** If it comes grilled, that means buttered and heated on a grill. Ask for it dry toasted without any fat.
  • Leave off the cheese in sandwiches or ask for half. **Ask for less meat and more veggies** like lettuce, sprouts, tomatoes, onions, green pepper and pickles. **Skip mayonnaise-based fillings such as ham salad.**
  • Include mustard, BBQ sauce or just a little mayonnaise. Any filling called "salad," as chicken salad or ham salad, means mixed with large amounts of mayonnaise. Most mayonnaise used in restaurants or delis is made with soybean oil, and each tablespoon has 100 calories and 11 grams of fat, although only 1-1/2 grams are saturated fat. Mayonnaise spread on a sandwich is much less than the amounts used when mixed with the filling. Request "light on the mayonnaise" to reduce calories.
  • Breads/buns that are rye, multigrain or wheat often has only a hint of whole grain. Tortilla wraps may contain partially hydrogenated fats with mostly refined, white flour.

Salads/Salad Bars

Salads may offer some healthy options. Dark green romaine lettuce or spinach is loaded with nutrients with very little calories. Load up the dressing and it may become a high-calorie splurge.

❖ Think dark green and bright colors for the most nutrients.

❖ Cooked dry beans/legumes, such as chick peas and kidney beans, are good plant protein, high-fiber choices.

❖ At the salad bar, look for items with vinaigrette-type dressings. This will drain off easier than creamy dressing.

❖ Go easy on the potato, ham and macaroni salads, as well as creamy coleslaw and pasta salads. If you really want them, stick to a small spoonful.

❖ Replace the croutons, typically refined carbohydrates with bad fats, and get a small sprinkle of sunflower seeds which, although high in fat, are a good fat with vitamin E and minerals.

❖ To dress your salad, try balsamic vinegar, rice wine vinegar or flavored vinegar like raspberry and just a touch of olive oil. This is also a good choice if you want to avoid the salt, sugars or high fructose corn syrup found in commercial dressings.

❖ Get a small container of dressing on the side and use sparingly. **Use the dip, spear, eat method. Dip fork into the dressing, spear a piece of your salad, then eat.** The fork holds just a taste of dressing without overdoing the calories. You eat so little that you may choose a regular dressing, which has more flavor. Regular dressings are also typically lower in sodium and added sugars than fat-free ones. With this method for controlling portions, you won't overdo the calorie intake.

❖ Load up on any fresh vegetables, including tomatoes, mushrooms, carrots, cucumbers, peppers, onions, radishes, cauliflower and broccoli.

Side Dishes/Vegetables/Starchy Sides

❖ Vegetables in a variety of colors, along with salads, should fill up half your plate. Order vegetables a la carte if not included or as an appetizer.

❖ Starches (rice, potato, noodles) should fill a fourth of your plate. You may need to leave part of what is served since portions are often large.

❖ Potatoes: choose baked, steamed or boiled and watch the portions. Remember, a serving looks like a small, round, new potato and most potatoes you are served will be three to five servings. **Potatoes are technically a vegetable, but nutritionally, they are closer to white bread, so count them as a starch.** Ask if the restaurant serves sweet potatoes, which may be quickly baked in the microwave. Ask for it plain, no butter. You may add a small amount of butter or chopped chives, lemon juice, balsamic vinegar, pepper, mustard, barbecue sauce or salsa. Watch portions as most sweet potatoes are quite large.

- ❖ Pasta: Portions are typically HUGE. One serving should be 1/2 cup.
- ❖ Ask how sides are prepared since they often include butter, oils or margarine. Find out if you can get plain, steamed, baked or boiled side dishes.
- ❖ Ask for mustard, salsa or low-fat yogurt, instead of sour cream or butter, to add to your sides.

Dessert

- ❖ You probably don't need the extra calories, but if you really want a dessert, split it with someone or even better with several people. Eat a few bites and leave the rest, remember waste it or "waist" it.
- ❖ Even if it is not on the menu, most restaurants have fresh fruit available. Try berries or sliced oranges, apples or pears served with a few chopped nuts and a drizzle of chocolate sauce.
- ❖ Try a low-fat or nonfat frozen yogurt in the smallest portion available with a sprinkle of chopped nuts or some fresh berries. Skip sherbert it is low fat but high in sugars.

Dining To Reduce Sodium

- ❖ Ask for meat that has not been marinated, brined or tenderized. Most pork and chicken is "tenderized," which makes it higher in sodium. Fish is a good choice if it is not breaded or fried; plain grilled is best.
- ❖ Skip soups, even low-fat broth types are high sodium. A cup is less sodium than a bowl.
- ❖ Instead of prepared salad dressing, stick to vinegar and oil from separate bottles.
- ❖ Choose a plain baked potato. All other starchy side dishes, such as rice, pasta, or potato other than baked, will have sodium added.
- ❖ When choosing fast-food sandwiches, the smallest plain hamburger will be the lowest in sodium. Skip the quarter-pounder. Skip cheese as most of it is processed and high in sodium.
- ❖ Skip the sauce, gravies, dressings, dipping sauces, ketchup and BBQ sauce or use about a teaspoon.
- ❖ Ask them to leave off the potato chips, tortilla chips, pickles and olives.
- ❖ Ask that salt, soy sauce and MSG be left off or get a small amount on the side.
- ❖ Avoid casseroles and dishes smothered with cheese, which increases the sodium, such as stuffed pasta, ravioli, manicotti and lasagna.

Dining Out Quiz

1. Foods fried in oils without trans fat are heart healthy.
   ❏ T ❏ F

2. Broth-based soups are lower in sodium than cream-based soups.
   ❏ T ❏ F

3. To limit the amount of food eaten, you can:
   a) Ask for a take-home bag at the beginning of your meal to put part of your meal before eating.
   b) Split an entrée or dessert.
   c) Order an appetizer and side vegetables instead of a main course.
   d) All of the above.

4. Vegetable portions tend to be too large when eating out.
   ❏ T ❏ F

5. Buffets are a good value and the recommended choice when eating out.
   ❏ T ❏ F

6. Asking for dressing and sauces on the side helps to control extra calories and sodium.
   ❏ T ❏ F

7. Choose the best choice for breakfast from the following:
   a) Egg white omelet with vegetables, lean ham, no cheese
   b) Pancakes and lean Canadian bacon
   c) Cornflakes and low-fat milk

8. Choose the best choice for lunch from the following:
   a) Fish sandwich
   b) Small roast beef sandwich
   c) Grilled vegetables with cheese on croissant

9. Choose the best choice for dinner from the following (lowest in saturated fat)
   a) Chicken Alfredo (3 ounces)
   b) Vegetable lasagna (1 cup)
   c) Petite beef tenderloin steak (3 ounces)

ANSWERS
On Page 281.

Smart 4 Your Heart

39

Physical Activity

The heart is a muscle. Like all muscles, the heart needs regular, moderate physical activity to be healthy. According to a 2006 Report by the U.S. Centers for Disease Control and Prevention (CDC) on Physical Activity and Nutrition, more than 50 percent of American adults do not get regular, daily exercise that is needed for health benefits and 24 percent of Americans are not active at all.[128]

Physical Activity

Any movement that is produced by moving the muscles and burns calories is a form of physical activity. It can be dancing, golfing, gardening or playing ball with the kids.

Exercise

Exercise is a specific type of activity that is planned. Exercise is designed to improve aerobic capacity, increase strength or improve flexibility. Examples are brisk walking, jogging, weight lifting, Pilates, kickboxing, yoga, etc.

Exercise and The Heart

Exercise improves the ability of the blood vessels to dilate and the heart to deliver oxygen to the working muscles. The heart is able to get more oxygen as exercise causes more blood vessels to develop. Chest pain called angina decreases when oxygen supply is improved.

❖ Exercise is one of the best things you may do for your heart, even if there is no direct affect on your cholesterol numbers.

❖ People who exercise regularly not only live longer, they live better.

❖ Before you begin any exercise program, it may be recommended that you first consult a physician or other qualified health care provider who can determine what is appropriate for you.

Physical Activity Affects Health

Being physically active on most days of the week reduces the risk of illness and death. According to the Surgeon General's report on Physical Activity and Health, physical activity improves health in the following ways:[129]

❖ Reduces the risk of early death from heart disease.

❖ Reduces the risk of developing diabetes and colon cancer.

❖ Reduces the risk of developing high blood pressure and reduces blood pressure in people who already have high blood pressure.

❖ Reduces feelings of depression and anxiety and improves our sense of well being.

❖ Helps control weight.

❖ Keeps our bones, muscles and joints healthy with lowered risk of osteoporosis.

❖ Helps prevent falls in the elderly.

According to research in Sweden, regular exercise in midlife reduces the risk of dementia by 50 percent or more and reduces the risk of Alzheimer's disease by more than 60 percent, particularly by carriers of the Apo E4 gene, a known genetic risk factor.[130] The researchers think it may be that the benefits came from an increased flow of blood to the brain. Any physical activity helped, as long as it caused an increase in breathing and sweating.

Take This Self-Assessment To Evaluate Your Physical Activity

Self-Assessment of Physical Activity — Part 1		
Circle yes or no to each question		
Yes	No	I get at least 30 minutes of moderate physical activity (see Page 255) on most days of the week in addition to daily activities. This does not have to be all at one time; it all adds up and counts. Any exercise is better than none. The goal, if you are just starting and were not exercising before, is to burn 1,000 calories a week (150 calories a day).
Yes	No	I find ways to incorporate activity into my daily routine by taking stairs instead of elevators, parking the car away from my destination so I can walk, and getting off public transportation early and walking part of the way.
Yes	No	I watch TV, play video games or surf the Web for less than an hour per day.
Yes	No	I monitor my activity with a pedometer, adding steps, with an ideal goal of at least 10,000 daily steps (point at which you are classified as "active").

If you answered "yes" to all of these questions, move on to the next set of questions on Page 255.

If you answered "no" to any of the above questions, work on making small changes until you can say yes. You might start by walking five to 10 minutes daily and increasing by a few minutes each week. Begin to limit sedentary behavior, such as TV and video watching and computer Web surfing. Those who watch three to four hours of TV a day have higher rates of obesity than those who watch less than an hour. Use some of the time you would usually spend on sedentary activities to do some physical activity. You might try to combine a normally sedentary activity such as TV viewing with walking on a treadmill. Tape your favorite programs or the news, and watch it while you exercise.

The best physical activity for someone who is sedentary, but capable of walking, is to begin to walk. Walking for most individuals is safe. Daily walking protects against heart disease and high blood pressure and reduces the risk of developing diabetes. Walking does not require any special skills or equipment other than a good pair of walking shoes. If you are very inactive, start with 10 minutes and do it daily. Add minutes when it seems too easy. As you continue to walk and your endurance increases, you may continue to gain benefits by increasing the pace or the time spent walking.

In the Nurses Health Study, it was found that those who walked briskly three to four hours a week cut their risk for major illness almost in half over the nonwalkers.[139]

Pedometers

A good way to motivate yourself and track your walking progress is to buy a pedometer and wear it every day. The small gadget is clipped to your belt or on the top of your waistband so it lines up directly above the knee. Pedometers are less accurate if you have a larger stomach. Try clipping it to the middle of your back on your belt where it may record more accurately. They also won't record cycling or swimming activities.

Reliable brands of pedometers are the *Accusplit Eagle, Digiwalker* and *Omron.* The basic models record your steps and are all you need. There are more expensive models that will do more, such as calculate calories and convert steps into miles. If you enjoy gadgets, you might consider one of those models, but they are more complicated to use and may be frustrating to some. The pedometer does record steps while jogging or running if you enjoy those activities.

For the first week, record your daily steps without attempting to make any changes. At the end of the week, add steps walked each day, divided by the number of days you recorded steps, to determine your daily average. If you are only doing routine daily activities, you will probably average 3,000 steps or less. When you reach 5,000 to 9,999 steps, you are "somewhat active," and 10,000 or more steps are needed to be "active."

EXERCISE NOTE

Of the 1,440 minutes in a day, make time for at least 30 of those minutes to be spent on some type of physical activity.

EXERCISE NOTE

- Walking 3,000 steps or less = AVERAGE

- Walking 5,000-9,999 steps = SOMEWHAT ACTIVE

- Walking 10,000 steps = ACTIVE

2,000 steps equals about a mile and burns 100 calories.

2,000 steps equals about a mile and burns about 100 calories.

PEDOMETER STEPS	
Day	Steps Recorded Daily
1	
2	
3	
4	
5	
6	
7	

Add steps recorded for total steps =_____ Divide by 7= _____daily average steps

Start with your daily average steps that you recorded for the week and increase it by 250 steps each day, or 1,750 steps each week, until you reach 10,000 steps over your starting steps. You will probably find that you need to include some specific time for walking to reach those goals. Example:

Week	Steps Added	Average Steps Per Day At End Of Week
1	None	1,500
2	250/day (1,750 per week)	3,250
3	250/day (1,750 per week)	5,000
4	250/day (1,750 per week)	6,750
5	250/day (1,750 per week)	8,500
6	250/day (1,750 per week)	10,250
7	250/day (1,750 per week)	12,000

Think of creative ways to add steps throughout the day, and you will see that every little bit adds up. If you find that at the end of the day you have not reached your goal, either walk in your neighborhood, or at a local school or mall, or take a walk on a treadmill. Checking the pedometer during the day is like having an exercise buddy that gives you a pat on the back for your efforts, as well as a gentle reminder that you need to get in more steps if needed.

The 10,000 mark is a minimum goal needed to maintain weight and the point at which you can classify yourself as "active." The best weight loss usually occurs at 12,000 steps or more. Walking 12,000 steps is equal to about 6 miles.

Amish adults, in spite of high-fat, high-calorie diets, have much lower rates of obesity than the average American, which is believed to be due to their more active lifestyles. In one study, Amish men averaged 18,000 steps and the women 14,000, compared to the average American adult who gets 3,000 to 4,000.[159]

When you can answer "yes" to all of the questions on Page 252, move on to the following set of questions. The goal is to increase intensity, or if that is not physically possible, to add more time.

Self-Assessment of Physical Activity – Part 2
Circle yes or no to each question

Yes	No	I include moderate aerobic exercise five or more days of 30 minutes or more; Or vigorous exercise three or more days of 20 minutes or more. Target range is to burn 150-400 calories each day.
Yes	No	I include strength training two to three times a week.
Yes	No	I include stretching or flexibility exercise daily.
Yes	No	I regularly alter my routine or activity to challenge my body.

Moderate Physical Activity

Moderate intensity activities are those that cause you to burn three to six times more energy than when sitting at rest or 4 to 7 calories per minute.

Examples of moderate activity according to NCEP ATP III guidelines are:

- ❖ Brisk walking (3 to 4 mph) for 30 to 40 minutes
- ❖ Swimming laps for 20 minutes
- ❖ Bicycling for pleasure or transportation, 5 miles in 30 minutes
- ❖ Volleyball (noncompetitive) for 45 minutes
- ❖ Raking leaves for 30 minutes
- ❖ Moderate lawn mowing (push a powered mower) for 30 minutes
- ❖ Home care (heavy cleaning)
- ❖ Basketball for 15 to 20 minutes
- ❖ Golf (pulling a cart or carrying clubs)
- ❖ Social dancing for 30 minutes

The number of calories burned varies by activity, intensity and how much you weigh. We each have unique physical activity needs based on our physical differences and goals. The amount of lean muscle compared to body fat, how many calories you eat, if you want to lose weight, your genes, and how physically fit you are, will all affect the amount of physical activity needed.

How Many Minutes A Day?

The 30-minute guideline is a starting point, not the maximum amount, as some individuals think. If you find you don't have a 30-minute block of time to get some physical activity into your day, then break it up into 10-minute segments. Aim to fit in as many 10-minute sessions as you can.

The Institute of Medicine found it took 60 minutes of moderate-intensity exercise (about 400 calories were burned) to maintain a healthy weight.[137]

The chart below is an example of moderate and vigorous intensity activities and the amount of calories a 140-pound person would burn in 30 minutes.

Calories Expended For 30 Minutes

Moderate- to Vigorous-intensity Activities	Calories burned in 30 min for 140 Pound (64 kg) Person
Biking, stationary	235
Biking, more than 12-14 mph	269
Dance, waltz, fox trot	101
Dance, polkas, square, line, disco	151
Running/jog 5 mph (1 mile in 12 minutes)	269
Sit, knit, sew,	50
Sit, desk, type	60
Sit, watch TV	34
Swim, slow, freestyle, laps	235
Walking, 3 mph	111
Walking, 3.5 mph	140
Walking, brisk, 4 mph	168

Source: Author calculated with Met levels obtained from Appendix A,
ACSM's Resource Manual for Guidelines for Exercise Testing and Prescription, Fifth edition.

Monitor Your Pulse

To get the most benefit, you should work at a level that is not too easy but also not so difficult that you risk getting injured.

The heart rate zone you want to be in for general health is 40 to 60 percent of your maximum heart rate. For fitness, 60 to 80 percent. For improving performance, greater than 80 percent.

To check your heart rate, place your index and middle finger on the inner part of your wrist or the side of neck. Press until you feel the pulse. Count beats for 10 seconds and multiply that number by six.

TABLE 39.1 Maximum Heart Rate By Age
(Number of Heart Beats in one Minute)

AGE	MAX HR	50% OF MAX HR	60% OF MAX HR	90% OF MAX HR
20	200	100	120	180
25	195	97	117	175
30	190	95	114	171
35	185	92	111	166
40	180	90	108	162
45	175	87	105	157
50	170	85	102	153
55	165	82	99	148
60	160	80	96	144
65	155	77	93	139
70	150	75	90	135
75	145	72	87	130
80	140	70	84	126

MAXIMUM HEART RATE

Beginner:	50%	**Fitness/Weight Loss:**	60-80%
General Health:	50-60%	**Improve Performance:**	80-90%

Maximum Heart Rate

To calculate your individual maximum heart rate range, follow the steps below.

STEP 1:

220 minus your age_____ = _____ Maximum Heart Rate (HR)

STEP 2 (50%):

Multiply the number from Step 1 by 0.5 if **just starting to exercise**.

_____ HR X .5 = _____ = HR for just starting to exercise

STEP 2 (60-80%):

Multiply the number from Step 1 by 0.6 or 0.8 if have been exercising regularly and are ready to **work on fitness**.

_____ HR X .6 = _____ = lower end of target HR zone for fitness

_____ HR X .8 = _____ = upper end of target HR zone for fitness

STEP 2 (90%):

Multiply the number from Step 1 by 0.9 to **improve performance**.

_____ HR X .9 = _____ = target HR zone for performance

EXERCISE NOTE

This formula may underestimate your target heart rate as you get older. Seek help from a fitness professional who may use the heart rate reserve and your perceived sense of exertion to calculate your specific target heart rate.

An example of a 52 year old with a maximum heart rate of 168 would be:
- ❖ 168 heart rate X 0.5 = 84 target heart rate for general health
- ❖ 168 heart rate X 0.6 = 100 target heart rate for fitness
- ❖ 168 X 0.9 = 151 target heart rate when ready to improve performance

The mathematical maximum heart rate has been questioned by some who feel it underestimates maximum heart rate for older adults. This is where the expertise of an exercise specialist trained by ACSM or another nationally recognized certification agency would be beneficial. They may use heart rate reserve. They can individualize the standard guidelines for you based on your fitness level and medications you may be taking that affect heart rate. This will minimize your risk for injury and help you reach your specific goals.

Medication May Affect Heart Rate

If you take medication such as a beta-blocker, which lowers your heart rate, instead of using a mathematical calculation, you may use how hard you feel your body is working as a guide. You want to exercise at a rate that feels somewhat hard but that you can still continue to exercise. Focus on how strenuous the exercise feels to you, how high your heart rate feels, how you are breathing, and how tired you feel, rather than focusing on only one concern, such as joint pain or shortness of breath.

If you are a heart patient who attended a cardiac rehabilitation program, you are probably familiar with the *Borg Scale*. The numbers on this scale relate to how difficult you perceive the exercise and how hard you feel you are working.

BORG RPE SCALE®

6	No exertion at all
7	Extremely light
8	
9	Very light
10	
11	Light
12	
13	Somewhat hard
14	
15	Hard (heavy)
16	
17	Very hard
18	
19	Extremely hard
20	Maximal exertion

For correct usage of the scale(s), the exact design and instructions given by Borg must be followed. Borg RPE Scale®, © Gunnar Borg, 1970, 1985, 1998

Weight Loss Or Optimal Fitness Levels

As fitness level improves, you are encouraged to move toward the upper end of calories expended on exercise and increased physical activity. To achieve optimal levels of fitness or weight loss, you will need to expend 1,000 to 2,000 calories weekly or about 150 to 290 calories on exercise a day. This may be accomplished in a variety of ways. Being more active in your daily activities counts, as well as walking or going to the gym. Daily sessions to burn 150 to 290 calories, or three sessions a week that burn 335 to 650 calories, or any other combination that fits into your lifestyle will help you lose weight or achieve optimal fitness.

If you lose a significant amount of weight, it requires 60 minutes daily or 2,800 calories of physical activity a week to maintain your new lower weight.

EXERCISE NOTE

Weight loss: Aim to burn 150 to 290 calories from exercise daily (1,000 to 2,000 per week).

Exercise Guidelines For Improving Lipids

To improve blood lipids, it takes regular, consistent amounts of exercise. Physical activity may significantly improve insulin sensitivity even without a change in body weight.

To raise HDL 2 to 8 mg/dl and lower triglycerides 5 to 38 mg/dl you need to burn 1,200 to 2,200 calories a week in exercise. If you walked, that would require about 24 miles a week for about nine to 12 months to see that benefit. If enough minutes are spent at a high enough intensity to burn 1,000 to 1,200 calories, benefits of exercise will occur even without a rise in HDL.

For sedentary or obese individuals or those with other health problems, the guidelines would require modification to gradually reach those levels over a period of time, as well as health care provider approval.

EXERCISE NOTE

To raise HDL and lower triglycerides, burn 1,200 to 2,200 calories a week from exercise.

Fat-Burning Mode

There are some who incorrectly advise that the heart rate stay at a lower intensity in a range that is considered to burn fat. The calories that are used in this range are supplied from the fat tissues. If you work at a higher heart rate range, some of the calories you use come from the glycogen reserves stored in the muscles and the liver, with less coming from fat stores.

The fuel you burn is less important in weight loss than the total calories you burn. The percent of calories burned from fat is greater during a slow walk than the percent of calories burned from carbohydrate, but the total calories burned are greater for a power walk.

An individual who is just starting to exercise or who is in poor health needs to work at low intensity, because higher levels are not possible and could be harmful. The advantage to a less-intense workout is that, for the beginner, it is at a pace that can be maintained for a much longer period of time. As you become better conditioned, you are encouraged to increase the intensity gradually.

In most cases, the time you have to exercise is limited; the higher target heart range will burn more calories so you lose more weight for a given amount of exercise time.

EXERCISE MYTH

Greater weight loss occurs at low-intensity workouts than at higher intensity because you are in the "fat-burning" mode.

Burning more calories per minute is your goal when you want weight loss. An added benefit of a more intense workout is that it takes longer for the body to return to baseline metabolism. Therefore, you will continue to burn more calories in the recovery phase after the intense exercise. It is the final balance between calories burned from any source and those eaten that determines weight loss or gain.

For weight loss, as your fitness improves, work at an aerobic capacity that is moderately hard and one that you can maintain for the desired length of time, 60 minutes on most days of the week.

Cool Down

After aerobic activity that has raised your heart rate, don't stop suddenly after you have completed your workout. It is best to slow the activity to a pace that is less intense before you stop, to allow your heart rate to drop gradually. As an example, you might walk or stretch for a few minutes until your body can cool down. Don't get into a hot shower until you have cooled down completely since exercise has expanded your blood vessels and has lowered your blood pressure. A hot shower could expand them even more, resulting in dizziness or fainting.

Stretching

Stretching at the end of a workout, when your muscles are warm from exercise, is the best time. Stretching after a workout also helps to reduce the buildup of lactic acid, which may cause muscle soreness.

Hold the stretch between 10 and 30 seconds. Don't bounce or force the stretch. If performed correctly, there is no such thing as too much stretching.

Aim to stretch all your major muscle groups at least once a day. Stretching will increase the blood flow to muscles and lubricate joints so you feel less stiff. A morning stretch is a good way to start the day. Go slowly since cold muscles may be injured more easily and don't stretch as much as when they are warm. Stretch several times a day if you can.

Strength Training

In addition to aerobic activity and stretching, weight training, also called strength training, is recommended for all adults, to reverse the muscle loss that occurs naturally with age. People in their late 30s and early 40s, begin to lose about a quarter pound of muscle every year. By age 80, people have typically lost a third of their muscle mass.

Strength training two or three times a week is recommended. Strength training builds muscle, which will help with weight management. You use more calories throughout the day when you have more muscle and less fat.

Strength training reduces the risk of osteoporosis by helping maintain bone density. It also helps prevent falls, which allows us to maintain normal activities that may become difficult as we get older.

Strength training may also reduce the inner layer of abdominal fat, which is the fat that raises the risk of heart disease and diabetes.

To get started at home, the books by author Miriam Nelson are excellent choices, as well as the Web site www.strongwomen.com. The books and Web site are based on her research that has been published in the *Journal of the American Medical Association*. The information is effective for both men and women.

Personal Trainers

While it is not necessary for you to hire a trainer, in some cases, it may be useful to learn correct form and to get the most benefit from the time you spend exercising. Consider hiring an expert for a few sessions to get started, especially if you want to start strength or flexibility training and are unsure of how to begin. The machines may be intimidating and it helps to learn how to use them correctly. Trainers can also show you the variety of exercises available to target all the major muscle groups. Trainers may help you avoid injury or adapt an exercise to meet your physical limitations.

As you look for a trainer, ask about certification and training. Certification by the American College of Sports Medicine (ASCM); and National Strength and Conditioning Association (NSCA); or another reputable, nationally recognized organization is a good start. Be aware that there are Internet certificates from less-reputable organizations, so avoid these. Some private health clubs do not require any specific certification or have their own certification; therefore, their advice may be questionable. A degree from a university, in a field such as physical education or exercise physiology is a plus.

What is probably more important than degrees and certifications is the type of experience trainers have. Look for someone who has worked with a variety of people and someone who can adapt the training to your unique needs. Some trainers hand out the same plan to each one of their clients with no regard to an individual's unique needs.

Choose someone that you can work with. You need someone who pushes you, but not to the point of injury. You don't need a buddy, but you do need someone with whom you feel comfortable. If you believe that your trainer is not listening to your concerns and is not adjusting workouts properly, that trainer may not be a good fit for you. Get a personal recommendation from someone who has already worked with the trainer you are considering. Schedule one lesson with a trainer to check out their style before you commit.

RECORD YOUR EXERCISE WEEKLY, ADDING ACTIVITIES YOU ENJOY

	Sun	Mon	Tue	Wed	Thur	Fri	Sat
Walked 30 minutes today							
Stretched today							
Strength training							
Swimming							
Yoga							
Spin class							
Other:							

Physical Activity Quiz

1. Exercise must lower your cholesterol numbers to be providing heart benefits.

   ❏ T   ❏ F

2. It requires 10,000 step counts daily to be considered "active."

   ❏ T   ❏ F

3. If you are exercising 30 minutes daily, there is no need to do more.

   ❏ T   ❏ F

4. A mile has about 2,000 steps and will burn _____ calories.
   - a) 50
   - b) 100
   - c) 150
   - d) 200

5. It usually takes 12,000 step counts or more daily for the best weight loss.

   ❏ T   ❏ F

6. Moderate activity is which of the following:
   - a) brisk walking 3 to 4 mph
   - b) raking leaves for 30 minutes
   - c) social dancing 30 minutes
   - d) all of the above

7. To maintain weight loss, the IOM states that _____ minutes daily are necessary.
   - a) 30
   - b) 45
   - c) 60
   - d) 90

8. For weight loss to occur about how many calories do you need to burn in activity each week.
   - a) 500 to 1,000
   - b) 1,000 to 2,000
   - c) 3,500

9. To raise HDL and lower triglycerides requires 1,200 to 2,200 calories of activity weekly.

   ❏ T   ❏ F

ANSWERS
On Page 281.

Smart 4 Your Heart

40

A Healthy Weight

About 66 percent of Americans are overweight or obese.[136] This is probably not new information to most of us. We can see it as we look around. Excess weight has been linked to many health problems, including increased risk for heart disease, gout, osteoarthritis and some types of cancer.

Losing weight reduces the risk of developing heart disease, especially if you have the cluster of risk factors for metabolic syndrome that includes high triglycerides, low HDL and a large waist.

Weight gain is a result of taking in more energy than your can use. Anytime we want it, great-tasting food is everywhere. Too much food, even too much "healthy" food, causes weight gain. Increased physical activity is important, but most of us would not be able to simply "work off" the extra calories. An hour of working out at the gym may burn several hundred calories, but we can easily consume several thousand calories in a single eating session of less than an hour.

BMI (Body Mass Index)

Body mass index is an estimate of body fat with relation to your height. To calculate BMI, your weight is divided by a factor for height. Using the chart that follows, you can find your BMI. If you are over age 75, it overestimates risk. A better measure is the waist-to-hip ratio discussed later.

Adult BMI Chart

1. Find your height in the left column.

2. Read across to your weight (pick the closest number).

3. Then follow that up to the top row for BMI.

TABLE 40.1   ADULT BMI

BMI	Normal						Overweight					Obese					
	19	20	21	22	23	24	25	26	27	28	29	30	31	32	33	34	35+
Height	Weight in pounds																
4'10"	91	96	100	105	110	115	119	124	129	134	138	143	148	153	158	162	167+
4'11"	94	99	104	109	114	119	124	128	133	138	143	148	153	158	163	168	173+
5'	97	102	107	112	118	123	128	133	138	143	148	153	158	163	168	174	179+
5'1"	100	106	111	116	122	127	132	137	143	148	153	158	164	169	174	180	185+
5'2"	104	109	115	120	126	131	136	142	147	153	158	164	169	175	180	186	191+
5'3"	107	113	118	124	130	135	141	146	152	158	163	169	175	180	186	191	197+
5'4"	110	116	122	128	134	140	145	151	157	163	169	174	180	186	192	197	204+
5'5"	114	120	126	132	138	144	150	156	162	168	174	180	186	192	198	204	210+
5'6"	118	124	130	136	142	148	155	161	167	173	179	186	192	198	204	210	216+
5'7"	121	127	134	140	146	153	159	166	172	178	185	191	198	204	211	217	223+
5'8"	125	131	138	144	151	158	164	171	177	184	190	197	203	210	216	223	230+
5'9"	128	135	142	149	155	162	169	176	182	189	196	203	209	216	223	230	236+
5'10"	132	139	146	153	160	167	174	181	188	195	202	209	216	222	229	236	243+
5'11"	136	143	150	157	165	172	179	186	193	200	208	215	222	229	236	243	250+
6'	140	147	154	162	169	177	184	191	199	206	213	221	228	235	242	250	258+
6'1"	144	151	159	166	174	182	189	197	204	212	219	227	235	242	250	257	265+
6'2"	148	155	163	171	179	186	194	202	210	218	225	233	241	249	256	264	272+
6'3"	152	160	168	176	184	192	200	208	216	224	232	240	248	256	264	272	279+
6'4"	156	164	172	180	189	197	205	213	221	230	238	246	254	263	271	279	287+

BMI table adapted from Nutrition and Your Health: Dietary Guidelines for Americans (1995): www.nhlbi.nih.gov/guidelines/obesity/bmi_tbl.htm

❖ A healthy range is a BMI between 18.5 and 24.9
❖ Overweight is defined as having a BMI of 25 to 29.9.
❖ Obesity is defined as having a BMI of 30 or more.

MY BMI IS _____

Healthy Weight Smart 4 Your Heart

Your Body Shape May Put You At Risk

As your belly size gets closer to your hip size, or if larger than your hips, your heart is at more risk. Waist circumference and waist-to-hip ratio have been found to be better associated with increased risk for heart attack than BMI. NHANES III found that for every inch a man's waist size increased, blood cholesterol level increases 8 percent and blood fat (triglycerides) increases 18 percent.[139]

Abdominal fat is different than fat found in other parts of the body. It is much more harmful and metabolically active, causing an increase in inflammation. Extra fat in the abdominal area increases your risk of heart disease, Type 2 diabetes, metabolic syndrome and hypertension. The fat that is located just below the skin, called subcutaneous, is less harmful.

Waist Circumference (WC)

To determine your waist circumference, place a tape measure on bare skin just above the navel, at the level even with your hip bone, horizontal to the floor. Where some people typically measure their waist is not the correct waist circumference. The tape measure should not slip into the indent at the navel and should not go under the belly. It should be snug, but should not compress the skin or sink into the navel depression. Relax, measure as you breathe out, not while inhaling or holding your breath.

❖ Men: waist greater than 35* inches (90 cm) puts you at greater health risk.
❖ Women: waist greater than 33* inches (83cm) puts you at greater health risk.

Note: You may find references that use waist greater than 35 for women and 40 for men. They use the BMI that corresponded to being overweight. Some studies find risk starts at the lower numbers used here.

My WC measurement is _____

Waist-To-Hip Ratio

Some believe the waist-to-hip ratio is a better way than waist circumference to predict risk of heart disease as we get older and for those individuals that have a BMI lower than 30 or 35, yet carry excess fat in the abdominal area.[140, 141]

After measuring your waist, measure your hips at the widest part of the buttocks. To determine your ratio, divide your waist measurement by your hip measurement.

Waist measurement _____ ÷ by hip measurement_____ = _____waist-to-hip ratio

A waist-to-hip ratio of 0.83 or less for women and 0.9 or less for men is desired.

Make weight loss a priority if: overweight with a high triglyceride level and low HDL.

Percent Body Fat

Your body weight includes lean muscle, fat and water. The percent of body fat is a measure of what percent of your weight is fat. When losing weight, you want to lose body fat while keeping lean muscle. A scale does not differentiate between whether you are losing fat, water or muscle. Therefore, it is important to measure body fat as you lose weight.

The average adult body fat is 15 to 18 percent for men and 22 to 25 percent for women. Men who have more than 25 percent fat and women with more than 32 percent fat have a much higher rate of illness and disease.

There are several ways to obtain your body fat. Your local fitness club or clinic will have a method to measure your body fat. It is often measured with either a skin caliper or a bioelectrical impedance device, such as a machine or a scale. If you do not belong to a club, there are calipers designed to allow self-measurement. One type of caliper is *Accu-measure* body fat calipers: www.accumeasurefitness.com.

If you track your body fat, a monthly check is all that is needed, since body fat percentages change slowly.

Daily Calorie Needs

According to exercise physiologists William McArdle and Frank Katch, authors of the textbook, *Essentials of Exercise Physiology*, the average calories consumed for women in the United States is 2,000 to 2,100 calories per day, and the average calories for men is 2,700 to 2,900 per day.[142] For a more individualized calculation, see below.

Adjust Calorie Intake

No matter how healthy your food is or what the combination of foods are, you must eat less, or burn more calories, to lose weight.

It takes a decrease of 3,500 calories to lose one pound of body fat. To lose one pound a week, divide the 3,500 calories by seven days in a week, which equals 500 calories less a day. You may be tempted to decrease the calories further, but too few calories may cause your metabolism to slow and increase loss of muscle. Reducing calories by 500, but not more than 1,000, is the most common guideline. The ACSM (American College of Sports Medicine) recommends that calories never drop below 1,200 for women or 1,800 for men. If you decrease your calories too much, your body will defend itself from starvation by slowing metabolism and increasing enzymes that store fat.

Daily Calorie Allowance For Weight Loss

Your current weight _____ X 12 = _____ minus 500
= _____ calories* for weight loss.

* not less than 1,200 for women or 1,800 for men or lower than your calculated RMR.

Healthy Weight Smart 4 Your Heart

Do Diets Work?

They work to take off weight while you stick to them. They don't work in the long run because they don't fit our lives. A study of four popular diets found there was no difference for weight loss after one year between the different diets, and the dropout rate was high for all of them because they were too difficult to follow or did not produce results.[143]

All the diets raised the good HDL cholesterol, except for a very low fat diet. None had any effect on triglyceride level, blood pressure or fasting blood sugar levels. However, c-reactive protein, a measure of inflammation, fell by 15 to 20 percent for all groups.

What Happens After The Diet?

When you quit the diet, it is likely that you will return to your usual way of eating. The problem with most diets is that you probably can't or don't want to follow the restrictions for the rest of your life. This means you won't keep the pounds off, no matter how well it worked. For example, if you followed a low-carbohydrate diet and gave up all the bread, crackers and cereal, once you can add back those foods, you do the same type of eating that caused your initial weight gain. If the weight is gained back, a search for another diet ensues and the cycle repeats itself.

Lifestyle Not A Diet

To lose and keep off weight requires small lifestyle changes that add up to habits you can keep for a lifetime. If you lose weight by making a few lifestyle changes, weight loss is typically slow. You might only lose one-half to 1 pound a week. If you did make a few changes and lost only a half a pound a week, that would be 26 pounds in a year. For some people, that is painfully slow. There are no quick fixes. Most people know that the only effective way to lose weight, and keep it off, is to eat only when hungry, not for all the other reasons we eat. It's also important to stop eating when satisfied, not stuffed, and to include regular exercise. But it is so boring and hard to do when a shiny new book shows up on the shelf, offering a quick and easy plan to follow. Every diet book assures you that they have found the answer or the "secret" combination or regimen that, when followed, closely allows you to eat as much as you want. You get your hopes up that this one will be different, this one will work. But diets are all the same.

If Diets Don't Work, What Does?

To succeed at weight loss, you must first determine what you need to do differently. One of the best tools to find out is a food journal.

Food Journals

Studies have proven that a food journal really works. If you are truthful and record at the time you eat or drink, even the spoonful of this or a couple of bites of that, you will become aware of things you need to change to succeed at weight loss. Start asking how hungry you are when you are eating and make a note. It will help you discover if you are eating for reasons other than true hunger.

Use your food journal to determine what might need to change. For example, are you doing very well all day but eating nonstop in the evening? Are you skipping meals or eating very small meals during the day? Are you grabbing whatever is available because you don't take the time to plan ahead? Perhaps you find that when you are home you eat well, but at work, the goodies are always tempting you, so you might want to do something different such as:

❖ Take a little of whatever is available and set it aside to eat with your lunch, rather than eating an undetermined amount every time you pass by the goodies.

❖ Bring a healthy snack from home, and when you get hungry, you won't be tempted to look for food.

❖ Take the treat home or save it for the next day, when you plan it into a meal, rather than adding it on to what you will already be eating.

❖ Don't eat all of the lunch you took to work, saving part of it for the next day, to compensate for the treat.

If you find yourself making poor choices when you are delayed at the office and get hungry, consider keeping frozen leftovers, a packet of salmon, or some unsalted nuts at the office to have available, in place of the vending machine offerings.

Do you restrict all the foods you like and then find that you overeat them later? Is there a way you could include foods you enjoy in smaller amounts?

At the end of the day or after a week, look at the journal and think about what you could do differently.

Daily Food Journal

Food eaten and where you ate it (home, restaurant, at your desk)	How hungry are you?	Time	Amount	Notes (optional)

Healthy Weight Smart 4 Your Heart

Change To Lower Calorie Choice	Amount	Calories Saved
Switch from whole milk to skim	8 oz.	46
Eat berries instead of angel food cake	1/2 cup 1 slice	35
Switch from 2% milk to skim	8 oz.	36
Choose unsweetened iced tea instead of lemonade or punch	8 oz.	90
Use sour cream instead of butter	1 Tbsp.	70
Replace butter with plain low-fat yogurt	1 Tbsp.	91
Switch from butter to light butter	1 Tbsp.	50
Replace some of the pasta with vegetables	1 cup	190
Eat raw veggies instead of cut-up fruit	1 cup	55

Change To Smaller Portion	Amount Decreased by	Calories Saved
Drink a smaller glass of juice	4 oz.	51
Have a smaller bowl berries	1/2 cup	35
Eat half a banana	4" piece	52
Have a smaller portion dried fruit	2 Tbsp.	50
Drink one less glass of wine	5 oz.	100
Have one beer instead of two	12 oz.	150
Eat a smaller handful nuts	1/4 cup	130 to 190
Eat half of a grilled chicken breast	3 oz.	100
Eat half a baked potato	3 oz.	93

Stop When You Are Full

Children before the age of 5 seem to follow internal signals of fullness better than adults. If allowed to serve themselves and eat without coaxing, children tend to eat amounts that meet their needs. By age 5, when served portions larger than they need, children begin to overeat. Before that age, they are better at eating only what they need, no matter the amount served. Coercing children into cleaning their plates and bribery to finish their vegetables before they leave the table will cause them to lose their internal satiety signals.

Knowing when you are hungry and when you are full are important signals that you may have to relearn. If you wait until your stomach is growling or you get a headache, you are too hungry. Ideally you want to eat before you reach that point. When you are over hungry, you tend to overeat.

To lose weight, you want to stop when you are feeling almost full, since you continue to get full after eating. In some cases, we have trained ourselves to ignore satiety signals and do not feel satisfied unless consuming excess amounts of food to the point of feeling stuffed. You may feel it is important to get large amounts of food for a low cost, even if you feel uncomfortably full. If you are served a 3-ounce burger, do you perceive this as a poor value? If you are served a 6-ounce burger, which is more than you need, you may be content that you received a good value, yet unhappy that you can't seem to lose weight. If you continue to seek out restaurants that serve large portions at reasonable prices, and all-you-can-eat buffets, you may be frustrated as your efforts to lose weight fail.

Why You May Not Lose Weight

It is possible to eat right, exercise and still not lose weight because you are taking in more calories than you realize.

Are you underestimating your calorie intake? Healthy foods like nuts, avocado, whole grains and dried fruits do have calories. Do you forget to include a bite or small handfuls of foods. Liquid calories, such as sports drinks, smoothies, all fruit drinks and coffee beverages, all add up. You can eat too much "healthy" food. On average when overweight we underestimate our calorie intake by 30 percent.

You may be eating too little healthy fat or too many processed "low-fat" diet-type foods without enough protein. Are you eating too few calories? If you are burning muscle instead of fat, your resting metabolic rate is lowered, making weight loss, even at low calorie intakes, impossible.

Do you have splurge days? If the calorie intake is very low during the day or for a few days, you may "blow it" when you get over hungry at night or on the weekend. Then, with your lowered metabolism, those extra calories quickly add back pounds. What might seem like an occasional treat that you deserve may slow your progress.

Do you eat too little for breakfast and lunch? Do you skip meals? Have you tried eating smaller, more frequent meals, about every four hours? Are you over-exercising or not doing resistance training? Do you vary your exercise routine, or do you do the same thing each time you work out? Adding more calories and including strength or resistance training or interval training in a healthy balance may be helpful. Seek professional help if you are stuck.

Active and Overweight

There has been some research that indicates that some individuals who are "fit and fat" are at less risk for developing disease than those who are naturally thin but not fit. If you are overweight and not able to reach your ideal BMI, staying physically active is your best protection against disease

NUTRITION NOTE

To lose weight, it's as important how much you eat, as it is what you eat.

Portions

Portion sizes need special attention. It may be helpful to measure your food to reinforce portion sizes, which are often blurred by the huge portions typically served today. Restaurant portion sizes are now two to five times larger than in 1970. When you see muffins the size of baseballs on a regular basis, that 500-calorie muffin looks average, not large. When given a normal serving size, many people feel cheated by the small size. Only by weighing these huge muffins do you realize how large it is compared to a standard-sized serving.

As the amount of food you are served increases, it acts as a cue for you to overeat, regardless of hunger or fullness. We know from studies that the larger the sandwich, the more is eaten – sometimes up to 50 percent more.

Use smaller plates, ideally, not more than 9 inches across. Review chapter 12 (Page 49) on how you fill your plate. Then fill a quarter of your plate with whole, intact grains and the other quarter with a lean protein, with the largest section being vegetables and salads. Eating this way gives you less calorie-dense, but higher nutrient-dense foods to keep you healthy, without hunger.

What Is A Serving?

The amount of food you serve yourself at one time is a portion of food. Serving sizes have been established for food groups. The portion of a food you eat during a particular eating occasion may be more or less than the established serving size for that food. You may not be aware of how much is considered a serving. For example, if you typically eat half of a bag of pretzels or the entire bag of microwave popcorn, your portion is more than one serving. If you count that portion as one serving, you are underestimating how many calories you really eat.

It is okay to have more than one serving if your nutritional needs require more. When putting gas in your car, which is measured in gallons, you are not restricted to one gallon. You may put in as many gallons as your tank holds. The same is true with food. Your servings can be as much as you need nutritionally.

Portion control is a key to weight management. If we are served large portions and eat them, as most adults will, it causes us to slowly gain weight, even if the food is healthy.

It takes practice to better judge what an appropriate serving looks like. Practice measuring food several times until you become aware of how much you are eating. Eventually, you will be able to estimate what an appropriate serving size looks like. Use the following chart to help you picture in your mind what a normal serving size is for some of your favorite foods.

NUTRITION NOTE

As little as an extra 100 calories per day will cause a 10-pound weight gain in one year.

WHAT IS A SERVING?

PROTEIN	**SERVING IS EQUAL TO:**
	1 oz. of fish, poultry or meat
	1/2 cup canned tuna or salmon
	1 oz. cheese or 1/4 cup shredded cheese
	1/4 cup cottage cheese or ricotta
	1 oz. tempeh
	2 oz. tofu (1/4 cup)
	1/4 cup dry textured vegetable protein or frozen soy crumbles
	1/2 veggie burger
	1/2 cup cooked legumes (dry beans, lentils or peas)
	1 whole egg, 2 egg whites, 1/4 cup egg substitute
	2 Tbsp. nut butter (1 protein + 2 fat)
	2 Tbsp. soy or whey protein powder
VEGETABLES *Note: Some vegetables are in grain group*	1 cup raw vegetables
	1/2 cup cooked or frozen vegetables
	2 cups leafy salad greens
	1 medium tomato
	1/2 cucumber
	1 stalk celery
	1/2 cup low-sodium vegetable juice (limit 1/2 cup per day)
FRUITS *Eat whole fruit rather than juices. Limit juice to 1/2 cup*	1/2 cup cut-up fruit
	1 cup berries or melon
	2 Tbsp. dried fruit (raisins, craisins, cherries, apricots)
	1 medium piece or 1/2 large (orange, kiwi, apple, peach, pear, nectarine)
	1/2 banana, mango, papaya, grapefruit
	2 small apricots, plums, tangerines, figs
	12 cherries
	17 grapes
STARCH/GRAIN *Intact grains*	1/2 cup cooked, intact grains (oat kernels, quinoa, wheat kernels, spelt, barley, bulgur, farro)
	1/3 cup brown rice, wild rice
	1/2 cup oatmeal, steel-cut or old-fashioned
	1/4 cup dry, rolled oats, barley, wheat, etc.
	3 cups popcorn, air popped
	1/2 cup pasta sauce

NOTE

See Page 351 to 368 for information on vegetables and recipes

STARCH/GRAIN

Starch vegetables

1/2 cup corn, peas
1/2 cup root vegetables (parsnip, turnip, rutabagas)
3 oz. baked or boiled red, Yukon or new potato
(size of golf ball)
1 cup mixed vegetables (corn, peas, beans)
1/3 cup baked beans

Grains processed into flour

Choose the following less often than intact grains:
1/2 cup whole-wheat pasta
1/2 hamburger bun, 1/2 whole-wheat English
muffin, 1/2 whole-wheat pita pocket
1 slice whole-wheat bread, whole-wheat tortilla
1 oz. whole-grain, low-sugar cold cereal

FAT

(a portion that has 5 grams fat)

1 tsp. liquid oil (olive and canola preferred)
1 Tbsp. regular salad dressing or cream cheese
1 tsp. regular mayonnaise or 1 Tbsp. light
1 Tbsp. nuts or seeds, raw, plain (no sugar; no added
oils, salt, flavorings)
2 tsp. nut butters, natural
1/8 or 1-ounce avocado

Choose the following less often:
2 Tbsp. half-and-half
1 tsp. butter
1 Tbsp. cream cheese
2 Tbsp. sour cream
2 tsp. sauce on foods (cheese, cream, hollandaise,
béarnaise, etc.)
2 Tbsp. shredded, unsweetened coconut
1/2 oz. *Dagoba* 73% chocolate or cocoa nibs
2 pieces *Dove* dark chocolate (2/3 starch + 1 fat)
16 chocolate chips, 60% cocoa (1 fat+ 1/2 starch)

**DAIRY OR
300 MG CALCIUM**

8 ounces nonfat milk
8 ounces soy, rice, oat, almond milk
1 cup nonfat or low-fat yogurt (plain or fruit
flavored with nonnutritive sweetener) or kefir
1-1/2 ounces cheese (reduced-fat)
1-1/2 cup cottage cheese (nonfat or 1%)
Calcium supplement containing 300 mg

Extras

All the "fun" foods fit in this area: cakes, cookies, pies, soda and alcohol. The healthiest way to reduce calorie intake is to eat smaller servings of the foods that provide little nutrition for the calories they contain. Even healthy versions that are low in fat and sugars provide little nutrition. To give them up all the time is not realistic, which is what many diets do, and the reason why they eventually fail. Balance is the key; have some of these foods, but in smaller amounts and less often. Limit this to about 100 to 150 calories.

Serving Size Practice

The following exercise will give you a chance to practice managing your serving sizes.

Equipment Needed

❖ Scale that can weigh in ounces, such as a postage scale or kitchen scale
❖ Liquid measuring cup with ounce markings
❖ Measuring spoons
❖ Glass, cup, bowl that you typically use
❖ Food items: Whatever is available in your cupboards and refrigerator

1. Start with your favorite cup or glass; if you have a variety of different glasses, gather them all. Fill them with water to where you normally fill them. Next, pour water into the measuring cup to see how many ounces you served yourself. Compare that to the serving size listed for the liquids you normally drink, such as milk or juice. The serving size for juice is 8 ounces, which is a cup serving according to the food guide pyramid. Juice serving size is 4 ounces for a diabetic food exchange serving. You may notice that food packages use a variety of serving sizes that are different from the pyramid or diabetic exchange serving sizes.

2. Using the scale, weigh several foods, such as a slice of bread. The standard serving is a slice that weighs 1 ounce. If you cut a piece of bread from a loaf, you will find that your serving of bread is probably several ounces, depending upon how thick the slice is. Wide pan slices are more than an ounce. Dense breads weigh more than diet breads.

3. If you eat cereal, fill your usual cereal bowl to the level in the bowl you typically do. Using the measuring cups or the scale, compare that amount to what is listed on the box as a serving. If you eat more than one variety of cereal, notice that the serving size and calorie amount varies. Most people typically pour out the same amount, regardless of the serving size indicated on the label.

4. Take a look in the refrigerator for any pieces of meat, chicken, tofu or cheese. Weigh it and then divide or portion it out until you have a 1- or 3-ounce portion. You will see that slices of deli meat look different than a piece of chicken or a serving of ground meat.

5. Using your measuring spoons, fill the teaspoon with butter, mayonnaise or nut butter and level it off. It is not how much you can hold in a teaspoon, but rather a level amount that is considered a serving. See how far it spreads. If it looks skimpy, see how much more it takes to get it the way you like it. If you used more, note how many more servings you used.

6. To determine a serving of ice cream, use a one-half cup dry measuring cup. Spoon the ice cream to a level amount. That is one serving. Although we may want to pile as much ice cream into the measuring cup as we can, it is only a level half cup that is a serving. You may think there is no need to be concerned if the ice cream is fat free or sugar free. The problem is that it is not calorie free and all of the calories quickly add up.

7. Potato serving size always seems to amaze people. Pick out a potato the size you would usually eat. Weigh it and compare it to the pyramid serving of 3 ounces. A serving is about the size of a golf ball or a small new potato, much smaller than the average-sized baked potato.

8. Measure out a food you eat by the handful into your cupped hand, such as nuts, chips, popcorn or pretzels. Now, put it on the scale and see how much it weighs. You will see that even healthy fat items, such as nuts, may add up quickly, so moderation is important if your goal is to lose weight.

You have the idea now; continue with foods that you normally eat. Take a day to measure different meals after you have portioned out what you would normally eat. Make your comparison and adjust your servings where necessary. After some practice, you will get better at estimating the correct amounts by simply looking at them. Repeat occasionally, as we tend to forget, and your servings may get larger.

Meal Planning (Plate Method)

Use the diagram on the next page to plan your meals in advance, using portions from Page 272 (What is a Serving). Spend some time in advance to create a meal plan with foods you enjoy. You can take items from the meals to create snacks if there are more than four hours between meals.

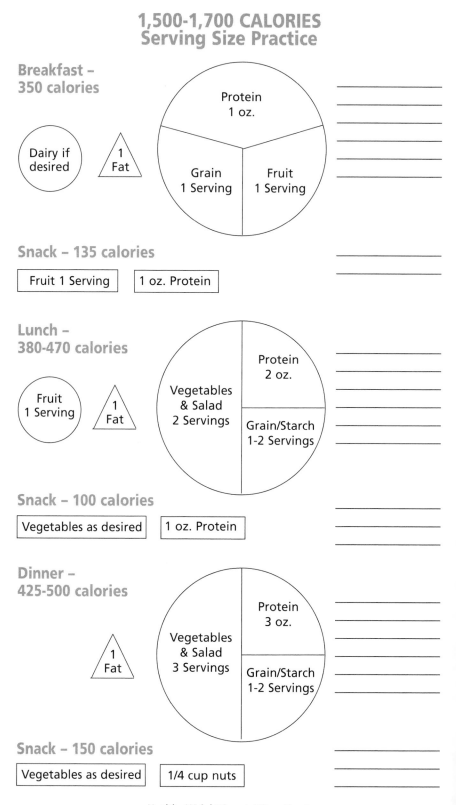

•For 1,500 calories, choose the smaller servings or calories when a range is given.

•For 1,700 calories, choose the higher calorie or larger serving when a range is given.

Dairy:
•May take a calcium supplement.

•May substitute soy or rice milk for dairy.

•If desired replace a grain/starch serving with milk.

•See Page 221 for calcium-rich foods.

**Breakfast –
350 calories**

Dairy if desired

1 Fat

Protein 1 oz.

Grain 1 Serving

Fruit 1 Serving

Snack – 135 calories

Fruit 1 Serving

1 oz. Protein

**Lunch –
380-470 calories**

Fruit 1 Serving

1 Fat

Protein 2 oz.

Vegetables & Salad 2 Servings

Grain/Starch 1-2 Servings

Snack – 100 calories

Vegetables as desired

1 oz. Protein

**Dinner –
425-500 calories**

1 Fat

Protein 3 oz.

Vegetables & Salad 3 Servings

Grain/Starch 1-2 Servings

Snack – 150 calories

Vegetables as desired

1/4 cup nuts

If Keeping A Journal Is Not Working

If you are not losing weight by keeping a food journal, then start writing down the calories for the food you are eating. Total it up at the end of the day, and compare that to Daily Calorie Allowance for Weight Loss which you calculated on Page 15.

Keep a running total. When you have a total of 3,500 calories less than what you need to maintain your weight, you will have lost a pound of body fat. What your scale says may not always reflect that since water fluctuations and the weight of muscle is not separated from fat weight.

Electronic Logs For Tracking Calories

An alternative to the pen and paper method is to use electronic logs. You can create a spreadsheet to track this information. There are free Web-based food journals such as the one at www.mypyramidtracker.gov or www.fitday.com. You may also purchase software for your computer or PDA.

Additional Resources

Seek out the help of a registered nutrition professional if you have difficulty making sense of your food records or are stuck as to how to fix problem areas you've identified.

Arm yourself with books that promote healthy ways to lose weight. The following are books you may find helpful:

❖ *Mindless Eating, Why We Eat More Than We Think* by Brian Wansink, Ph.D. (October 2006)
❖ *Eat, Drink and Weigh Less* by Mollie Katzen and Walter Willett, MD. Hyperion Books. First edition, (April 11, 2006)
❖ *The EatingWell Diet* by Jean Harvey-Berino, Joyce Hendley and the editors of *EatingWell* (April 16, 2007)
❖ *The Beck Diet Solution* (workbook also available) by Judith S. Beck, Ph.D. (2007)

Online Weight Loss

Divided into 64 lessons that you complete in 16 weeks. You will learn to develop your own personal plan at www.healthyweight4life.net.

National Weight Control Registry

To try to understand what works, the National Weight Control Registry gathers data on individuals who have maintained at least a 30 pound weight loss for at least one year. Researchers tracked more than 5,000 successful losers. There was not a common diet they followed, although the majority used diet and exercise together to lose the weight. The dieters shared these common strategies to keep their weight off:

❖ Eight out of 10 ate breakfast daily.
❖ They paid attention to total calories, no matter where they come from.
❖ They weighed themselves at least once a week. They had a plan of what they would do if the scale reached a certain number.
❖ They spent 2,500 calories for women and 3,300 calories for men per week in moderate physical activity.

BOTTOM LINE

Even small losses of 10 pounds, or a 5- to 10- percent loss of initial body weight, will decrease your risk for heart disease. Work toward a lifestyle you can stick to and that fits your lifestyle.

QUIZ ANSWERS

Fat Quiz (Page 66)
1. Olive, canola
2. True
3. False. Moderate in fat is best
4. False. They are still high in calories and high heat breaks down oils and may contain the toxin HNE.
5. In the cupboard
6. True
7. False. No amount is healthy
8. corn, soybean, safflower, grapeseed, sunflower
9. Saturated
10. Monounsaturated

Saturated Fat, Meat, Poultry Quiz (Page 82)
1. Cheddar with 6 grams saturated fat (Ounce of prime rib beef has 4 grams saturated fat; ounce of salmon has less than 1 gram saturated fat.).
2. False. 3 oz. salmon has 1 gram saturated fat.
3. Beef, pork, veal, lamb
4. True
5. Round and loin (sirloin) are the leanest cuts.
6. False. Meat, even the leanest, should not be more than 1/4 of your plate.
7. False. Organic has nothing to do with feeding grass and is typically fed organic grains
8. Hormones
9. False. Natural has nothing to do with what the chickens are fed.
10. True
11. False. The brining process adds sodium to the flesh.
12. True
13. Poultry

Trans Fat Quiz (Page 88)
1. False. They may still have up to a half gram.
2. True
3. True
4. False
5. False. Some have trans fats.
6. False. They have saturated fat which should be eaten in moderation.
7. True
8. False. They may be low or high in saturated fats, check the nutrition labels.
9. True
10. Oat bran muffin, donuts, fish sticks, oatmeal cookies, wheat crackers, granola bars, whole-wheat bread, popcorn.

Cholesterol Quiz (Page 91)
1. True
2. True
3. Animals
4. False
5. Chicken breast, hot dog, skim milk
6. False
7. 200 mg
8. True
9. What your body makes
10. True

Fish Quiz (Page 102)
1. False
2. True
3. False. It is EPA and DHA from fish oil that is FDA approved.
4. All except salmon
5. True
6. False. Smoked fish have less omega-3 and are high in sodium.
7. True. Buy canned with no salt added if you want lower sodium.
8. False. But farmed is higher in PCBs which are suspected to cause cancer.
9. True. Unless you buy troll-caught albacore tuna, which is lower in mercury.
10. True

Fish Oil Supplement Quiz (Page 108)
1. False. Only part of fish oil is EPA and DHA, so you will need more than one capsule with most brands.
2. True
3. False. Only a small amount of flax is converted into EPA and DHA.
4. True. Check www.consumerlab.com for more recent information.
5. False. Cod liver oil may contain too much vitamin A if taken in the amounts needed for cholesterol benefits.
6. True
7. False. They are safe to take with all drugs other than *Coumadin,* which may require a decrease in dose.
8. False
9. True for those with heart disease.
10. True

Flaxseed Quiz (Page 118)
1. True
2. d) milled or ground flax
3. False
4. b) frozen and c) refrigerated
5. False. The oil is fragile and should not be heated.
6. False. Omega-3 in whole flaxseed remains intact even after baking.
7. False. There is no difference.

Flaxseed Quiz (Continued)

8. False. While that is ideal, it may be ground and stored in the refrigerator or freezer for three months.
9. True
10. True

Nut Quiz (Page 124)

1. False. If weight management is a goal, they must be eaten in a moderate amount like all foods.
2. c) 1-1/2 ounces
3. True
4. c) walnuts
5 a) almonds
6. c) frozen up to a year
7. True
8. c) However, peanuts cannot be eaten raw.
9. a) almonds, c) hazelnuts, e) peanuts, f) pecans, h) pistachios, i) walnuts, j) some pine nuts
10. False. Although some are high in calories.

Soluble Fiber Quiz (Page 141)

1. True
2. b) oats, d) psyllium, e) barley pilaf
3. False
4. True
5. True
6. False
7. True
8. False
9. True
10. False

Whole-Grain Quiz (Page 150)

1. True
2. True. There is no established amount of whole grains that must be in a product for it to make the statement "made with whole grains,"

3. Answer B is correct. Although Choice A has more fiber, it includes refined flour. Choice B is made entirely with whole grains.
4. False. There are gluten-free whole grains such as brown rice, quinoa, wild rice, teff, etc.
5. f) steel-cut oats
6. False. Organic means the grain was grown without conventional pesticides, artificial fertilizers, sewage, sludge or human waste. Organic grains may be whole or refined into white flour.
7. False. A grain that has been separated and then parts added is not nutritionally the same as an intact grain.
8. False. Rye does not contain as much gluten as wheat so white flour is often added to give it the same texture as wheat breads. If the bread lists whole rye as the only ingredient, it will be a dense loaf with little if any rise.
9. d) woven wheat cracker
10. b) quinoa

Beans & Legumes Quiz (Page 156)

1. True
2. True
3. False. They are high in fiber, making them a low-glycemic food.
4. False. There are canned with no added salt varieties or they may be drained and rinsed to remove some of the sodium.
5. False. The added sugars make them a less desirable choice.

6. True. Peas are one of the few members of the legume family that are cooked as fresh vegetables.
7. True
8. False. It should be taken at the same time you eat the beans.
9. True. A half banana has 200 mg and beans average 310 mg.
10. True

Soy Quiz (Page 161)

1. True
2. False. Taking isoflavones supplements is not recommended.
3. True
4. False. There is little to support the idea that fermented soy is different.
5. a) soy milk, d) soy nuts, f) tempeh
6. b) soy crumbles to replace ground beef
7. True
8. True
9. True
10. True

Carbohydrates & Sugars Quiz (Page 176)

1. b) apple, c) 100% whole-wheat bread, e) broccoli
2. True
3. True
4. True
5. c) cannot be assigned a value since they have no carbohydrates.
6. False. All carbohydrates, if more than 5 grams per serving, "count."
7. True
8. True. Do not assume that organic contain no HFCS .
9. True
10. True

11. False
12. False. Sugar alcohols have half the calories.
13. False
14. True

Sodium Quiz (Page 187)
Higher sodium choice listed first:
1. a) chicken 410, olives 190
2. a) soup 810, pickle 330
3. b) bran muffin 320, french fries 190
4. a) bread 320, peanuts 230
5. a) macaroni and cheese 750, ham 480
6. a) bran flakes 460, bacon 290

Blood Pressure Quiz (Page 196)
1. True
2. True
3. True
4. b) less than 120 systolic and less than 80 diastolic
5. False. Fish oil lowers blood pressure.
6. True
7. a) 4-5 servings of vegetables 4-5 servings of fruit daily.
8. False
9. True
10. All are correct

Beverage Quiz (Page 202)
1. False
2. False. It is the same.
3. True
4. False. It can raise blood pressure.
5. True. Paper filters remove the chemicals.
6. True
7. False. The best source is freshly brewed tea.
8. True. It has twice as much as red wine and three times as much as green tea.
9. d) all are true

10. False. One for women and two for men.
11. False. Alcohol raises HDL but also raises triglycerides.

Vitamin K Quiz (Page 210)
1. True
2. False. Not all are high and only those very high in vitamin K need to be limited, not avoided.
3. a) cooked leafy greens
4. True
5. True
6. True
7. True
8. True
9. False

Vitamin/Mineral Quiz (Page 222)
1. False
2. f) all of the above
3. False. Most have very small amounts of herbs that will do little to provide benefits.
4. False
5. False. High intake increases risk for bone fractures.
6. True
7. True
8. False. We have conflicting evidence.
9. False. It is a well-absorbed form.
10. False. Additional iron is not recommended.

Supplements Quiz (Page 234)
1. False. FDA does not regulate supplements.
2. b) sterols
3. True
4. True
5. True
6. False. No-flush niacin does not work in humans.
7. False. It does not lower cholesterol.
8. False. It does not work.

9. False. FDA prohibits red yeast products from having lovastatin, which it considers a drug.

Niacin Quiz (Page 240)
1. b) niacin
2. b) niacin
3. True
4. True
5. True
6. False. Flushing for most will diminish with time
7. d) all of the above

Dining Out Quiz (Page 250)
1. False. Fried foods are still high in calories and fat.
2. False. Broth based may be low fat but high sodium.
3. d) all of the above
4. False.
5. False. Buffets tend to encourage overeating.
6. True
7. a) Egg white omelet with vegetables, lean ham, no cheese
8. b) Small roast beef sandwich
9. c) Petite beef tenderloin steak. Adding cream and cheese to chicken and vegetables makes them less healthy options.

Physical Activity Quiz (Page 262)
1. False. It is heart healthy and one of the best things, even without any change in cholesterol.
2. True
3. False. 30 minutes is the minimum needed.
4. b) 100
5. True
6. d) all of the above
7. c) 60
8. b) 1,000 to 2,000
9. True

RECIPES

he recipes that follow have been taste tested by family, friends and individuals who have attended cooking classes and cooking demos. I included the ones that most people found enjoyable, and I hope some of them become your favorites as well.

NUTRITION FACTS: The *Food Processor Software* by ESHA research was used to analyze recipes. If data for nutrients was missing especially soluble fiber and omega-3, that information was added from other sources, such as the USDA nutrient data base. Only the added sugars are listed, not the grams of sugar that exist naturally in foods, such as the natural sugars in fruit, dairy or grains.

Some of the ingredients specify brand names and are explained in the notes with the recipe. A summary of ingredients is also provided below. A large, well-stocked grocery store will have most of the items. A few might require a trip to a local health food store or a chain, such as *Trader Joe's* or *Whole Foods*. When brand names are suggested, they were used to determine the nutritional analysis. There may be other brands that would be similar in the stores where you shop. If you substitute another brand, it may change the nutritional analysis. In some recipes, the use of no-salt-added ingredients, along with a small amount of sea salt, resulted in better tasting, lower sodium dishes than if regular canned-with-salt items had been used and the salt omitted.

INGREDIENTS

- **Butter/Margarine.** Use extra-virgin olive oil, expeller-pressed canola oil or high oleic safflower oil when possible instead of margarine or shortening. If you want the flavor of butter, try using a teaspoon or two for flavor. In baking, use half butter and half oil, or use products that do not have partially hydrogenated oils and do not use the process of "interesterification." These include *Smart Balance* (regular tubs or sticks work best for baking) and *Earth Balance* (found in health food stores). The light versions have air and water whipped into them and work best as a spread for table use instead of cooking.

- **Bouillon/Broth.** Paste-type bouillon bases have better flavor than dry, granular types. Some are high in sodium. There are very low sodium types which don't have much flavor. The solution is to use the best flavored ones in half or one-third of the amount suggested on the container. This reduces the sodium but allows for plenty of flavor. For example, *Organic Better Than Bouillon Chicken Base* or *Penzeys Spices' Chicken Base* has good flavor even

OIL TIP

See Page 63 for explanation of expeller-pressed oils.

when used in half the recommended amount. This reduces sodium to 375 mg per cup. *Imagine Low-Sodium Vegetable Broth*, 140 mg sodium per cup, sold in aseptic boxes, is another option if you want a ready-to-use product. If your diet requires very low sodium, dry cubes such as *Rapunzel No Salt Added* has 65 mg per cup of prepared broth. *Organic Gourmet Low Sodium* has 133 mg sodium in 1 cup prepared.

- **Bread Crumbs.** Make your own from leftover dried pieces of bread, or start with fresh bread, such as 100% whole-wheat bread (one made from sprouted grain if possible). Pulse in a food processor until broken into crumbs. Then, bake in 250°F oven to dry out (stir after 10 minutes) and continue to bake until dry. If you have time, air dry instead of baking. Spread crumbs on a pan, cover with a paper towel or dish towel. Allow to dry several days. When dry, place in food processor and process into fine crumbs. Store leftover crumbs in freezer. If you want to purchase ready-to-use crumbs try *Ian's Whole Wheat Panko Bread Crumbs*.

- **Cake Mixes.** *Bob's Red Mill Cake Mix* has whole wheat as the first ingredient. Use in moderation; it is not a low-sugar item as is true with all cakes unless artificial sugars are used. *Dr. Oetker Organics Cake Mixes* do not have partially hydrogenated fats in them but are not whole wheat.

- **Cheese.** Fat-free cheese tends to have little taste and higher sodium. Try half the amount the recipe suggests, or choose a cheese made from 2% milk or part-skim milk, often labeled as reduced fat. *Cabot* makes a reduced-fat cheddar cheese with 75% less fat that has good flavor and works well in cooking. It can be purchased on their Web site. *Cabot* also has a 50% *Reduced-Fat Cheddar Cheese*. Swiss cheese is often the lowest in sodium, but Baby Swiss is not low in sodium.

- **Cottage Cheese.** In recipes, use 1% low-fat, no-salt-added cottage cheese. You will not notice the lack of salt when combined with other ingredients. You can add additional herbs and seasoning for flavor if desired.

- **Cocoa.** Use natural. Dutched has been treated with alkali, destroying some of the flavanoids, which are compounds that provide health benefits in cocoa and chocolate. See Page 436 for information on chocolate.

- **Creamer.** Choose products that do not have partially hydrogenated fat or high fructose corn syrup in the ingredient list. Many fat free products have those ingredients. One option is soy creamers such as *White Wave Silk Creamer*. Another option is to use 2% milk.

- **Date Sugar.** It is made from finely ground dates. It can be substituted for brown sugar. It does not dissolve as well, and can make some items grainy.

- **Eggs.** Free-range eggs from a local source are ideal. If buying at the store, choose eggs that are omega-3 enriched. Special diets fed to the chicken increase the omega-3 content in brands such as *Gold Circle Farms* or *Eggland*.

- **Edamame (ay-duh-MAH-may).** Immature green soybeans. Often found in frozen section, shelled or still in pods. Some require cooking while others are ready to eat.

- **Ground Meat (meatless).** Soy meat products such as *Morningstar Farms Meal Starters Recipe Crumbles*, *Lightlife Gimme Lean* or *Quorn Grounds* (meatless and soy free) are easy to use products which can replace ground meat. Look for them in the frozen or refrigerated sections of the store.

- **Ketchup.** Choose an organic brand to avoid high fructose corn syrup.

- *Lundberg* **Rice.** This brand has several different varieties of brown rice and wild rice blends. If unavailable, combine brown and wild rice.

- **Mayonnaise.** Check the ingredients and avoid those with high fructose corn syrup. Brands to look for include: *Ojai Cook Lemonaise Light, Smart Balance Omega*; *Spectrum Light*; *Trader Joe's Light Mayonnaise*; *Kraft Mayo With Olive Oil, Reduced Fat*; or *Nayonaise*.

- **Mustard.** There are mustards with no sodium such as *East Shore Sweet and Tangy* or *Westbrae Natural Stoneground Mustard, No Salt Added*.

- **Nuts (toasted).** Store nuts in freezer. Toast nuts for deeper, richer flavor so you can use less. If toasting a small amount, use a dry pan over medium heat, stirring until slightly golden. Set aside in a separate dish to avoid heat from the pan which would continue to cook the nuts. If toasting a larger amount, set the oven or toaster oven at 275°F. Spread nuts on a pan in a single layer. Use whole pieces, as small or chopped pieces tend to burn easily. Watch carefully as they should take only 10 to 15 minutes to become golden. If they get too dark, they will not taste good. It is best to buy nuts without any added salt or fats. To remove salt from nuts, drop them into boiling water for a couple minutes, stir and drain. Spread nuts on a pan, and dry in a 200°F oven about 15 to 20 minutes.

- **Oils.** Extra-virgin olive oil, organic or expeller-pressed canola oil or high oleic safflower oil are preferred. It is best not to use high heat; instead use medium or medium-high heat to avoid breaking down oils. See Page 63.

- **Pasta.** Whole wheat listed as the first ingredient is preferred. Some brands have ground flaxseed added. Start with thin varieties such as angel hair or rotini, which are less chewy and dense than penne or lasagna. Try brands such as *Hodgson Mills*, *Bella Terra Racoonto*, *Bionature* and *Vita Spelt*.

MAYO TIP

- Choose a mayonnaise that is made with canola or olive oil.

- Fat free may be higher in added sugars and salt.

PASTA TIP

Durum wheat is a species of wheat that is high in protein and gluten, which makes it ideal for pasta. Choose 100% whole durum.

Semolina is coarsely ground endosperm of durum wheat. May also be called durum semolina. It is not whole wheat unless the word *whole* is stated as in whole-wheat durum semolina.

- **Parmesan Cheese.** Buy a chunk and grate as you need it for the best flavor. You won't need much to add a lot of flavor. Skip the cheese sauce and add a light sprinkle of freshly grated Parmesan to vegetables to save 30 calories for every tablespoon. See Page 390.

- **Rice.** Instead of white rice, choose brown. It takes longer to cook but has more minerals and fiber. To cook rice on stove top, bring 2 cups of water to a boil, add rice, then drop temperature to a simmer and cover tightly. Cook 45 minutes without peeking or stirring. Remove from heat and let set 10 minutes. A rice cooker or steamer is another option.

- **Roasted Red Peppers.** These can be purchased in jars, or make your own according to the recipe on Page 355.

- **Salmon.** Canned, wild salmon is an economical source of omega-3 fats. If you cannot find it in a store near you, canned, no-salt-added, wild Alaskan salmon is available at www.vitalchoice.com

- **Salsa.** Sodium varies widely. *Frog Ranch Salsa* has 40 mg sodium in 2 tablespoons.

- **Soups.** The best are the ones you make. If buying them canned or boxed, avoid ones with high fructose corn syrup or partially hydrogenated fat. Choose those that are lower in sodium. One of the lowest sodium canned soups that still tastes good is *Amy's Light In Sodium*. Butternut squash, cream of tomato, and chunky tomato bisque can be thickened with arrowroot or cornstarch to make into a quick sauce. *Trader Joe's Low-Sodium Roasted Red Pepper* and *Tomato* is also great. *Pacific Foods* is another good brand.

- **Soy Sauce or Tamari.** Look for a reduced-sodium variety and use sparingly to keep sodium reasonable. Some brands of tamari are wheat free.

- **Spices and Seasonings.** A wonderful source of flavor in healthy cooking comes from herbs and spices and using salt sparingly. Any plain herb or spice can be used. A great mail-order source is *Penzeys Spices* at www.penzeys.com. Check the salt free section on their Web site if you want more than a single spice or herb.
  - **Aleppo Pepper.** It has more heat than chili powder but less than crushed red peppers with cumin-like undertones. It is available from *Penzeys Spices.*
  - **Lemon pepper.** A salt free variety such as *Penzeys Spices' Sunny Spain.*
  - **Salt.** When cooking, buy fresh, frozen or no-salt-added ingredients, and add small amounts of sea salt that has not been refined and still contains minerals, such as *Redmond Real Salt.* Some sea salts are highly refined.

- *Pleasoning Mini-Mini Salt.* This has no potassium and only 110 mg of sodium. It is a good choice for use at the table if you need to follow a very low sodium diet that is also low in potassium. It is available from www.pleasoning.com.
- *Veg-It* and *Spike Salt Free.* These work to add additional flavoring when using smaller amounts of salt. They work best when added to foods during cooking.

- **Sun-Dried Tomatoes.** If soft, they do not need soaking. You can chop by pulsing them in a food processor. If sundried tomatoes are dry and hard, rehydrate them by covering them with 1/2 cup boiling water and allowing them to stand 10 minutes. Reserve the soaking liquid to use in the recipe to replace another liquid or use to sauté vegetables.

- **Stevia.** Several different companies make stevia. The quality, flavor and sweetness varies. Some companies combine pure stevia powder with inulin, maltodextrin, erythritol or another filler. These are sweet but not as sweet as the pure powder, so the amount needed will vary. Try several different brands and choose what you like best. If you use too much, it will be excessively sweet with an aftertaste. Mixing stevia with sugar or other sweeteners is a good way to start to reduce the amount of sweeteners you use while learning how to bake with stevia. Stevia is also available as a liquid with a dropper to measure quantity.

- **Tomatoes.** Choose canned tomatoes with no-salt-added when fresh are not in season.

- **Tofu.** For firm tofu, use the basic preparation method from Page 395. Once prepared, you can add it to recipes to replace strips or pieces of chicken or meat for a meatless version. For silken tofu, use brand such as *Mori-Nu.*

SPROUTED GRAIN

Sprouting a grain produces more slowly absorbed sugars, lowers the glycemic index and increases the vitamins, minerals and the protein quality.

- **Tortillas.** Choose whole-grain varieties that do not contain any partially hydrogenated oils. Brands such as *La Tortilla Factory Smart and Delicious Low-carb High Fiber* or sprouted-wheat varieties such as *Alvarado Street, Food for Life* or *French Meadow Fat Flush* are recommended. Choose sprouted grain if possible.

- **Tuna.** Look for troll-caught varieties. Canned, troll-caught albacore tuna contains about one-third the mercury and four times more omega-3 than conventional canned albacore and is fished in a sustainable manner. Brands such as *Mary Lu Seafoods* (www.maryluseafoods.com) are troll caught. If you cannot find a similar product, substitute wild, canned salmon or canned mackerel for tuna.

- **Whey Protein.** This is a dry powder, usually plain, vanilla or chocolate flavored that is made from cow's milk. The powder has very little carbohydrate or fat. Look for it anywhere supplements are sold.

- **Whole-Wheat Pastry Flour.** Use instead of white flour. For more information, see Page 319.

- **Worcestershire Sauce.** Choose an organic brand, such as *Annie's,* which does not use high fructose corn syrup. While high in sodium, a small amount can add flavor without exceeding your sodium allowance.

- **Yogurt.** Avoid those that have sugars added or use artificial sweeteners. Greek yogurt has been drained and is thick, with a rich flavor. It is lower in carbohydrates and higher in protein than other yogurts. The first choice is *FAGE Total 0%* Greek Yogurt. Another is *Oikos Organic 0% fat Greek Yogurt.* Any plain nonfat yogurt is a good choice. If you find the nonfat too tangy, try *Stonyfield Low-Fat Plain Yogurt.* It has a little less saturated fat than other brands of low-fat yogurt and is less tangy..

- **Yogurt Cheese.** This is a way to make your own "Greek-like" yogurt. Start with plain yogurt. Place yogurt into a mesh strainer lined with a paper coffee filter or cheesecloth. To thicken, let it drain, covered, in the refrigerator. The longer it drains, the thicker it becomes. After 24 hours, it will be thick enough to spread.

TIPS FOR BEING SUCCESSFUL WITH A RECIPE

Before you start do the following.

1. Read through the recipe so you have an understanding of what is needed and the steps involved.
2. Assemble all the tools and prepare all ingredients required for the recipe before starting to cook.
3. If chopping, place a wet cloth under the cutting board to prevent its movement on the counter.
4. Fill your sink with hot, soapy water, and clean up as you go.
5. To make a double recipe, simply measure the ingredient twice. For example, if you need 1/3 cup of chopped tomatoes, add two 1/3 cups of chopped tomatoes.

HELPFUL TOOLS AND EQUIPMENT

Some of the items you may find useful in your kitchen are listed below.

Box-Style Grater. Useful for grating Parmesan cheese and shredding vegetables such a carrots. See Mandolin and Microplane grater on the next page.

Chef's Knife and Paring Knife. These are the two essential knifes you need. You can purchase a good quality knife for a reasonable price from *Forschner/Victorinox*. Another good quality but more expensive brand is *Wusthof*.

Coffee Grinder. Useful for grinding whole flaxseed and spices.

Food Processor. This will allow you to chop nuts, make sauces and puree a variety of ingredients quickly.

Freezer. Having a separate freezer will allow you to stock up on bargains. It will also allow you to prepare foods in large batches when you have the time to cook. Portion food into the size you need and store in the freezer for quick meals. It is also a great place to store whole grains and nuts. Freezers come in a variety of sizes. Buy one that is right for your needs.

Ginger Grater. Allows you to quickly grate fresh ginger root. Choose one with a ceramic grating surface and rubber base to grip the counter. To remove the peel from ginger root, gently scrape with a knife or a serrated grapefruit spoon to remove the thin skin. To preserve ginger root, place the peeled root in a jar and cover completely with vodka or rice wine vinegar.

Handheld Blender. These blenders can be placed into foods, such as a pot of soup, rather than transporting foods to a blender container.

Mandolin Slicer. Allows you to make thin, uniform slices of vegetables and fruits.

Microplane Graters. Originally a wood working tool, this has become a useful kitchen tool. There are a variety of sizes. The fine-grind style can be used for zesting peel from citrus or grating ginger, nutmeg and chocolate.

Mortar and Pestle. Helpful to grind fennel and crack rosemary into smaller pieces.

Oil Pump Sprayer. A nonaerosol spray pump that is pressurized by pumping the cap. It allows you to spray a mist of any oil you prefer. Some are easily clogged. The *MISTO Oil Sprayer* has provided the best results.

Pans. A skillet/fry and sauté pan can be interchangeable. The basic differences are:
- A skillet or fry pan has sloped sides to allow for easy turning. They often do not have a lid.
- A sauté pan has 90 degree (square) edges from the bottom to side, along with deeper sides. They come with lids. The pan works best for braising or those recipes that have liquids or require covering. Compared to a skillet they have a little more flat cooking surface for the same size pan.

Nonstick Pans. These are not great for your health or the environment. Stick to stainless steel or cast iron. If you have always cooked with nonstick, spend some time relearning to cook without it. To do this, preheat the pan on medium about 2 minutes and keep heat medium. If browning food such a meat, chicken or tofu, add a bit of oil to the food itself rather than into the pan. Next, place the oiled food in the preheated pan and allow to cook without attempting to move it for 3 to 4 minutes. This is the hard part, as most people like to push or move the food. Be patient and turn only at the end to allow the item to brown and then release from the pan. *Cybernox Sitram* has a stick-resistant stainless steel pan (not coated) that when seasoned works well for most foods. It is not as stick resistant as nonstick pans, but it is better than regular stainless steel.

Rice Cooker. These can range from inexpensive to pricey, depending upon the features they have. The most basic model will allow cooking rice or any grain easily.

Rubber Mallet. The type you find in a hardware store with a black rubber head attached to a wooden handle works well for pounding meat thinly without tearing. It also works well to split squash as you tap a cleaver or the back of a knife with the mallet.

Zester. A handheld tool that allows the removal of the outside rind of citrus, removing the flavorful colored part and leaving the white bitter part behind. See Microplane Grater above.

SAFE COOKING TEMPERATURES:

Do not rely on color or other methods for determining if food is cooked. A thermometer is much more reliable.

Safe Temperatures for Beef, Lamb, Veal
Cook roasts and steaks to an internal temperature of at least 145°F (63°C). For medium cook to 160°F (71°C), well done to 170°F (77°C).

Safe Temperatures for Pork; Ground Beef, Ground Pork, Ground Veal, Ground Lamb; Injected Meat
Cook to 160°F (71°C).

Safe Temperatures for Poultry (including Ground Poultry)
Cook to 165°F (74°C).

Safe Temperatures for Fish
Cook until fish flakes or reaches 145°F (63°C). However, remove fish from the heat when it reaches 130°F (54°C), as it continues to cook off the heat. This prevents overcooked, dry fish.

SAFE TEMPERATURES
Egg dishes
160°F (71°C).

Casseroles and leftovers
165°F (74°C).

VEGETABLE PREPARATION

Asparagus. Hold each stalk in one hand and use the other to snap off the bottom. It will naturally break where it becomes tough. Not all pieces will be uniform, but they will all be edible.

Broccoli and Cauliflower. Break off florets and cut into desired size. Peel and dice the stalk if desired.

Bell Pepper. Cut bell pepper in half, remove and discard top stems and inside white veins and seeds.

Beets. The entire beet plant is edible. Remove the stalks and leaves, and wash well to remove dirt. The unpeeled bulbs can be wrapped in foil and baked or boiled in a pot of water. Slip off the skins after they are cooked and cooled, then cut into pieces. Remove stalks from leaves and cut into 1-inch pieces. Sauté stalks with a little oil until almost tender, and then add the leaves that have been cut into strips. Toss with vinaigrette from Page 371.

Bok Choy. Separate leaf from stalk and slice or chop into chunks. Stir-fry stems for a few minutes before adding leaves, which cook quickly.

Brussel Sprouts. Choose those that are tightly closed and without yellow or brown leaves. Cut off a thin slice from the bottom. Cut in half if large or cut an "X" into the base to speed cooking. They taste best when roasted.

Cucumber, Summer Squash, Zucchini. These have edible peels. Cut off the ends and then cut in half lengthwise. Lay on cutting board and slice across into uniform pieces.

Diced Onion. First, cut off the top end (not the bottom root end). Then peel off skin. Make crosswise cuts, almost to the bottom. Cut in half and lay the flat cut side down on a cutting board. Make cuts from the root end to the top, without cutting through the bottom root end. Slice across in the opposite direction for evenly diced onion.

Eggplant. The peel is edible. Eggplant is always cooked to eliminate a toxic substance that exists only in the raw form. Recipes often call for salting, but this is not necessary.

Fennel. It makes a good substitute for celery. It can be eaten raw or grilled, roasted, stir-fried or steamed. It has a woody core that can be cut out after slicing. Remove any parts of the stalks that are woody. Use the feathery leaves like dill. Slice or dice the bulb.

Jicama. Use a paring knife to peel brown outer skin. Slice into pieces.

Kale, Collards, Turnip or Other Greens. Strip leaves from the stems. If stems are thin, they may be cooked and then the leaves added during the last few minutes. If woody, discard stems. See basic recipe, Page 363.

Parsnip or Rutabaga. Scrub well and eat peel unless they have been waxed, which will require peeling. They can be eaten raw or grated into a salad. They may also be steamed, roasted or baked.

Spaghetti Squash. Cut in half and remove seeds. Then microwave or bake until you can rake the flesh into spaghetti-like strings.

Squash, Butternut. This squash can be easily peeled with a sturdy peeler such as an *Oxo Peeler*. It makes an excellent substitute for canned pumpkin. It is also good pureed into a soup or cut in cubes and roasted.

Squash, Hubbard, Kabocha, Buttercup. Cut into pieces with a heavy chef's knife. Tapping the knife with a rubber mallet makes it easier to cut through the tough skin. Remove the seeds. Use a small, sharp paring knife to peel off skin. Alternatively, bake and scoop the cooked pulp from the peel.

EGGPLANT TIP

Eggplant has a tendency to soak up a lot of oil; therefore, it is best grilled or roasted after lightly brushing or spraying with olive oil.

A heart healthy diet should supply you with calories that are packed with nutrients, such as vitamins, minerals, phytochemicals and fiber. It should be enjoyable and fit your budget and your taste preferences. A wide variety of fresh, unprocessed foods, especially vegetables, is best. The following menus are a guide to help you design meal plans that work for you.

As you plan your menu, refer back to the diagram on Page 51 as a guide.

1. **Breakfast** can be the same every morning. If you like variety, rotate between two or three favorites. Use the weekends to make a batch of steel-cut oats, muesli or veggie egg muffins for the week so you can reheat and eat quickly.

2. **Pack your lunch** if you eat away from home. You are in control of what you are eating rather than relying on the usual unhealthy choices that are available. If you find mornings hectic, make your lunch for the next day BEFORE you go to bed. Make up baggies of raw, cut-up vegetables for several days at one time. Then your baggies are ready to grab and go the rest of the week.

   If you typically take sandwiches, rotate the fillings and think beyond deli meat and cheese sandwiches. Check out the recipe section for ideas. If you prefer hot food, plan to prepare extra at dinner so that you have leftovers for the next day. If you can get great salads out, you could take your own protein (legumes or leftover salmon) and dressing to add to them.

There is no menu that works for everyone, so change it to suit your needs.

For example, substitute a different vegetable based on what is in season or what you like.

3. What's for **dinner**? Think about what you will have for dinner the day before in case it requires you to thaw or prep items. It will also allow you to shop on your way home. Even better is to plan the entire week so you can shop once for the entire week. This may seem like a lot of work, but you will find that once you start doing it, your life will be less stressful and eating healthier will be easier as it takes less effort. You will save many hours a week not having to think about what to have for dinner or by having to make fewer trips to the store. The menu plans/ideas can be saved and used again.

Your Top 10. If you have 10 healthy recipes for your main meal, you will have enough for two weeks without repeating an item since you will probably have leftovers and perhaps eat out during that time. You may even want to take a day for trying out new recipes. You can modify favorites that you already have, or you can find 10 in the recipe section of this book. Once you have your top 10, you can add new ones, drop others or rotate them by season. For example, in the summer, your favorites might include salad main courses with grilled items. In the winter, it may include stews, soups and chili. Decide how much variety you like to have. For some families, eating the same thing every couple of weeks is fine, while others want more variety. Keep adding weeks of meal plans until you find the level of variety that works best for you.

Have a list of some simple, quick ideas that you can make when there is no time to cook. See Page 299 for some ideas

wheat free, lower-carbohydrate, low-glycemic, no refined grains menu plan

If you have high triglycerides, elevated blood sugars or are trying to lose weight, this sample meal plan is suggested.

	Day 1	Day 2	Day 3
Breakfast	♥ Veggie Egg Muffin (Page 309) ♥ Strawberries ♥ Water or tea	♥ Yogurt parfait, layer the following in a dish: • Greek yogurt, *Fage Total 0%* or low-fat plain yogurt • Toasted Grain Granola (Page 316) • Ground flaxseed • Berries	♥ Smoothie, whey protein powder mixed with water ♥ Nectarine ♥ Water or Tea
Snack	♥ 1/4 cup walnuts ♥ Apple ♥ Water	♥ 1/3 cup dry-roasted soy nuts ♥ Orange ♥ Water	♥ 1 ounce raw or dry-roasted almonds ♥ String cheese ♥ Water
Lunch	♥ Creamy Vegetable Soup (Page 347) ♥ 1 kiwifruit ♥ Water	♥ Garden Salad (Page 369) topped with • Salad Dressing (Page 371) and pieces of • Grilled chicken, leftover salmon or tempeh ♥ Water	♥ Cottage cheese, 1%, no-salt-added, topped wit • 1/2 cup crushed pineapple canned in juice ♥ Raw vegetables (broccoli, cauliflower, grape tomato bell pepper, cucumber) dipped into • Hummus (Page 428) ♥ Water
Snack	♥ Low-fat string cheese ♥ Raw veggies (baby carrots, pea pods, grape tomato, etc.) ♥ Water	♥ Celery sticks or broccoli stalks dipped into • 1 tablespoon almond butter ♥ Water	♥ Hard-cooked egg ♥ Baby carrots and grape tomatoes ♥ Water
Dinner	♥ Walnut-Crusted Salmon (Page 410) (*note: replace bread crumbs with more walnuts*) ♥ Kale (Page 375) ♥ Sweet Potato Fries (Page 366) ♥ Salad and dressing ♥ Water	♥ Chicken Beany Burger (Page 408) ♥ Sage Green Beans With Walnuts (Page 357) ♥ Ginger-Roasted Carrots (Page 357) ♥ Water	♥ Garden Salad (Page 369) topped with steamed or grilled shrimp ♥ Cut-up fruit with Chocolate Sauce (Page 437) ♥ Water

7-DAY MENU PLAN (no wheat or refined grains)

Day 4	Day 5	Day 6	Day 7
♥ Breakfast Quinoa (Page 314) ♥ Mixed berries ♥ Water or Tea	♥ Salmon Beef Burger (Page 406) or purchase *Shelton Free-Range*, or *Jennie-O All-Natural Turkey Burgers* ♥ Strawberries ♥ Water or Tea	♥ Scrambled Egg (Page 307) ♥ Turkey Sausage (Page 310) ♥ Peach slices or half grapefruit ♥ Water or Tea	♥ Omelet with veggies, such as asparagus, mushrooms, bell pepper (Page 307) ♥ Pear slices ♥ Water or Tea
♥ 1 ounce raw or dry-roasted nuts (almond, soy, walnut, etc.) ♥ Pear or papaya slices ♥ Water	♥ 1 ounce raw or dry-roasted nuts (almond, soy, walnut, etc.) ♥ Kiwi or mango ♥ Water	♥ 1 ounce raw or dry-roasted nuts (almond, soy, walnut, etc.) ♥ Cantaloupe or watermelon ♥ Water	♥ 1 tablespoon natural peanut butter or almond butter spread on ♥ Apple slices ♥ Water
♥ Salmon Spread (Page 341) rolled up in lettuce leaf ♥ Broccoli and cauliflower with ♥ Garden Herbed Dip (Page 430) ♥ Water	♥ Leafy green salad topped with • Hard-cooked egg • Chopped walnuts • 1 tablespoon crumbled feta or blue cheese • 1 tablespoon Salad Dressing (Page 371) ♥ Water	♥ Portobello Mushroom Melt (Page 342) ♥ Raw veggies (broccoli, cauliflower, grape tomatoes, bell pepper, cucumber) ♥ Grapes ♥ Water	♥ Large tossed salad with • raw, chopped veggies • 1 tablespoon Salad Dressing (Page 371) topped with • Nutty Fruity Salmon (Page 338) ♥ Water
♥ Baby spinach with • 1 ounce turkey breast or boiled shrimp or string cheese • 1/2 tablespoon Vinaigrette Dressing (Page 371) ♥ Water	♥ Roasted Red Pepper Dip (Page 430) with ♥ 1 cup raw veggies (baby carrots, celery, kohlrabi, radishes, etc.) ♥ Water	♥ Apples with • Pumpkin Dip (Page 431) ♥ Water	♥ Hummus (Page 428) or bean dip with • 1 cup raw veggies (baby carrots, jicama, daikon, etc.) ♥ Water
♥ Spaghetti squash, with • Pasta Sauce (Page 388) • and ground soy crumbles or red lentils • Parmesan cheese ♥ Oven-Roasted Vegetables (Page 356) ♥ Water	♥ Poached Fish (Page 414) ♥ Spinach Parmesan (Page 364) ♥ Salad and dressing ♥ Water	♥ Vegetarian Chili (Page 383) ♥ Steamed broccoli ♥ Salad and dressing ♥ Water	♥ Chicken Rolls (Page 401) ♥ Roasted Vegetables (Page 354) ♥ Black Bean Salad (Page 378) ♥ Water

7-DAY MENU PLAN (with whole grains)

	Day 1	Day 2	Day 3
Breakfast	♥ Steel-Cut Oats (Page 312) topped with grated apple, cinnamon, chopped walnuts, ground flaxseed, skim or unsweetened soy or rice milk ♥ Hot Chocolate *Teecino* (Page 303)	♥ Breakfast Burrito To Go (Page 308) ♥ Orange slices ♥ 1 ounce Brazil nuts ♥ Water	♥ Fruity Cinnamon Rolled Oats With Oat Groats (Page 313) topped with nuts and milk ♥ Water

Snack	♥ Raw vegetables with
	  • Roasted Red Pepper and Bean Dip (Page 430)
	♥ Water
		♥ Raw vegetables with
		  • Spinach Dip (Page 431)
		♥ Water
			♥ Edamame, steamed
			♥ 1 ounce raw almonds
			♥ Water

Lunch	♥ Green Salad With Salmon And Vinaigrette Dressing (Page 377) ♥ Blueberry Walnut Bran Muffin (Page 322) ♥ Water	♥ Portobello Mushroom Melts (Page 342) ♥ Roasted asparagus spears ♥ Salad and dressing ♥ Water	♥ Creamy Vegetable Soup (Page 347) ♥ Sandwich Spread (Page 341) on 100% whole-wheat bread ♥ Water
Snack	♥ Hard-cooked egg ♥ Granola Bar (Page 426) ♥ Water	♥ Part-skim mozzarella stick ♥ 15 grapes ♥ Water	♥ Hummus (Page 428) ♥ Baby carrots ♥ Water
Dinner	♥ Lemon-Baked Tempeh (Page 397) ♥ Nutty Rotini (Page 335) ♥ Crumb-Topped, Oven-Roasted Vegetables (Page 356) ♥ Water	♥ Walnut-Crusted Salmon (Page 410) ♥ Quinoa Pilaf with Red and Yellow Peppers (Page 330) ♥ Summer Vegetable Medley (Page 360) ♥ Water	♥ Crispy Baked Fish (Page 413) ♥ Quick Multi-Grain Mix (Page 328) ♥ Sage Green Beans With Walnuts (Page 357) ♥ Salad and dressing ♥ Water

Menu Planning Smart 4 Your Heart

7-DAY MENU PLAN (with whole grains)

Day 4	Day 5	Day 6	Day 7
♥ Banana Blueberry Smoothie (Page 305) ♥ Pumpkin Maple Pecan Oat Bran Muffin (Page 321) ♥ Water	♥ *Fage Total 0% Yogurt* topped with • Muesli (Page 315) • Frozen mixed berries ♥ Water	♥ Cheese Toast (Page 317) ♥ Kiwi slices ♥ Water	♥ Cottage cheese with 1 tablespoon oat bran topped with ♥ Blueberries and a sprinkle of cinnamon ♥ Water
♥ Greek yogurt topped with chopped walnuts ♥ Orange slices ♥ Water	♥ Apple, sliced ♥ Pumpkin dip (Page 431) ♥ Heart Fuel Nutty Snack Mix (Page 427) ♥ Water	♥ Frozen grapes ♥ 1 ounce walnuts ♥ Water	♥ 1 ounce dark chocolate ♥ Water
♥ Grilled nut butter sandwich ♥ Green Salad with Dressing (Page 369) ♥ Water	♥ Cottage Cheese Spread (Page 339) on toasted sprouted-grain bread ♥ Roasted Vegetables (Page 354) ♥ Water	♥ Whole-Wheat Veggie Wrap (Page 343) ♥ Roasted Vegetables And Orzo (Page 334) served over green salad ♥ Water	♥ Parmesan Pesto Pizza (Page 346) ♥ Green Salad with dressing (Page 369) ♥ Water
♥ Steamed shrimp with 2 tablespoons organic ketchup mixed with 1 teaspoon horseradish ♥ Water	♥ Smoked salmon wrapped around cooked asparagus spear ♥ 1 ounce raw almonds ♥ Water	♥ Leftover cooked chicken ♥ 1 ounce raw pecans ♥ Zucchini Julienne with Lemon and Chives (Page 380) ♥ Water	♥ Leftover salmon or Nutty Fruity Salmon (Page 338) in pita pocket with spinach, tomato slices and sprouts ♥ Apple ♥ Raw, cut-up vegetables ♥ Water
♥ Oven–Fried Parmesan Chicken Nuggets (Page 404) ♥ Sweet Potato Fries (Page 366) ♥ Roasted asparagus ♥ Water	♥ Asian Chicken (Page 402) ♥ Wild Rice Spinach Salad (Page 374) ♥ Basic Kale (Page 363) ♥ Water	♥ Simply-Seasoned Grilled Salmon (Page 418) ♥ Broccoli Couscous (Page 333) ♥ Water	♥ Spinach Parmesan (Page 364) ♥ Chicken Beany Burgers (Page 408) ♥ Creamy Butternut Squash Sauce (Page 367) over ♥ Multi-Grain Mix (Page 327) ♥ Water

GENERAL PLANNING TIPS

- Eat breakfast every day.
- Eat every three to four hours to avoid extreme hunger.
- Have lean protein or healthy fats with every meal.
- Never eat carbohydrates alone, whether as a snack or meal.
- Include soluble fiber from flaxseed, oat bran or legumes daily.
- Fill half your plate with brightly colored vegetables.
- Drink mostly water or tea (green, white, red, herbal).
- Avoid processed foods with high fructose corn syrup, partially hydrogenated oil, artificial sweeteners, diet drinks, junk food and fried foods.
- Snack on real foods (vegetables, nuts, fruit) instead of packaged, processed, boxed, manufactured snack foods.
- Watch portions if weight loss is a goal.

QUICK BREAKFAST IDEAS

- Yogurt (plain low-fat), frozen berries, topped with flaxseed and chopped nuts
- Baked tofu (*White Wave, Wildwood, Soy Delicious*)
- Baked Lemon Tempeh (Page 397)
- Hard cooked eggs
- Veggie Egg Muffins (Page 309) (make ahead and freeze)
- Sliced apple spread with nut butter and chopped nuts
- Smoked salmon
- Sardines in mustard or tomato sauce
- Smoothie (Page 304-306)
- Whey protein powder, frozen mixed berries and soy or rice milk blended into a shake
- Steel-Cut Oats (Page 312) (reheat in microwave)
- Baked Steel Cut Oats (Page 312) or Baked Oatmeal (Page 315)
- Toasted sprouted-grain bread with a slice of veggie soy cheese or ricotta cheese
- Cottage cheese (nonfat or 1%) with frozen thawed berries
- Leftovers
- Cooked chicken or turkey breast

- **Pinto Beans and Rice:** Combine 2 cups leftover rice or Multi-Grain Mix (Page 327) with a can of drained and rinsed pinto beans and package of frozen mixed vegetables that have been thawed. Heat. Add leftover cooked chicken if desired.

- **Black Beans and Brown Rice:** Combine and heat a can of black beans drained and rinsed, 1/2 cup frozen corn, 1/2 cup salsa (or more if desired), 1/2 cup instant brown rice made according to package directions, and chipotle chili powder.

- **Stuffed Peppers:** Cut bell peppers in half and remove the stem, seeds and membrane. Add leftover black beans and rice from above and microwave until pepper is softened.

- **Pita Pocket Pizza:** Lay pita pocket (separate if you prefer a thinner crust) on baking sheet, spread with tomato sauce and, top with mozzarella cheese and leftover chopped vegetables. Bake 10 minutes at 375°F.

- **Tamale Pie:** Prepare *Bob's Red Mill Cornbread Mix*. Spread a can of *Amy's Light In Sodium Chili* in baking dish and drop cornbread on top. Sprinkle a few tablespoons of shredded reduced-fat cheddar on top and bake about 15 minutes.

- **Shephards Pie:** Mix a can of reduced-sodium chili or 2 cups leftover chili with 1 cup frozen mixed vegetables and place in baking dish. Microwave sweet potato, remove pulp, mash and place on chili mixture. Bake until warmed through.

- **Chili Sweet Potato:** Baked sweet potato topped with chili and low-fat sour cream or *Fage Total 0% Yogurt*.

- **Cheesy Sweet Potato:** Baked sweet potato topped with 1/4 cup nonfat or 1% cottage cheese, 2 tablespoons each salsa and black beans, 1 tablespoon frozen corn, and 1 tablespoon reduced-fat cheddar cheese. Microwave 1 minute or until cheese is melted.

- **Hummus Wrap:** Spread hummus on a whole-wheat tortilla, add any leftover vegetables or chopped raw vegetables, roll and eat.

- **Quick Soup:** Start with a can of reduced-sodium soup, add a can of drained and rinsed black beans (or your favorite bean such as northern, kidney or lentils), and 2 cups of frozen or leftover vegetables (mixed or stir-fry, etc). Add reduced-sodium broth to desired consistency.

- **Creamy Soup:** Cook peeled and diced carrots, sweet potatoes or butternut squash in enough reduced-sodium chicken broth to cover until tender. Add 1/2 package silken tofu and purée with immersion hand blender. Season with curry powder or grated fresh ginger or roasted garlic for whichever flavor you prefer.

- **Macaroni and Cheese:** Prepare box of whole-wheat macaroni and cheese, along with an extra cup of plain shell or macaroni pasta. While pasta is cooking, microwave frozen broccoli and chopped red bell peppers for a few minutes. Stir into cooked and drained macaroni, along with the cheese packet, adding about 1/4 cup of milk and a dollop of fat-free sour cream or plain low-fat yogurt.

- **Main Meal Salad:** Start with 2 to 3 cups of salad greens on each plate. Add canned tuna or salmon or baked tofu for protein and any vegetables you like, such as roasted red pepper, cucumber, bell pepper, tomatoes, mushrooms, shredded carrots, artichoke hearts, walnuts, feta cheese.

- **Quick Pasta Sauce:** Cook whole-wheat rotini or microwave spaghetti squash. Combine jar of pasta sauce with 1 can crushed, no-salt-added tomatoes; a tablespoon of red wine; 1/2 teaspoon Italian seasoning. Add 1 cup of frozen meatless crumbles such as *Morningstar Farms Meal Starter Recipe Crumbles,* if desired, and heat. Serve over pasta or squash.

- **Double-Baked Potatoes:** Microwave sweet potato, remove pulp to bowl and add for each potato, 1/2 cup low-fat cottage cheese, 2 tablespoons frozen cut-leaf spinach, and 1 tablespoon feta or grated Parmesan cheese. Mash together, put back into potato shell, and bake or microwave to heat.

- **Frozen Turkey Burger:** Cook *Shelton's Free-Range Turkey Burger* or *Jennie-O Turkey All Natural Burger* on an indoor grill and top it with a thin slice of reduced-fat, reduced-sodium Swiss cheese. Top with a dollop of salsa or chutney.

- **Meatless Burgers:** Choose from frozen food section brands such as *Bocca, Morningstar* Farms or *Dr. Praeger.* Cut into strips after cooked. Add salsa; corn; black beans; cooked, frozen, or stir-fried vegetables; and microwaved sweet potato that has been diced. Combine and serve in a pita pocket.

- **Veggie Burger Ideas:** Thaw in microwave about a minute, then heat in toaster to crisp outside slightly. Top with salsa (black bean and corn, peach, etc.), chutney, corn and chili relish, pesto, peanut or teriyaki sauce, or BBQ sauce. Then add some feta cheese, red onions, black olives, roasted red peppers, sliced avocado or hummus. The possibilities are endless.

- **Vegetarian Wrap:** Cook veggie burger, cut into strips. Saute fresh or frozen bell pepper strips. Heat a whole-wheat tortilla and top with burger, bell pepper and a spoonful of salsa. Roll up and eat.

- **Crock Pot Lasagna:** In four-quart crock pot, layer the following into three layers: 1 jar pasta sauce; 1/2 of an 8-ounce box no-boil, whole-wheat lasagna broken into large pieces; 1 cup low-fat ricotta and 1 cup reduced-fat mozzarella cheese. Cook on low for 3 to 4 hours. If desired, sprinkle top with 2 tablespoons Parmesan cheese.

- **Lemon Fish:** Squeeze juice from fresh lemon over fish fillet such as barramundi, cod, catfish, etc. Sprinkle with *Penzeys Spices' Sunny Spain* (salt-free lemon pepper). Spray fish with cooking spray and cook in sauté pan for about 5 minutes. Turn and cook the other side until it flakes.

- **Quick Baked Fish (from frozen):** Place a block of frozen fish in a shallow baking dish. Rub with oil and sprinkle with seasoning. Peel and cube a sweet potato, add to baking dish along with cubed bell pepper and zucchini. Rub or spray oil on the vegetables and spread out on the dish. Bake at 450°F. for 20 minutes or until fish flakes easily and vegetables are soft. May also use individual frozen fillets and cut vegetables into smaller-pieces. Reduce cooking time since smaller, thinner pieces will cook faster.

- **Salmon with Black Bean Salasa:** Rub oil on salmon and sprinkle with chili powder and cumin. Broil salmon. Drain and rinse a can of black beans, add a couple spoonfuls of salsa, half a cup of diced mandarin oranges (may use fresh oranges if desired), a tablespoon of lime juice and a half teaspoon of cumin.

- **Tarragon Baked Fish:** Place fish in shallow casserole dish. Squeeze lemon juice over fish then sprinkle with dry tarragon and dried mustard. Bake at 400°F. until fish flakes about 10 minutes for thin fillets.

- **Quick Stir-Fry:** Sauté a pound of chicken breast tenders in a tablespoon of oil. Add frozen stir-fry vegetables, a can of reduced-sodium chicken noodle soup, and a tablespoon of reduced-sodium soy sauce. Heat until vegetables are thawed.

- **Quick Grilled or Baked Chicken:** Season chicken breasts with one of the following before cooking on a grill or baking in oven. Also works well on fish, tofu or tempeh.
  - Lemon pepper and chipotle chili powder
  - Reduced-sodium taco seasoning
  - Italian seasoning, such as *Penzeys Spices' Tuscan Sunset or Mural of Flavor*

Quick Meal Ideas

- **Debbies Easy Chicken Bake:** Place frozen chicken breasts, chop green onion and fresh pea pods on sheet of aluminum foil. Sprinkle with desired seasoning such as *Penzeys Spices' Tuscan Sunset or Mural of Flavor.* Wrap up and bake at 250°F. for 1 1/2 hours. Serve over brown rice.

- **Chicken and Baby Carrots:** Brown chicken breast in pan. Add baby carrots to pan along with a half cup of apple juice, cover and simmer 10 minutes until all is tender. Stir in two teaspoons of honey mustard and serve.

- **Rosemary Baked Chicken:** In covered baking dish place chicken breasts, about a half cup of white wine and chopped fresh rosemary or dry cracked rosemary. Marinate in refrigerator overnight if you have time. Bake at 350°F. for 1 hour.

- **Yogurt Chicken:** Cut two boneless, skinless chicken breasts into chunks. Brown in skillet. Combine a container of plain, non-fat yogurt with a teaspoon of cumin and two tablespoons of chutney or apricot jam. Add to pan with browned chicken and cook about 5 minutes longer.

- **Quick Stir-Fry:** Sauté a pound of chicken breast tenders in a tablespoon of oil. Add frozen stir-fry vegetables, a can of reduced-sodium chicken noodle soup, and a tablespoon of reduced-sodium soy sauce. Heat until vegetables are thawed.

- **Chicken and Rice Bake:** To reduce the sodium in packaged rice mixtures, add some plain rice. For example, to a box of *Uncle Ben's Whole Grain And Wild Rice*, add 1 cup instant brown rice and increase the water on the package by 1 cup; then add 2 cups of frozen broccoli florets and prepare as directed. Meanwhile, brown 2 boneless, skinless chicken breasts or use leftover chicken from recipe on Page 400. Cube and stir into rice mixture when done. Serve with a green, leafy salad or a frozen vegetable.

- **Beef and Salsa:** Brown a pound of 100% grass-fed beef, buffalo or venison, drain, and add a 16-ounce jar of your favorite salsa. Allow to simmer or put in crock pot and cook several hours. Works well to make tacos or make a taco salad by adding to the top of a large, green, leafy salad.

Hot Chocolate

Most hot cocoa mixes are made from cocoa that has been treated with alkali. This reduces the health benefits of the cocoa. The fat free varieties add artificial sugar substitutes and are high in sodium. Instead, make your own using **natural** *cocoa powder for a healthier, less sweet beverage. If you want a fat free version, omit the chocolate.*

1	cup unsweetened soy milk (almond milk, rice milk or skim milk)
1	tablespoon dark chocolate chips (1/2 ounce) such as *Ghirardelli 60% Cacao*
1	tablespoon unsweetened cocoa powder (natural, not dutched)
1/4	packet of stevia herbal sweetener (if more sweetness is desired)

1. Heat 1/2 cup milk on high for 1 minute in microwave.
2. Add chocolate chips and cocoa, then stir.
3. Add the remaining cold milk and stevia to taste.

FLAVOR VARIATIONS
- ❖ add 1/8 teaspoon cinnamon
- ❖ add 1/2 teaspoon instant espresso
- ❖ add 1/4 teaspoon coconut, orange, almond or peppermint extract

Chocolate is heart healthy because it has flavanoids, a type of antioxidant which may protect your heart. The more cocoa in chocolate, the higher the antioxidants. Dark chocolate has more cocoa. Antioxidants prevent oxidation of LDL cholesterol, which protects against heart disease.

Hot Chocolate Teeccino

1	cup brewed *Teeccino* according to package directions. Store leftovers in refrigerator and reheat as needed.

Add:

1	tablespoon dry soy milk (*Better Than Milk* is one brand), vanilla whey protein or nonfat dry milk
1	tablespoon dark chocolate chips such as *Ghirardelli 60% Cacao*
1	tablespoon unsweetened cocoa powder (not dutched)

Stir until chocolate has melted and well blended. Serve.

Teeccino is a dark, rich, full-bodied herbal coffee. It contains a blend of herbs, grains, fruits and nuts that are roasted and ground. It brews like coffee. Teeccino has no caffeine. It has a mild, sweet taste from dates and figs, but only has 15 calories per cup. It has 65 mg of potassium and 3 grams of carbohydrates per cup. It comes in almond amaretto, chocolate mint, hazelnut, mocha, java, vanilla nut and original flavors. See www.teeccino.com for more information.

NUTRITION NOTE
Omega-3 from soy milk.

Servings: 1

NUTRITION PER SERVING

Serving size	8 ounces
Calories	163
Protein	11 g
Carbohydrate*	16 g
(*5 g sugars from chocolate)	
Fiber	8 g
Soluble fiber	0.4 g
Fat	11 g
Saturated fat	3 g
Cholesterol	0 mg
Sodium	31 mg
Potassium	82 mg
Calcium	47 mg
Omega-3 ALA	210 mg

NUTRITION NOTE
Dutch-processed or **alkalized** cocoa has a lot less health benefit because it has been treated with an alkali that reduces the flavanoids.
A more healthy choice is one that is natural, unsweetened cocoa.

Servings: 1

NUTRITION PER SERVING

Serving size	8 ounces
Calories	131
Protein	3 g
Carbohydrate*	21 g
(*5 g added sugars from chocolate)	
Fiber	3 g
Soluble fiber	0.23 g
Fat	8 g
Saturated fat	3 g
Cholesterol	0 mg
Sodium	51 mg
Potassium	239 mg
Calcium	46 mg
Omega-3 ALA	105 mg

Breakfast In A Glass

NUTRITION NOTE
Chocolate soy milk will
have added sugars.

You can put the ingredients for a smoothie into a blender, blend, and then drink. It can be as simple as a scoop of whey protein; or soy protein with water, milk or juice that you shake in a jar; or more involved like the following smoothie recipes. Adding yogurt or whey protein powder adds protein to keep you satisfied for a longer time.

Choco-Berry Smoothie

Servings: 2

NUTRITION PER SERVING

Serving size	1-1/2 cup
Calories	190
Protein	19 g
Carbohydrate*	23 g
(*no added sugars)	
Fiber	5 g
Soluble fiber	1 g
Fat	5 g
Saturated fat	1 g
Cholesterol	5mg
Sodium	84 mg
Potassium	462 mg
Calcium	268 mg
Omega-3 ALA	1,890mg

Bonus:	
Magnesium	9% DV)
Selenium	16% DV)
Copper	(9% DV)
Zinc	(9% DV)

1/4	cup oat bran
2	tablespoon ground or milled flaxseed
1/2	cup frozen blueberries
1	cup plain, unsweetened soy milk, rice milk, skim milk or chocolate soy milk
1	cup water
2	ice cubes
1/4	cup chocolate whey protein

1. Place all ingredients in blender.
2. Blend on high until smooth and creamy.
3. Pour into glass and serve.

Blueberries: *Eat a half cup of blueberries daily to get heart and cancer protection, as well as possible brain health and vision benefits.*

HELPFUL HINT
Peel ripe banana, cut in
chunks and freeze for
later use in smoothies.

Orange Banana Smoothie

Servings: 2

NUTRITION PER SERVING

Serving size	1 cup
Calories	121
Protein	18 g
Carbohydrate*	25 g
(*no added sugars)	
Fiber	1.7 g
Soluble fiber	0.7 g
Fat	0.7 g
Saturated fat	0.2 g
Cholesterol	3 mg
Sodium	86 mg
Potassium	392 mg
Calcium	236 mg
Omega-3 ALA	20 mg

Bonus:	
Vitamin C	(35% DV)
Selenium	(9% DV)
Folate	(6% DV)
Vitamin D	(140 IU)

1/2	cup yogurt, plain, nonfat or low-fat
1/4	cup orange juice
1/2	banana (frozen preferred)
1	cup nonfat milk or plain, unsweetened soy milk
2	tablespoon oat bran
1	teaspoon vanilla extract
1/2	teaspoon banana extract
1	packet stevia herbal sweetener, if desired

1. Blend until smooth.
2. Refrigerate leftovers and shake before serving. Best if used within two days.

Orange Juice: *Contains the flavanoids hesperidin and naringenin, along with vitamin C. The white membrane called albedo is very rich in pectin and the phytochemicals limonin and glucarates. The pectin of the albedo lowers your cholesterol, curbs appetite and suppresses your hunger for a few hours. The white albedo is sweet and neutral tasting, unlike the colored part that is quite bitter.*

Banana Blueberry Smoothie

1/2	banana (if frozen will make smoothie thicker)
1/2	cup blueberries or frozen berry mix
1	pitted date or a teaspoon of date sugar (optional)
1	tablespoon ground or milled flaxseed
1/2	cup orange juice
1/2	cup nonfat or nondairy milk (soy, rice, almond milk, etc.)
4	ice cubes

1. Place all ingredients in blender.
2. Blend until smooth.

Blueberries: *Blueberries contain an antioxidant, pterostilbene, which may help lower LDL cholesterol, may protect against cancer, and may help maintain memory. It also gives them a dark midnight blue color. The antioxidant power is measured by an ORAC score. The ORAC score ranks wild blueberries as the fruit with the highest score. Cultivated blueberries have less antioxidants than wild blueberies but still score high.*

HELPFUL HINT
• Date sugar can be found in health food stores. It is made from dried dates finely ground into a sugar-like consistency.

Servings: 2

NUTRITION PER SERVING

Serving size	1 cup
Calories	130
Protein	3.8 g
Carbohydrate*	26 g
(*no added sugars)	
Fiber	3.2 g
Soluble fiber	1 g
Fat	2 g
Saturated fat	0.2 g
Cholesterol	3 mg
Sodium	28 mg
Potassium	407 mg
Calcium	97 mg
Omega-3 ALA	965 mg

Bonus:	
Vitamin C	(12% DV)
Magnesium	(12% DV)
Folate	(9% DV)
Copper	(7% DV)
Selenium	(7% DV)
Zinc	(5% DV)

Tropical Smoothie

1/2	cup ice cubes (or 1/2 cup water)
1/2	cup carrot juice (chilled) or pineapple juice
1/4	cup crushed pineapple (packed in water) with juice (chilled)
1	cup chilled vanilla soy milk (unsweetened) or low-fat coconut milk
1/4	package (about 4 ounces) chilled silken tofu (*Organic Silken Mori-Nu Soft*)
1/2	teaspoon coconut extract
1/4	teaspoon rum extract
1/4	teaspoon cinnamon
1/2	packet stevia herbal sweetener or sweeten to your taste

1. Combine all ingredients in blender and blend until smooth.
2. May refrigerate leftovers, and shake well before serving.

Servings: 2

NUTRITION PER SERVING

Serving size	1-1/2cup
Calories	112
Protein	9 g
Carbohydrate*	12 g
(*no added sugars)	
Fiber	1.3 g
Soluble fiber	0.5 g
Fat	3.5 g
Saturated fat	0.5 g
Cholesterol	0 mg
Sodium	57 mg
Potassium	469 mg
Calcium	63 mg
Omega-3 ALA	207 mg

Bonus:	
Magnesium	(13% DV)
Vitamin C	(12% DV)
Copper	(11% DV)
Iron	(10% DV)
Zinc	(6% DV)

Heart Smoothie

1/2	cup frozen blueberries or mixed berries
1/4	cup whey protein powder
1	cup milk (skim, soy, rice, oat)
1	tablespoon psyllium husk (natural food stores)
1	teaspoon liquid fish oil

1. Place all ingredients in blender. Cover with lid.
2. Blend on high until smooth and serve. May also use immersion blender

Good source of heart protective antioxidants, soluble fiber and omega-3.

Avocado Fruit Smoothie

1/2	cup frozen, unsweetened strawberries
1/2	cup frozen blueberry or mixed berry
1/4	avocado, peeled and pit removed
1	scoop vanilla whey protein powder
1	cup water
	sweetener, if desired

1. Place all ingredients in blender. Cover with lid.
2. Blend on high speed for 2 minutes or until smooth and creamy.

Avocados: *An avocado, while high in fat, contains mostly good fat called oleic fatty acid, a type of monounsaturated fat also found in olive oil. This heart healthy fat can raise HDL and lower LDL when it replaces saturated fat. Like all plant foods, avocados don't have cholesterol.*

Avocado is rich in glutathione, a powerful antioxidant that blocks intestinal absorption of certain fats. They are also a good source of potassium, which can lower blood pressure. One medium avocado contains 10 grams of fiber. Avocados contain betasitosterol, a phytosterol that reduces the amount of cholesterol absorbed from foods. Research shows that avocados boost the absorption of other healthy things found in foods such as carotenoids.

Scrambled Eggs

   1   egg (omega-3 enriched)
   2   egg whites or 1/4 cup egg substitute

1. Place egg and whites in a small dish. Blend together with a fork.
2. Heat small sauté or fry pan on medium-low heat for 1 minute. Spray pan with cooking spray. Add eggs.
3. As egg sets, push cooked edges to center, continue until all of the egg is set.

VARIATION: OMELET

❖ Use egg mixture from above.
❖ As edges set, lift to allow liquid to run under and cook until set.
❖ Add reduced-fat cheese or sautéed veggies if desired, then fold in half and continue to cook another minute to allow cheese to melt.

VEGGIE SUGGESTION

❖ Before cooking the eggs, microwave or sauté diced onion, bell pepper, mixed veggies, broccoli or spinach. Fresh, frozen or leftover vegetables may be used. Keep warm until eggs have set.

OMEGA-3 ENRICHED EGGS VS. ORDINARY EGG

Per 1 large egg (50 g)	Eggland's Best (omega-3 enriched)	Gold Circle Farm DHA eggs	Ordinary large egg
Omega-3 total (mg)	100	225	37
DHA (mg)	50	150	18
EPA (mg)	20	nd	2
Cholesterol (mg)	175	nd	213
Vitamin E	25% DV	20% DV	3% DV
Lutein (mg)	200	nd	145

nd – no data available

NOTE: *Omega-3 from DHA and EPA are allowed by the FDA to make a health claim about benefits for heart health. One ounce of salmon has 300-613 mg of DHA + EPA. Omega-3 enriched eggs are not all the same. Eggs don't have much omega-3 compared to salmon, but these brands have more than an ordinary egg and more than some fish, such as tilapia which has only 5 mg per ounce.*

Servings: 1

NUTRITION PER SERVING

Serving size	1/2 cup
Calories	105
Protein	13 g
Carbohydrate*	0.5 g
(*no added sugars)	
Fiber	0 g
Fat	5 g
Saturated fat	1.5 g
Cholesterol	180 mg
Sodium	171 mg
Potassium	176 mg
Calcium	31 mg
Omega-3	
EPA+DHA	20-150 mg

Scrambled Tofu Egg

Servings: 1

NUTRITION PER SERVING

Serving size	1/2 cup
Calories	130
Protein	18 g
Carbohydrate*	0.5 g
(*no added sugars)	
Fiber	0 g
Fat	7 g
Saturated fat	1.8 g
Cholesterol	180 mg
Sodium	100 mg
Calcium	20 mg
Potassium	232 mg
Omega-3	
EPA+DHA	20-150 mg

1	egg (omega-3 enriched)
1/4	box (or 3 ounces) silken tofu (*Organic Silken Mori-Nu Soft*)

1. Open tofu package and drain off water. Blend with small food processor. Remove 1/4 of package, reserving the rest for later use. Place tofu in small bowl, add egg and blend. You can skip the puree step and mash tofu with a fork. The mixture will have lumps, but once it's cooked they blend in.
2. Heat small sauté pan over medium-low heat for 1-minute. Spray with cooking spray or add a teaspoon of oil. Pour in egg mixture and cook stirring until eggs begin to set. If any water is released while cooking, soak it up with a paper towel or drain.

NOTE: This may look strange while cooking, but the result is a light and fluffy mixture.

VARIATION

❖ Before adding egg/tofu mixture, sauté 1/4 cup vegetables. Suggested vegetables include: chopped onion, chopped bell peppers (green, red, yellow, etc.), sliced mushrooms, thawed frozen vegetables such as cut-leaf spinach, Asian vegetable mix, frozen stir-fry vegetables or bell pepper strips.

Breakfast Burrito To Go

Servings: 1

NUTRITION PER SERVING

Serving size	1 filled burrito
Calories	185
Protein	21 g
Carbohydrate*	19 g
(*no added sugars)	
Fiber	14 g
Fat	7 g
Saturated fat	1 g
Cholesterol	180 mg
Sodium*	470 mg
(*300 mg from tortilla)	
Potassium	110 mg
Calcium	5 mg
Omega-3	
EPA+DHA	20-150 mg

1	whole-wheat tortilla (such as *LaTortilla Factory Low Carb High Fiber Smart & Delicious*) or flourless, sprouted-wheat tortilla
1	scrambled egg or scrambled tofu egg mixture
	Salsa, if desired

1. Heat tortilla in microwave or skillet.
2. Add scrambled egg or scrambled egg tofu mixture
3. Top with salsa, if desired.
4. Fold in sides and roll up.

For lower sodium:

French Meadow Fat Flush Organic Sprouted Tortilla 6" has 105 mg sodium. See www.frenchmeadow.com.

Tumaro's Soy-full Heart Flatbread Wheat, Soy & Flax has 65 mg sodium. See www.tumaros.com

Veggie Egg Muffin

Prepare and refrigerate for a great grab-and-go breakfast.

2	cup frozen broccoli florets, thawed and chopped (may use fresh, cooked and chopped)
1	cup frozen cut-leaf spinach, thawed (may use fresh baby spinach, chopped)
1/4	cup diced sun-dried tomatoes or roasted red bell pepper or 1/4 cup finely diced bell pepper
1/2	cup soy sausage or turkey sausage (Page 310) or chopped smoked salmon (may omit and use extra vegetables)
1/2	cup shredded *Cabot 75% Reduced-Fat Cheddar Cheese* (2 ounces)
2	cup egg substitute or 16 egg whites
4	eggs (omega-3 enriched)
1/4	teaspoon freshly ground black pepper
1/2	teaspoon onion powder (may use 1/4 cup finely chopped red onion)

1. Preheat oven to 350°F.
2. Prepare a 12-cup muffin pan by spraying with cooking spray. If using a silicon muffin pan, no pan preparation is required.
3. Combine broccoli, spinach, tomatoes, sausage and cheese. Divide evenly into muffin pans (about 1/4 cup each).
4. Combine egg substitute, eggs, pepper and onion powder in large measuring cup. Whisk with fork to blend. Pour a small amount (1/4 cup) into each muffin well, over top of broccoli mixture, dividing as equally as possible.
5. Bake 30 minutes or until center is almost firm. Remove from pan and eat hot or warm.

Refrigerate leftovers up to a week. Microwave wrapped in paper towel 30 seconds or until warm. For longer storage freeze. When ready to eat thaw overnight and heat.

VARIATION

❖ Vary vegetables to include any that you enjoy or have leftover, such as roasted vegetables, sautéed onion, mushrooms, green onion, mixed vegetables, cooked kale, cooked asparagus or shredded zucchini. Chop vegetables into small pieces if large.

❖ Replace part of the cheese with feta, reduced-fat Swiss, or grated Parmesan.

❖ Use soy sausage, such as *Morningstar Farms Meal Starter Recipe Crumbles Sausage-Style*, right from the bag; or *Gimme Lean Ground* Sausage Style that has been crumbled and sautéed first. Use a potato masher to break *Gimme Lean* apart.

NUTRITION NOTES
Most of the sodium is found in egg whites, not yolks.

SODIUM:
1 whole egg – 65 mg
2 egg whites – 110 mg
1/4 cup egg substitute – 115 mg

Servings: 12

NUTRITION PER SERVING

Serving size	1 muffin
Calories	70
Protein	9 g
Carbohydrate*	3 g
(*no added sugars)	
Fiber	1.3 g
Soluble fiber	0.4 g
Fat	2 g
Saturated fat	0.7 g
Cholesterol	61 mg
Sodium	146 mg
Potassium	182 mg
Calcium	81 mg
Omega-3	
EPA+DHA	33 mg

Turkey Sausage

1-1/4	pounds ground turkey breast or turkey white meat
1/3	cup oat bran or quinoa flakes
1/4	cup plain, unsweetened soy milk, skim milk or water
1	teaspoon rubbed sage (or more to your taste)
1	pinch each paprika, black pepper, thyme, nutmeg
1/2	teaspoon no-salt seasoned salt substitute (optional)

1. Mix all ingredients and refrigerate for 30 minutes or overnight if you have time.
2. Form into 8 flattened patties (about 1/4 cup each), unless you prefer to have crumbles.
3. Sauté in heavy skillet over medium heat until golden. Turn and cook other side.
4. Cook until a meat thermometer reads 165°F.

VARIATION

❖ Pizza sausage. For a "sausage" flavor substitute 1-1/2 teaspoon fennel that has been ground in a coffee mill for the sage. Most commercial sausage seasonings are primarily salt. Crumble and sauté for pizza topping or other uses.

HELPFUL HINTS
• May freeze cooked patties, if desired.

• Replace oat bran with dry oatmeal or rolled barley flakes, pulsed into flour in a coffee mill or blender.

Servings: 8

NUTRITION PER SERVING

Serving size	1/4 cup patty
Calories	90
Protein	18 g
Carbohydrate*	3 g
(*no added sugars)	
Fiber	1 g
Soluble fiber	0.2 g
Fat	1 g
Saturated fat	0.4 g
Cholesterol	35 mg
Sodium	51 mg
Potassium	396 mg
Calcium	14 mg
Omega-3 ALA	10 mg

NOTE: *Ground turkey breast or white meat is low in fat. Ground turkey can be dark meat and may also include the skin, which makes some products higher than ground round or ground sirloin! Check labels. If there is no label choose ones that state "breast" or "white."*

Salt substitute works well, as the "bitterness" of potassium gives the sausage a nice "bite" that works well with the seasonings.

Hot Oats

If you eat cereals for breakfast, choose oats or barley, which has soluble fiber. Soluble fiber is the type that lowers cholesterol. Choose steel-cut oats or old-fashioned oats instead of quick cooking or instant, since they have a lower glycemic index. Instant which are precooked and dried are the least nutritious. The instant packets of oatmeal are highly sweetened (some with high fructose corn syrup), often with added sodium and other things you don't get if you cook your own. You can make oats quickly without using instant.

1. *When you have time, cook a week's worth of rolled oats, thick-rolled oats, steel-cut or oat groats. Refrigerate, then microwave a portion each morning, thinning with milk and adding flavoring options (Page 312).*
2. *Make it in the microwave as follows:*

Microwaved Old-Fashioned Rolled Oatmeal

1/3	cup dry, old-fashioned rolled oats (not quick)
3/4	cup cold water

1. Combine in large 4-cup glass measuring cup or bowl (this prevents volcano-like boilover). Microwave for a minute, stir. Cook for 15 second intervals to avoid boilover. Repeat four times for total of 1 minute.
2. Remove and let stand 5 minutes, covered. Add flavoring options as desired (Page 312).

VARIATION
❖ Use rolled barley; or rolled rye; or a combination of rolled oats, rolled barley and rolled rye.

FOR CREAMIER OATS
❖ Use 1 part milk to 3 parts water. Or add them to cold water rather than adding to boiling water.

KNOW YOUR OATS
❖ Grocery stores usually stock old-fashioned rolled oats. If you don't find the other forms of oats discussed below, look for them at a health food store.
  - **Oat groats,** whole kernels of oats with only tough outer husk removed, then toasted. Keeps all the nutrition and has a lower glycemic index. Can be cooked and used like rice.
  - **Steel-cut oats**, also called Irish oats or Scottish oats, are whole kernels that have been cut into several pieces. Some Irish or Scottish varieties have the pieces rolled flat, creating quick oats. Choose those that are not rolled flat. The less you break down the grains, the lower the glycemic response.
  - **Thick rolled oats** are like old-fashioned oats but are thicker flakes.
  - **Old-fashioned rolled oats**, kernels of oats that have been steamed and flattened into flakes.
  - **Quick oats** smaller pieces, higher glycemic index. Old-fashioned is preferred.
  - **Instant oats** typically have added sugars, salts, etc. Skip these.
  - **Cold oat cereals** made from flour are often shaped in circles. They have added salt in most cases and some have modified cornstarch. They have a high glycemic index and are often low in fiber. It is better to choose a less processed cereal.

Servings: 1

NUTRITION PER SERVING

Serving size	1/3 cup dry about 3/4 cup cooked
Calories	140
Protein	5 g
Carbohydrate*	25 g
(*no added sugars)	
Fiber	4 g
Soluble fiber	2 g
Fat	2.5 g
Saturated fat	0.5 g
Cholesterol	0 mg
Sodium	1 mg
Potassium	143 mg
Calcium	19 mg
Omega-3 ALA	10 mg

Bonus:	
Magnesium	(27% DV)
Thiamin	(15% DV)
Zinc	(9% DV)

Steel-Cut Oats

1/2   cup steel-cut oats
1-1/2   cups water (2 cups if you prefer softer oats with less texture)
1   teaspoon cinnamon, if desired

NUTRITION PER SERVING

Serving size	3/4 cup
Calories	148
Protein	5 g
Carbohydrate*	27 g
(*no added sugars)	
Fiber	4 g
Soluble fiber	2 g
Fat	3 g
Saturated fat	0.5 g
Cholesterol	0 mg
Sodium	1 mg
Potassium	143 mg
Calcium	19 mg
Omega-3 ALA	10 mg

Bonus:	
Magnesium	(27% DV)
Thiamin	(15% DV)
Zinc	(9% DV)

NUTRITION NOTE
Steel-cut oats are less gelatinous than rolled oats when cooked. They have a lower glycemic index, which causes less of a rise in blood sugars and less of an insulin surge.

Buy them from the bulk bin at a health food store for a better price.

1. (Optional step) Toast steel-cut oats. Place oats in dry pan over medium heat, stirring occasionally until slightly golden. In the beginning, you won't need to stir as often but once they begin to turn color, stir constantly.
2. Bring water to boil (add 1 teaspoon cinnamon, if desired).
3. Stir in oats, boil for 5 minutes. Cover, let stand off heat for 10 minutes. Alternatively, simmer for 15 minutes.
4. Add flavoring options as desired.

NOTE: *Make this in a crock pot overnight, if desired. It will form a crust on the edges that can be stirred in.*

FLAVORING OPTIONS
To 1/2 cup of cooked grain, add one or several of the following:
- Option 1: Add 1/4 teaspoon cinnamon, milk, soy, grain, nut or nonfat dairy. If you want it sweeter, use a half packet of stevia, vanilla soy milk or *White Wave's French Vanilla Soy Creamer, Fruit Sweet by Wax Orchards,* or maple syrup or raw honey.
- Option 2: Half an apple, grated; 1/2 teaspoon cinnamon or pumpkin pie spice, tablespoon of raisins and milk.
- Option 3: Add 1/2 tablespoon natural peanut butter or almond butter to any option.
- Option 4: Add 1 teaspoon dried fruit such as raisins, currants, dried blueberries, dried cherries or craisins.
- Option 5: Add 1 teaspoon chopped walnuts, almonds or any other nut.

Baked Steel-Cut Oats

1   recipe steel-cut oats from above or 1-1/2 cups leftover cooked steel-cut oats

Prepare steel cut oats as above. Let cool for 15 minutes then add the following:

2   tablespoons currants
2   tablespoons walnuts, toasted and chopped
1/2   apple, grated or pear chopped
1   teaspoon vanilla extract
1/4   cup egg substitute or 1 egg

NUTRITION PER SERVING

Serving size	1 piece
Calories	198
Protein	7 g
Carbohydrate*	33 g
(*3 g added sugars)	
Fiber	5 g
Soluble fiber	2.2 g
Fat	5 g
Saturated fat	0.7 g
Cholesterol	0 mg
Sodium	23 mg
Potassium	196 mg
Calcium	33 mg
Omega-3 ALA	333 mg

Stir to combine. Place in a glass loaf pan and bake in toaster oven or oven for 30 minutes. Sprinkle the top with 1 tablespoon of brown sugar. Broil 3-5 minutes. Cut into 4 servings. Eat as is or add milk and berries if desired. Tastes good cold.

Fruity Cinnamon Rolled Oats With Oat Groats

Combining both rolled oats and whole oat groats is a great way of getting more texture and soluble fiber for a tasty breakfast.

2	cups water
1	cup old-fashioned oats (thick-cut if you can find them)
1	cup cooked whole oat groats (see below)
1/2	cup dried fruit, if desired (raisins, golden raisins, dried currents, blueberries, cherries) or grated apple or pear
2	teaspoons honey
1	teaspoon cinnamon

Topping:

❖ Milk, soy, grain, nut or nonfat dairy.

❖ Nuts, such as almonds or walnuts, or seeds, like sunflower or ground flaxseed.

❖ Natural peanut butter or any other nut butter (almond, sunflower, cashew, etc.)

1. Bring water to a boil and add remaining ingredients except toppings. Reduce to simmer and cook uncovered for 5 minutes. Let stand 2 minutes. Add toppings and serve.
2. Store leftovers in refrigerator, and reheat in microwave or on stove top.

NUTRITION NOTES
- Rolled barley is a great substitute for the rolled oats.

- Substitute hulled barley, rye or wheat berries for the oat groats.

Servings: 8

NUTRITION PER SERVING

Serving size	1/2 cup
Calories	169
Protein	5 g
Carbohydrate*	35 g
(*1.5 g added sugars)	
Fiber	6 g
Soluble fiber	2 g
Fat	1.5 g
Saturated fat	0.5 g
Cholesterol	0 mg
Sodium	7 mg
Potassium	231 mg
Calcium	22 mg
Omega-3 ALA	3 mg

Bonus:	
Selenium	(12% DV)
Thiamin	(11% DV)
Iron	(10% DV)

Whole Oat Groats

If you don't like the gummy texture of rolled oats, then cook the whole oat kernels for a less sticky product and eat them as a hot cereal.

1	cup whole oat kernels (oat groats)
2	cups water

1. Place oats and water in rice cooker and cook until done. A vegetable steamer may also be used.
2. To cook on stove top, bring water to boil, add oats, reduce heat to simmer for 45 minutes. Refrigerate the extra and reheat as needed.

NUTRITION NOTES
Any whole grain can be cooked and eaten as a breakfast cereal. See next page for some suggestions.

Add flavoring options, if desired (Page 312).

Barley In A Rice Cooker

Barley is also high in soluble fiber (see Page 127). To prepare hulled barley using a rice cooker:

1. Place 1 cup of barley and 2 cups of water in a rice cooker.
2. Place the rice cooker in a sink as the barley tends to create a lot of foaming, which can make a mess on your counters.
3. You can also cook barley in a saucepan on the stove about 45 minutes.

Oat Groats Or Hulled Barley In Vegetable Steamer

1. Place 1 cup of grain and 1 cup of water in steaming bowl, filling the base to the highest level with water, and steam for 75 minutes.
2. If water remains in steaming bowl, drain after finished cooking.

Breakfast Amaranth

1. Place 1/2 cup amaranthwith 1-1/2 cups water or apple juice in pan.
2. Bring to boil, reduce to simmer and cook 20 minutes or until liquid is absorbed.

Breakfast Quinoa

1	cup water
1/2	cup quinoa, rinsed and drained
1/2	apple, grated
1/2	teaspoon cinnamon
1/3	cup dried fruit (craisins, raisins, dates, currants)
2	tablespoons chopped toasted walnuts

1. Combine all ingredients and bring to boil, reduce and simmer for 15 minutes or until water is absorbed.
2. Allow to stand 5 minutes. Serve with milk or low-fat yogurt if desired.

NUTRITION NOTES
Walnuts add omega-3

Servings: 2.

NUTRITION PER SERVING

Serving size	1 cup
Calories	279
Protein	7 g
Carbohydrate*	51 g
(*no added sugars)	
Fiber	6 g
Soluble fiber	0.8 g
Fat	6 g
Saturated fat	0.5 g
Cholesterol	0 mg
Sodium	13 mg
Potassium	414 mg
Calcium	23 mg
Omega-3 ALA	643 mg

Bonus:
Magnesium	(28% DV)
Iron	(27% DV)
Copper	(23% DV)
Vitamin E	(19% DV)

Muesli (Uncooked Rolled Oats)

1   cup rolled grain (flakes)
   • rolled oats, rolled barley or rye flakes, or combination of several different flakes
   • toasted, if desired (Page 316)
1/2 cup plain, nonfat yogurt
1/2 teaspoon cinnamon
     sweetener, if desired (stevia, honey, brown sugar, etc.)
1/2 cup liquid
   • milk (soy, rice, nonfat dairy)
   • fruit juice, such as apple juice
2   tablespoons nuts
   • slivered almonds, chopped walnuts, sunflower seeds
1   tablespoon ground flaxseed or oat bran
2   tablespoons dried fruit
   • craisins, currants, dried blueberries, apricots, figs, cherries
1/2 cup fresh fruit
   • 1/2 apple with peel, grated
   • diced fruit, such as pears, peaches, mango
   • berries

1. Place ingredients in a bowl in the order listed. Mixture can be eaten immediately, or if you like it softer, allow to sit overnight, refrigerated.
2. Alter to suit your particular tastes or to use fruits that are in season.

Servings: 3

NUTRITION PER SERVING

Serving size	1/2 cup
Calories	246
Protein	9 g
Carbohydrate*	40 g
(*no added sugars)	
Fiber	6.5 g
Soluble fiber	2.6 g
Fat	6 g
Saturated fat	1 g
Cholesterol	2 mg
Sodium	43 mg
Potassium	282 mg
Calcium	150 mg
Omega-3 ALA	640 mg

Betty's Baked Oatmeal

This is one of the ways that Betty Holloway, a registered dietitian, encourages her clients to prepare rolled oats. A small amount of sugar added to the top and carmelized under the broiler makes it seem decadent yet it only has 3 grams of sugar per serving.

2   eggs (omega-3 enriched) or 1/2 cup egg substitute
2   cups low-fat milk (almond, rice or soy milk may be used)
1   teaspoon vanilla extract
1   teaspoon cinnamon
1   tablespoon brown sugar (maple syrup, date sugar or sucanat may be used)
2   cups old-fashioned rolled oats
2   tablespoons dried fruit (cherries, craisins or raisins)
Topping: 1 tablespoon brown sugar

1. Preheat oven to 350°F.
2. Combine eeg, milk, vanilla, cinnamon and sugar. Add oats and dried fruit.
3. Pour into oiled 8 inch square pan.
4. Bake 30 min. Sprinkle 1 tablespoon brown sugar over the top and broil 3 to 5 minutes or just until sugar melts and bubbles.
5. Cut into 8 pieces. Serve with milk, toasted walnuts or almonds and berries.

Variations: replace half of the milk with an equal amount of apple cider and add a grated or diced apple or pear before baking.

Servings: 8

NUTRITION PER SERVING

Serving size	1 piece
	2 inch X 4 inch
Calories	162
Protein	7 g
Carbohydrate*	26 g
(*3 g added sugars)	
Fiber	3 g
Soluble fiber	1 g
Fat	2.8 g
Saturated fat	0.6 g
Cholesterol	46 mg
Sodium	43 mg
Potassium	204 mg
Calcium	93 mg
Omega-3 ALA	25 mg

Toasted Grain Granola

3/4	cup rolled, toasted grains in any combination (oats, barley, wheat, rye, etc.), see below
1	tablespoon date pieces
1	tablespoon craisins
1	tablespoon raisins
1/2	tablespoon walnut pieces
1/2	tablespoon sliced almonds
1	tablespoon sunflower seeds

1. Combine all and store leftovers in refrigerator.
2. Serve with milk or soy milk or with yogurt and fruit.

For a gluten free version use certified gluten-free oats and quinoa flakes.

TOASTED ROLLED GRAINS

❖ **Oven method**
1. Preheat oven to 350°F. Spread 2 cups of rolled oats (or rolled barley, rolled rye, rolled wheat or quinoa flakes) on a jellyroll pan or large cookie sheet. Do not oil pan. If using quinoa flakes watch carefully so they don't burn.
2. Bake for 15 to 20 minutes until slightly golden. Stir after 10 minutes.
3. Remove and allow to cool. Store in refrigerator or freezer.
4. Use any time you use oats.

❖ **Pan method** (If you want to toast a small amount, do it in a pan.)
1. Place oats in dry pan over medium heat.
2. Stir until slightly golden. At first, you do not need to stir often, but as the grain starts to change color, stir continuously to avoid burning.

Servings: 4

NUTRITION PER SERVING

Serving size	1/4 cup
Calories	103
Protein	3 g
Carbohydrate*	19 g
(*no added sugars)	
Fiber	3 g
Soluble fiber	1 g
Fat	2.8 g
Saturated fat	0.3 g
Cholesterol	0 mg
Sodium	0 mg
Potassium	138 mg
Calcium	12 mg
Omega-3 ALA	90 mg

Bonus:	
Iron	(11% DV)
Selenium	(7% DV)
Magnesium	(6% DV)

Cheese Toast

1   slice sprouted-grain, flourless, whole-grain bread
1   tablespoon yogurt cheese or nonfat Greek yogurt (*Fage Total Greek Yogurt 0%*) or low-fat ricotta
1/4   teaspoon honey (easier to use a squeeze bottle than to try to measure)
1/8   teaspoon cinnamon, as desired
1   teaspoon ground flaxseed or oat bran

1. Toast the bread.
2. Spread with yogurt cheese.
3. Drizzle with honey, sprinkle with cinnamon, and swirl with a knife to blend.
4. Top with flaxseed or oat bran and enjoy.

YOGURT CHEESE

❖ To make yogurt cheese, start with plain, fat-free or low-fat yogurt. Purchase a brand that does not add stabilizers, such as gelatin, as they will not drain as well.

❖ Place a coffee filter or several layers of cheesecloth inside a mesh strainer set over a bowl. Stir yogurt until smooth, then scoop into strainer. Cover with plastic wrap or bag, put in refrigerator, and let stand 12 to 24 hours. The longer it stands, the thicker it becomes. It will reduce by about half the amount you started with. Remove yogurt cheese and stir in other ingredients as desired. As an alternative, use yogurt cheese plain like cream cheese.

FLAVORED SPREADS

To make flavored spreads, stir into 1 cup of yogurt cheese any of the following:

❖ **Nutty fruit spread:** 2 tablespoons golden raisins, chopped; 1 tablespoon pecans, chopped; 1 teaspoon grated orange rind; and 1 packet stevia or other sweetener

❖ **Herbed spread:** 1 teaspoon dill weed, 1 teaspoon thyme, pinch of sea salt and white pepper

❖ **Maple spread:** 1/8 teaspoon cinnamon, 2 teaspoons honey, 3 drops maple extract flavoring

❖ **Fruity spread:** 3 tablespoons mixed dried diced fruit, 1 teaspoon honey, 1/2 teaspoon cinnamon

❖ **Peanut butter:** Mix 1 tablespoon natural peanut butter with 1 or 2 tablespoons of yogurt cheese

FLAXSEEDS

❖ Flaxseeds are a good source of lignans, a soluble fiber, and plant *omega-3* fat in the form of alpha-linolenic acid (ALA). The omega-3 in flaxseed cannot carry a health claim about lowering cholesterol like omega-3 in fish. However, flax has benefits to heart health. The lignans in flax may act as antioxidants to reduce inflammation and block the oxidation of LDL cholesterol, a key to preventing heart disease.

NUTRITION NOTE
Has omega-3 from flax.

Servings: 1

NUTRITION PER SERVING

Serving size	1 slice
Calories	107
Protein	6 g
Carbohydrate*	17 g
(*1.5 g added sugar from honey)	
Fiber	5 g
Soluble fiber	0.5 g
Fat	2 g
Saturated fat	0.1 g
Cholesterol	0 mg
Sodium	141 mg
Potassium	53 mg
Calcium	180 mg
Omega-3 ALA	532 mg

Oven-Baked French Toast

NUTRITION NOTES
Use slices of flourless, sprouted, cinnamon raisin, whole-wheat bread.

1/2   cup (or 4 ounces) refrigerated or thawed frozen egg substitute product
1/2   cup skim milk, vanilla soy milk or *White Wave Silk Soy Creamer*
2   teaspoons vanilla
2   cups oat bran flake cereal, finely crushed to about 3/4 cup
1/2   loaf whole-grain French bread (diagonally sliced 1/2-inch thick)
    Nonstick cooking spray or oil in pump sprayer

1. In shallow bowl or pie pan, combine egg product, milk and vanilla; mix well.
2. Crush cereal using a blender or food processor. Place crushed cereal in another shallow bowl or pie pan.
3. Dip each slice of bread in egg mixture, turning to coat both sides. If you have leftover egg mixture, evenly divide and spoon over each piece.
4. Dip egg soaked bread in crushed cereal, turning to coat both sides. Place on baking sheet and spray bread with cooking spray, turn and spray other side.
5. Cover with foil; refrigerate at least 1 hour or overnight. When ready to serve, heat oven to 425°F. and remove foil. Bake 10 minutes or until golden brown, turn slices and bake 10 minutes more.
6. Serve with unsweetened applesauce or mashed berries and greek-style yogurt.

Servings: 8

NUTRITION PER SERVING

Serving size	1 slice (1 ounce)
Calories	120
Protein	5 g
Carbohydrate*	22 g
(*no added sugars)	
Fiber	2 g
Soluble fiber	0.6 g
Fat	1 g
Saturated fat	0 g
Cholesterol	0 mg
Sodium	185 mg
Potassium	107 mg
Calcium	41 mg
Omega-3 ALA	10 mg

Whole-Grain Flours

WHOLE-WHEAT FLOUR

Whole-wheat flour is made from hard, red wheat and contains the bran and the germ along with the endosperm. Whole-wheat flour should be stored in the refrigerator or freezer to prevent rancidity.

WHITE WHOLE-WHEAT FLOUR

This is a general classification for a variety of wheat that includes hard, white, winter wheat; hard, white, spring wheat; and soft, white wheat. It has a slightly tan or golden color, lighter than traditional red whole-wheat flour, but contains all the nutrients of the whole grain, which includes the bran and germ. White wheat does not contain the tannins or phenolic acid, which are bitter; therefore, the taste is milder.

If you make yeast breads with white whole-wheat flour, they will rise higher, have a lighter color, and taste milder than traditional whole-wheat flour. It is also a good substitute for whole-wheat pastry flour and all-purpose flour.

You can purchase white whole-wheat flour at some stores or find it at www.bobsredmill.com. The *King Arthur* brand is available at www.kingarthurflour.com.

GRAIN MILL

While not many people mill their own flour, you can purchase a mill designed for home use to grind wheat berries into flour as needed. With a home mill, you can adjust how coarse or fine you want to grind your flour. You will be amazed by the fresh taste of foods made with freshly milled flour. Whole-wheat bread will have a lighter texture and higher rise when using freshly ground flour. The *Prairie Gold Hard, White, Spring Wheat* berries (www.wheatmontana.com) are my favorite for making bread. Wheat berries can be purchased through food buying clubs or health food stores

WHOLE-WHEAT PASTRY FLOUR

Whole-wheat pastry flour is made from a soft winter wheat, which has lower gluten content. It works well in items such as cakes, cookies, muffins and pie crusts. I recommend whole-wheat pastry flour to people who are at the early stages of switching from eating refined foods to whole grain. Use it to make healthier baked goods. Start with half all-purpose white flour and half whole-wheat pastry flour, and gradually increase the amount of whole-wheat pastry flour. You will find the switch is easier if you do it gradually. Do not substitute whole-wheat pastry flour for bread flour in yeast recipes. You can grind your own pastry flour from soft wheat berries.

HELPFUL HINT
Wheat berries are whole kernels of wheat. When ground they become whole wheat flour.

Butternut Squash Rolls

1	cup cooked, pureed butternut squash
3/4	cup skim milk heated to 110°F
1/4	cup canola oil
1/4	cup brown sugar
3	cups white whole-wheat flour
2	teaspoons instant dry yeast
1	cup whole-wheat pastry flour or all-purpose flour (more or less)
1/4	teaspoon sea salt

1. Cut butternut squash in half, remove seeds, and microwave cut side down until soft. Remove pulp and measure out 1 cup, reserving the rest for another use.
2. Combine milk, oil, squash and brown sugar. If using leftover cold squash, heat the mixture so it is at 110°F. Combine whole-wheat flour and yeast. Stir in and beat smooth.
3. Add 1/2 cup pastry flour and salt, adding more flour as needed until stiff enough to knead. Turn out onto counter and knead for 5 minutes or use heavy-duty mixer with dough hook.
4. Return dough to bowl. Oil top, cover with a cloth, and allow to rise at room temperature until doubled.
5. Spray muffin tins (18 cups) with cooking spray.
6. Divide dough into 18 pieces. Then, divide each of the 18 into 3 pieces for a total of 54 pieces. Roll each piece into balls by placing the dough into the palm of your well-oiled hand. Using your fingers, tuck dough into tight balls. Place 3 balls of dough into each muffin cup.
7. Preheat oven to 400°F. Cover with cloth and allow to rise until doubled.
8. Bake for 15 to 20 minutes.

Servings: 18

NUTRITION PER SERVING

Serving size	1 roll
Calories	138
Protein	4 g
Carbohydrate*	24 g
(*2 g added sugar)	
Fiber	3 g
Soluble fiber	0.5 g
Fat	3.6 g
Saturated fat	0.3 g
Cholesterol	0.2 mg
Sodium	39 mg
Potassium	137 mg
Calcium	25 mg
Omega-3 ALA	300 mg

Bonus:

Selenium	(31% DV)
Iron	(15% DV)
Copper	(11% DV)
Beta-carotene	(10% DV)
Magnesium	(8% DV)
Zinc	(7% DV)

SAF Perfect Rise Yeast is one brand of instant dry yeast. Instant yeast does not require hydrating with warm water prior to use as is required by active dry yeast.

Pumpkin Maple Pecan Oat Bran Muffins

Bowl One:
2	cups dry oat bran
1/2	teaspoon baking powder
1	teaspoon baking soda
1	teaspoon cinnamon
1/3	cup pecans, toasted, chopped

Bowl Two:
1	cup plain, unsweetened soy milk, rice milk, skim milk, etc.
1	tablespoon lemon juice or white vinegar
2/3	cup canned pumpkin
1/3	cup maple syrup
1	teaspoon vanilla extract
2	eggs (omega-3 enriched)
2	tablespoons canola oil

1. Preheat oven to 400°F. Spray mini muffin pan (30 muffins) with nonstick cooking spray.
2. Combine all dry ingredients in Bowl One.
3. In Bowl Two, combine soy milk and lemon juice. Let stand 5 minutes. Then add remaining wet ingredients. Stir to combine.
4. Add dry ingredients from Bowl One to Bowl Two, and stir with spoon until just combined.
5. Place 3 tablespoon batter into mini muffin pans.
6. Bake for 15 minutes or until center springs back when pressed with finger. If indent remains, bake 2 minutes longer and test again.
7. Remove from pan and let cool completely. Store in freezer.

NUTRITION NOTES
May use buttermilk instead of milk and lemon juice.

Servings: 15

NUTRITION PER SERVING

Serving size	2 mini muffins
Calories	103
Protein	4 g
Carbohydrate*	24 g
(*2 g added sugar)	
Fiber	3 g
Soluble fiber	0.9 g
Fat	5.6 g
Saturated fat	0.7 g
Cholesterol	28 mg
Sodium	113 mg
Potassium	127 mg
Calcium	32 mg
Omega-3 ALA	220 mg
Bonus:	
Beta-carotene	(34% DV)
Selenium	(11% DV)
Magnesium	(9% DV)
Zinc	(6% DV)
Copper	(5% DV)
Vitamin K	(4 mcg)

Blueberry Walnut Bran Muffins

Bowl One:

1-1/3	cup plain, unsweetened soy milk, rice milk or skim milk
1	tablespoon lemon juice or white vinegar
2/3	cups water
2	cups unprocessed or millers wheat bran
1/2	cup date sugar or brown sugar
2	eggs (omega-3 enriched)
1/4	cup dried currants
2	tablespoons canola oil
1	teaspoon vanilla extract

Bowl Two:

1/3	cup ground or milled flaxseed
1-1/3	cup whole-wheat pastry flour
1-1/2	teaspoon baking soda
1/2	cup chopped walnuts
1	cup wild blueberries (if canned, drained)

1. Preheat oven to 400°F. Spray muffin pan (12 muffins) plus three (6-ounce size) custard cups or ramekins with nonstick cooking spray.
2. In Bowl One, combine soy milk and lemon juice, allowing to stand 5 minutes. Add remaining ingredients listed for Bowl One. Allow to stand 30 minutes to soften bran.
3. In Bowl Two, combine flaxseed, flour, baking soda and nuts. Stir to combine.
4. Drain blueberries if canned.
5. Add dry ingredients from Bowl One to Bowl Two and stir with spoon until just combined. Add blueberries and quickly fold in, being careful not to overmix the batter.
6. Scoop 1/2 cup batter into prepared muffin pans.
7. Bake for 15 minutes or until center springs back when pressed with finger. If indent remains, bake 2 minutes longer and test again.
8. Remove from pan and let cool completely. These soften after being stored. Best stored in freezer if not using within a day or two.

NUTRITION NOTES

- Use low-fat buttermilk and omit lemon juice.

- Look for date sugar in a natural foods store.

- Millers bran is an inexpensive ingredient that can be found at any natural foods store.

Servings: 15

NUTRITION PER SERVING

Serving size	1 muffin
Calories	69
Protein	6.5 g
Carbohydrate*	23 g
(*4.8 g added sugar)	
Fiber	6.5 g
Soluble fiber	0.8 g
Fat	7 g
Saturated fat	0.6 g
Cholesterol	28 mg
Sodium	144 mg
Potassium	185 mg
Calcium	45 mg
Omega-3 ALA	151 mg

Bonus:

Thiamin	(17% DV)
Selenium	(4% DV)
Magnesium	(3% DV)
Iron	(8% DV)
Copper	(4% DV)
Vitamin K	(4 mcg)

Whole-Wheat Bread

1-3/4	cup water (110°F)
2	tablespoons extra-virgin olive oil
2	tablespoons honey (or half molasses and half honey)
4-1/2	cup white whole-wheat flour* or ideally 3 cups *Prairie Gold Hard, White, Spring Wheat* berries freshly milled into flour
1/2	teaspoon sea salt
2	tablespoons vital wheat gluten
1	tablespoon *SAF Perfect Rise Instant Yeast*
1/4	cup cracked 7-grain hot cereal (*Bob's Red Mill*); dry, not cooked
1/3	cup whole flaxseeds

1. If water is too cold, warm to 110°F.
2. If using a grain mill, grind wheat berries into flour. If flour has been stored in refrigerator or freezer, it must be at room temperature or the bread will not rise well. Grind flaxseed using coffee grinder. Combine flour, salt, gluten, yeast, 7-grain cereal and ground flaxseed.
3. Combine water, oil and honey in bowl.
4. Add the flour mixture to the liquid ingredients. If dough is too soft, add additional flour a tablespoon at a time. If it's too dry, add water a tablespoon at a time. Knead using a *KitchenAid Mixer* with dough hook for 15 minutes. It will take about 5 minutes before it gathers into a ball. Or, use a *Bosch Mixer* to knead for 8 minutes.
5. Preheat oven to 375°F.
6. Let dough rise for 10 minutes. Shape into one loaf (10 X 5-inch pan) or two smaller loaves (4-1/2 X 8-1/2 inch pan). Cover with cloth and allow to rise until doubled. If your kitchen is cool, you can set the bread in your oven with a shallow pan of boiling water. Place the pan of water on the rack below the loaves. Do not cover loaves inside the oven; the warm steam will keep them moist. When bread is almost doubled, remove and preheat oven.
7. Bake for 45 minutes.
8. When bread has cooled, slice into 20 slices. Place waxed or parchment paper between slices and freeze. Remove slices as needed. Do not store bread in the refrigerator, it will stale and become dry faster.

NOTE: If you are unable to find white whole-wheat flour, you will get a lighter loaf by using 1 cup all-purpose flour and 3-1/2 cups traditional whole-wheat flour.

*I have made this recipe for many years using a **KitchenAid** Mixer before I got a **Bosch Mixer**. I prefer the bread that I make from the Bosch. I have also tried to make this in a variety of brands of bread makers, none of which compare to the loaves made with the Bosch.*

White whole-wheat flour is milled from a variety of white whole-wheat rather than red. It has the same nutrition and fiber as traditional whole-wheat flour. It produces bread that is lighter in texture, flavor and color than traditional whole wheat.

HELPFUL HINTS

To make different varieties, try one of the following:
- Add 1/2 cup chopped sun-dried tomatoes, 1/2 teaspoon cracked rosemary, and 1/3 cup sunflower seeds
- Add 1 tablespoon cinnamon, 1/2 cup chopped walnuts, and 1/2 cup craisins, chopped
- Substitute kamut or spelt for the wheat
- Replace some of the wheat with rye, splet or kamut

Servings: 20
(1 large loaf with 20 slices each)

NUTRITION PER SERVING

Serving size	1-1/4 ounces
	(36 gram)
	1/2" thick slice
Calories	133
Protein	5 g
Carbohydrate*	23 g
(*1.7 g sugars added from honey)	
Fiber	4 g
Soluble fiber	0.6 g
Fat	3 g
Saturated fat	0.4 g
Cholesterol	0 mg
Sodium	60 mg
Potassium	144 mg
Calcium	16 mg
Omega-3 ALA	600 mg

Bonus:	
Selenium	(28% DV)
Magnesium	(12% DV)
Zinc	(6% DV)

Butternut Squash Bread with Fruit and Nuts

NUTRITION NOTES
To prepare squash, split in half and scoop out seeds. Bake or microwave until soft. Remove pulp from skin. Freeze extra for use later or use in recipe on Page 367.

Bowl One:

1	cup butternut squash, cooked and mashed
2	eggs (omega-3 enriched preferred)
1/2	cup date sugar (see Page 284) or brown sugar
1/3	cup buttermilk
1/4	cup canola oil
1	teaspoon vanilla extract

Bowl Two:

1/4	cup dried cherries, chopped
1/4	cup craisins
1/4	cup dried blueberries or raisins
1/4	cup currants
1/3	cup chopped pecans

Bowl Three:

1	cup whole-wheat pastry flour
1	cup all-purpose flour (or additional whole-wheat pastry flour)
1	teaspoon baking powder
1/4	teaspoon baking soda
1/2	teaspoon ground cinnamon

1. Preheat oven to 350°F
2. In three separate bowls, measure the ingredients listed and place in each bowl.
3. Spray a 9 X 5-inch loaf pan with cooking spray.
4. Starting with Bowl One, add the dried fruit from Bowl Two and stir. Add the dry ingredients from Bowl Three to Bowl One (all ingredients are now together in Bowl One).
   Stir only until combined.
5. Scrape batter into prepared loaf pan.
6. Bake for 45 to 55 minutes or until toothpick inserted into center comes out clean. When completely cooled, slice and serve.
7. Freezes well.

SUBSTITUTE

❖ May use canned pumpkin instead of squash. May vary dried fruit and nuts as desired.

Servings: 14

NUTRITION PER SERVING

Serving size	1 slice
Calories	184
Protein	3.8 g
Carbohydrate*	28 g
(*5 g added sugars)	
Fiber	3.3 g
Soluble fiber	0.7 g
Fat	7 g
Saturated fat	0.7 g
Cholesterol	26 mg
Sodium	78 mg
Potassium	102 mg
Calcium	32 mg
Omega-3 ALA	420 mg

Bonus:

Vitamin C	(15% DV)
Beta-carotene	(21% DV)

When you cook grain, cook extra since it will keep refrigerated for a week or can be frozen. It can then be used for quick meals. Cook grains in reduced-sodium chicken or vegetable broth/bouillon. This adds a reasonable amount of sodium acceptable for most individuals; however, you can use no-salt-added broth if necessary.

ON THE STOVE TOP

It may take some trial and error to figure out the best setting to use on your range to keep the liquid at a simmer, almost a boil, but not boiling. Use a medium-sized pot with a tight-fitting lid.

1. Bring liquid to a boil.
2. Add grain, reduce heat to achieve a simmer or "gentle" boil, and cook covered, without peaking, for the time suggested in the chart below. If temperature is too low, the grain will not be cooked in the amount of time suggested. If temperature it too high, the pot will boil over. Adjust as needed.
3. Without opening, let stand 10 to 15 minutes after finished cooking.
4. Now open. If the water has not been absorbed and the grain is too firm, simmer a little longer. However, if the grain is tender, simply drain off the excess liquid.

IN A RICE COOKER

These cookers use a sensor to determine when the liquid has been absorbed and then turn off. There is little guesswork as to when grains are done. You can adjust to your preference. Start with the same amount of water as if cooking on the stove top. If you want the grain to be firmer; the next time you make it add 1/2 cup less water. If it's too firm add more water.

GUIDE FOR STOVE TOP OR RICE COOKER

Use package directions if buying prepackaged grains. Use the cooking time as a guide since it will vary depending how you adjust the heat. The faster the grain simmers, the quicker it cooks. Grains should be allowed to stand 10 minutes after active cooking time.

GRAIN COOKING GUIDE

For 1 Cup Grain:	Amount of Liquid	Cooking Time	Cooked Yield
Amaranth	1-1/2 cups	20 minutes	1-1/2 cups
*Barley, whole, hulled	2-1/2 cups	45 minutes	3 cups
Barley, pearled	2 cups	30 minutes	3 cups
Bulgur	1-3/4 cups	20 to 25 minutes	2 cups
Couscous, whole-wheat	1-1/2 cups	2 to 5 minutes	4 cups
Cracked Wheat	1-1/2 cups	15 minutes	2-1/2 cups
*Kamut	2-1/2 cups	60 minutes	2-1/2 cups
Buckwheat Groats			
Kasha (dry toast first)	2 cups	15 minutes	4 cups
Millet (dry toast first)	2 cups	20 minutes	4 cups

HELPFUL HINTS
Amaranth can be cooked as a cereal. It can be added to other whole grains using 1 part to 3 parts other grains. Add to soups or stews to thicken them,.

Whole Grains - Smart 4 Your Heart

NUTRITION NOTE
Brown rice which
requires 45 minutes
to cook can be
soaked overnight to
shorten cooking time
to 17 minutes.

For 1 Cup Grain:	Amount of Liquid	Cooking Time	Cooked Yield
*Oat Groats	2 cups	45 minutes	3 cups
Oats, steel-cut	3 cup	15 minutes	4 cups
Quinoa	2 cups	15 minutes	3 cups
Rice, brown	2 cups	45 minutes	3 cups
*Rye	2 cups	30 minutes	2 cups
*Spelt	2-1/2 cups	60 minutes	2-1/2 cups
*Triticale	2-1/2 cups	45 to 50 minutes	3 cups
*Wheat Berries	2-1/2 cups	60 minutes	3 cups
Wild Rice, long-grain	3 cups	50 minutes	3-1/2 cups

*cooking time reduced when soaked overnight

ELECTRIC COUNTERTOP VEGETABLE STEAMER

These can also be used for grains. One popular model is made by *Black & Decker*. For every cup of grain, put 1 cup of water in the steamer basket. Less is required since the steam will provide some moisture. If the grain is tender at the end of the cooking time but water remains in the basket, drain it off.

Grains that require 60 to 75 minutes steaming: wheat berries, kamut, spelt, rye, triticale, oat groat, hulled barley, wild rice, brown rice.

Grains that require 30 to 40 minutes: amaranth, bulgur, millet, steel-cut oats, quinoa, teff.

MICROWAVE

You can cook whole grains in plastic rice steamers specifically designed for microwave use, but you won't save time since the grain has to absorb the water before it softens.

SOAKING GRAINS

To reduce cooking time, soak grains overnight. Do not drain or add additional water. Brown rice, which typically takes 45 minutes to cook, only needs about 17 minutes when it is soaked.

Multi-Grain Mix

Make several baggies of this grain mixture when you have all the grains out. Then use as needed whenever your recipe calls for long-cooking brown rice.

Grain mixture:

1/2	cup brown rice (not quick cooking)
1/2	cup mixture of grains such as:

      1 tablespoon wheat berries
      2 tablespoons rye berries
      1 tablespoon wild rice
      2 tablespoons whole oat groat
      2 tablespoons pearled, whole or hulled barley

. . . .

1	teaspoon *Organic Better Than Bouillon Chicken or Vegetable Base*
2-1/4	cups water

To cook on stove top

1. Bring 2 cups water and 1 teaspoon bouillon to a boil. Add 1 cup of grain mixture and reduce heat to simmer. Cover and cook without peeking for 45 minutes.
2. Remove from heat and allow to stand 10 minutes before uncovering. Fluff with fork and serve.
3. If you prefer this to be less chewy, cook everything except the rice for 15 minutes, Quickly dump in the rice, cover and continue cooking 45 minutes longer.

To cook in rice cooker

Place all ingredients in cooker and turn on. It's done when the rice cooker's l light goes off.

NOTE: Use any of the following whole, intact grains in the grain mixture:

❖ *Wheat berries, soft or hard, red or white*
❖ *Brown rice, regular (jasmine brown, basmati brown, Lundberg brown, etc.)*
❖ *Oat, whole groats*
❖ *Rye, berries*
❖ *Triticale, whole*
❖ *Barley, unhulled, whole*
❖ *Buckwheat, whole*

Servings: 7

NUTRITION PER SERVING	
Serving size	1/2 cup
Calories	87
Protein	2.5 g
Carbohydrate*	17 g
(*no added sugars)	
Fiber	1.5 g
Soluble fiber	0.2 g
Fat	0.7 g
Saturated fat	0 g
Cholesterol	0 mg
Sodium	108 mg
Potassium	75 mg
Calcium	6 mg
Omega-3 ALA	10 mg

Quick Multi-Grain Mix

1/4	cup instant brown rice
2	tablespoons quick-cooking barley
1/4	cup bulgur
1-1/2	ounces (about 1/3 cup) whole-wheat spaghetti broken into 1" pieces or whole-wheat orzo
1/2	teaspoon dried parsley flakes
1/2	teaspoon *Veg It Seasoning,* or *Mrs. Dash* or *Spike Salt Free* (optional)
2	cups reduced-sodium chicken broth or 2 cups water +1 teaspoon *Organic Better Than Bouillon Chicken Base*

1. Measure rice, barley, bulgur, spaghetti, parsley and seasoning into a bowl.
2. Bring broth or water and chicken base to boil in saucepan with tight-fitting lid.
3. When water begins to boil, add rice mixture to saucepan, reduce to simmer, cover, and cook 15 minutes – no peeking.
4. Remove from heat and let stand covered 10 minutes.

Barley Nut Pilaf

1	medium onion, chopped
1	stalk celery, diced
1	carrot, peeled and diced
1/2	cup slivered almonds
1	cup hulled, whole barley (may use pearled)
1	tablespoon extra-virgin olive oil
4	cups water
2	teaspoons *Organic Better Than Bouillon Chicken Base*
1	teaspoon turmeric (optional spice)
1/2	cup flat-leaf parsley, chopped

1. Peel and chop onion and carrot. Dice celery.
2. Sauté onion, celery, carrot, almonds and barley in olive oil for 5 minutes on medium-high heat.
3. Place sautéed mixture in 5-quart rice cooker, along with water, turmeric and chicken base. Cook until light goes out.
4. Stir in chopped parsley and serve.

NOTE: *Look for hulled or hulless barley in a natural food store. It is less refined than pearled barley. See Page 138 for more information on barley. May cook on stove top. Cover and simmer for 60 minutes or until water is absorbed.*

If using refined barley such as medium or pearled barley, decrease water to 2 cups. It will cook in less time.

NOTE: *Turmeric contains curcumin which lessens insulin resistance*

Oat Groat Pilaf

1	medium onion
1	stalk celery
1	medium carrot, peeled
1	teaspoon olive oil
1	cup whole oat groats
2	cups reduced-sodium chicken or vegetable broth
1/4	teaspoon freshly ground black pepper to taste
2	tablespoons minced, fresh flat-leaf parsley (optional)

1. Over medium-high heat, in a dry, heavy saucepan, cook oats, stirring for about 3 minutes until slightly golden. Set aside.
2. Peel and dice onion and carrot. Dice celery.
3. Add oil, onion, celery and carrot to saucepan. Sauté and stir 1 minute.
4. Add the broth and black pepper. Bring the mixture to a boil, reduce the heat, add the oats, cover the pan and simmer for about 40 minutes.
5. Remove from heat. Stir in the parsley.

NOTE: This can also be made in a rice cooker or steamer.

Oat groats *are the whole kernel of oats with only the fibrous hull removed; they are not cut or flattened. Look for them in the natural foods section of grocery stores or natural/health foods stores.*

Servings: 6

NUTRITION PER SERVING

Serving size	1/2 cup
Calories	125
Protein	4 g
Carbohydrate*	22 g
(*no added sugars)	
Fiber	3.4 g
Soluble fiber	1.5 g
Fat	2 g
Saturated fat	0.39 g
Cholesterol	0 mg
Sodium	46 mg
Potassium	84 mg
Calcium	18 mg
Omega-3	none

Bonus:	
Selenium	(18% DV)
Iron	(16% DV)
Magnesium	(12% DV)
Copper	(11% DV)
Zinc	(10% DV)

Quinoa Pilaf with Red and Yellow Peppers

1/2	each roasted red and yellow peppers, diced (Page 355)
1	tablespoon minced shallots or onion
1	tablespoon minced garlic
1	cup quinoa
2	cups reduced-sodium chicken broth or 2 cups water + 1 teaspoon chicken or vegetable base
1/8	teaspoon ground white pepper
1	bay leaf
1/2	teaspoon dry thyme or 1 sprig fresh thyme

1. Roast peppers, unless using already roasted from jar or your freezer. Dice. Chop shallots and garlic.
2. Place quinoa in mesh strainer and rinse well.
3. In a medium saucepan, add the quinoa, shallots, garlic, broth, pepper, bay leaf and thyme. Bring the liquid to a boil. Lower to simmer and cover the pot tightly. Cook 10 to 15 minutes.
4. Remove and discard the bay leaf and thyme if using a fresh sprig. Fluff the quinoa with a fork to separate the grains and release steam.
5. Fold in the peppers and serve.

Servings: 6

NUTRITION PER SERVING

Serving size	1/2 cup
Calories	129
Protein	5 g
Carbohydrate*	21 g
(*no added sugars)	
Fiber	7.5 g
Soluble fiber	0.7 g
Fat	2.4 g
Saturated fat	0.6 g
Cholesterol	0 mg
Sodium	101 mg
Potassium	204 mg
Calcium	14 mg
Omega-3 ALA	10 mg

Bonus:	
Magnesium	(15% DV)
Zinc	(15% DV)
Vitamin A	(10% DV)

Quinoa (KEEN-wah) is a gluten-free super grain, rich in protein and high fiber. It has the highest quality of protein of the grains. Look for it in the health food section of the grocery store, and cook and use it like you would rice. The seeds are usually white or ivory, but there are red and brown/black varieties.

Rainbow Veggie Rice

2 cups cooked or leftover brown rice or *Multi-Grain Pilaf* (Page 327) or *Lundberg Wild Rice Blend*
1 stalk celery, diced
1/2 medium red onion, peeled and diced
1 carrot, peeled and diced
1/4 red bell pepper

1/2 cup frozen cut-leaf spinach, thawed
1/2 cup frozen broccoli florets, thawed and chopped
1/4 cup frozen corn
1/2 cup frozen green peas

1/2 teaspoon onion powder
1/2 teaspoon tarragon
1/2 teaspoon *Mrs. Dash Tomato Basil Garlic Seasoning Blend* or another salt-free seasoning
1/4 teaspoon sea salt

1 tablespoon olive oil

1. Cook rice if you don't have leftover rice. (To cook 1 cup brown rice, use 2 cups water plus 1 teaspoon *Organic Better Than Bouillon Chicken Base*.)
2. Dice all of the fresh vegetables about the same size and place in bowl. Remove stem, seeds and membrane, and dice bell pepper.
3. In another bowl, measure out the frozen spinach, broccoli, corn and green peas.
4. In small dish, measure the onion powder, tarragon, seasoning and salt.
5. In skillet over medium heat, sauté celery, onion, carrot and bell pepper with a tablespoon of oil until tender.
6. Add spinach, broccoli, corn and peas. Sauté until heated. Add rice and seasoning, and sauté a few minutes more until warmed.

VARIATIONS

Add cubed, baked tofu; leftover chicken; or legumes/beans, such as garbanzo, black or kidney. Vary the vegetables to whatever you like or have available.

Servings: 9

NUTRITION PER SERVING

Serving size	3/4 cup
Calories	152
Protein	6.5 g
Carbohydrate*	22 g
(*no added sugars)	
Fiber	4.5 g
Soluble fiber	1 g
Fat	5 g
Saturated fat	0.8 g
Cholesterol	0 mg
Sodium	176 mg
Potassium	212 mg
Calcium	53 mg
Omega-3 ALA	21 mg
Bonus:	
Beta Carotene	(30% DV)
Vitamin C	(17% DV)
Magnesium	(13% DV)
Selenium	(10% DV)
Zinc	(8% DV)

Basmati Rice Pilaf

This recipe is from Dr. Majed Abuhajir, a compassionate and skilled hematologist oncologist, who is also an amazing cook. Be sure to buy aged basmati rice; it is key to the success of this recipe. The best place to buy it is at an Indian store.

1	cup aged basmati rice
1-1/2	cups water + 1 teaspoon *Penzeys Spices' Chicken Stock/Soup Base*
1	tablespoon olive oil
2	cloves garlic, chopped
2	medium onions, peeled and chopped
1	carrot, peeled, grated
1/2	cup frozen mixed vegetables or green peas (optional)
1/8	teaspoon cinnamon
1/2	teaspoon ground allspice, (whole can be used, if desired)
1/2	teaspoon (more or less to taste) freshly ground black pepper
1/2	teaspoon turmeric
	Toasted almonds and/or pine nuts (optional)

1. To wash rice, place 1 cup aged basmati rice in bowl, cover with water and swish rice, then drain off water. Continue this process until the water no longer looks cloudy and remains relatively clear. This usually takes 5 rinses or more
2. Cover washed rice with water and soak at room temperature for 30 minutes.
3. Toast slivered almonds or pine nuts in dry pan until golden, then set aside.
4. Drain rice in fine mesh strainer for a few minutes.
5. Prepare stock by mixing water and chicken base. Bring to a boil then set aside until needed.
6. Prepare the garlic, onion and carrot.
7. Heat 1 tablespoon olive oil in heavy pan with tight-fitting lid. Add vegetables to pan, adding optional vegetables, if using, such as mixed vegetables; green peas (frozen and thawed); or leftover cooked, diced vegetables. Sauté until soft.
8. Add soaked and drained rice and sauté until kernels are coated, but don't let rice brown.
9. Add cinnamon, allspice, black pepper and turmeric.
10. Add hot broth to pan, reduce to simmer, then cover and cook 10 minutes without lifting the lid.
11. Remove from heat and let stand covered 5 minutes. Uncover and fluff using a fork.
12. Sprinkle toasted nuts on rice before serving.

VARIATION
Use brown basmati rice (from any store) in place of aged white rice, and increase the cooking time to 25 minutes. I like to add a bay leaf and 4 whole cardamom seed pods, crushed to release the seeds. Discard the pods before serving. You can add lentils (brown, green or beluga) to this at step 7, since lentils will cook in the time needed for the brown rice.

Servings: 6

NUTRITION PER SERVING

Serving size	1/2 cup
Calories	145
Protein	6 g
Carbohydrate*	25 g
(*no added sugars)	
Fiber	3 g
Soluble fiber	0.2 g
Fat	2.5 g
Saturated fat	0.5 g
Cholesterol	0 mg
Sodium	190 mg
Potassium	43 mg
Calcium	7 mg
Omega-3 ALA	16 mg

Broccoli Couscous

2	cups frozen broccoli florets, thawed
1	cup low-sodium chicken broth (or 1 cup water + 1 teaspoon *Organic Better Than Bouillon Chicken or Vegetable Base*)
1	teaspoon Dijon mustard
1	teaspoon extra-virgin olive oil
2/3	cup whole-wheat couscous
2	tablespoons pine nuts, toasted (Page 285)

1. Chop broccoli florets in bite-size pieces. (If using fresh, steam or cook 3 to 4 minutes in microwave.)
2. Bring chicken broth, mustard, oil and chopped broccoli to a boil.
3. Add couscous to boiling liquid and cover. Let stand 5 minutes. Couscous will stick together as one clump.
4. Add pine nuts and use a fork to fluff while stirring in nuts.

Couscous is not a grain, it is tiny pasta. The whole-wheat variety of couscous is made from coarsely ground durum whole wheat, a high-protein, high-gluten variety of wheat. Choose the varieties that specify they are 100% whole durum. Most of what we buy in stores today has been pre-steamed and only requires adding hot water and a short cooking time. Cooking it with broth or a tiny amount of salt will add flavor to an otherwise bland-tasting product. The oil will help to keep the pieces separate.

NUTRITION NOTE
Broccoli is a source of omega-3.

Servings: 4

NUTRITION PER SERVING

Serving size	3/4 cup
Calories	148
Protein	6 g
Carbohydrate*	25 g
(*no added sugars)	
Fiber	5 g
Soluble fiber	0.6 g
Fat	3.6 g
Saturated fat	0.2 g
Cholesterol	0 mg
Sodium	181 mg
Potassium	110 mg
Calcium	34 mg
Omega-3 ALA	50 mg
Bonus:	
Vitamin C	(37% DV)
Vitamin K	(38 mcg)

Roasted Vegetable and Orzo

1   cup Roasted Vegetables (Page 354) or buy roasted red and yellow bell peppers sold in jars
1   cup dry whole-wheat orzo or whole-wheat pasta shells, rotini or whole-wheat bow ties
2   tablespoons pine nuts or slivered almonds, toasted (Page 285)
2   tablespoons finely chopped fresh flat-leaf parsley

2   tablespoons sliced basil leaves

1   tablespoon walnut oil or canola oil

1/8   teaspoon sea salt
      Few grinds freshly ground black pepper

1. Roast vegetables, dice and place in bowl. This step can be done ahead of time, refrigerate the vegetables until ready to make salad.
2. Cook pasta according to package directions.
3. Meanwhile, toast pine nuts, then add to bowl with vegetables.
4. Chop parsley, slice basil and add to bowl with the vegetables.
5. When orzo is cooked, drain well Add oil, salt and pepper into bowl with vegetables and nuts.
6. Toss and serve or chill until ready to serve.

NUTRITION NOTE

Orzo is a pasta shaped like rice. Look for whole wheat.

Servings: 4

NUTRITION PER SERVING

Serving size	1/2 cup
Calories	196
Protein	7 g
Carbohydrate*	25 g
(*no added sugars)	
Fiber	1.8 g
Soluble fiber	0.3 g
Fat	7 g
Saturated fat	0.5 g
Cholesterol	0 mg
Sodium	77 mg
Potassium	191 mg
Calcium	19 mg
Omega-3 ALA	390 mg
Bonus:	
Vitamin C	(54% DV)
Vitamin K	(39 mcg)

Nutty Rotini

1-1/2	cup dry, whole-wheat rotini pasta (about 3 cups cooked)
1/2	of a 15-ounce can northern beans, or white kidney beans (cannellini) no-salt-added preferred
2	tablespoons natural peanut butter or almond butter
2	teaspoons honey
1	teaspoon reduced-sodium soy or tamari sauce
1/4	teaspoon onion powder
1	clove garlic or 1/4 teaspoon garlic powder
3	tablespoons water
1	cup frozen mixed vegetables, thawed
1/2	cup frozen cut-leaf spinach, thawed

1. Cook pasta in boiling water, being careful not to overcook. While cooking, prepare remaining ingredients.
2. Drain and rinse beans, then mash with fork. Add peanut butter, honey, soy sauce, onion powder, garlic and water. You may also put everything into a small food processor to blend. Stir and microwave or heat until warm.
3. Microwave or cook mixed vegetables until desired tenderness. Add spinach and heat until warm.
4. Drain cooked pasta. Add warmed bean mixture and vegetables. Stir and serve.

Servings: 6

NUTRITION PER SERVING

Serving size	1/2 cup
Calories	155
Protein	6 g
Carbohydrate*	26 g
(*3 g sugars from honey)	
Fiber	3 g
Soluble fiber	1.2 g
Fat	3 g
Saturated fat	0.5 g
Cholesterol	0 mg
Sodium	65 mg
Potassium	111 mg
Calcium	35 mg
Omega-3 ALA	20 mg

Bonus:
Beta-carotene	(33% DV)
Folate	(14% DV)
Selenium	(18% DV)

Asian Noodles

Sauce ingredients: (makes 1 cup sauce)

1	large garlic clove, crushed or finely minced (or 1/4 teaspoon garlic powder)
1-1/2	tablespoons reduced-sodium soy sauce or tamari
2	teaspoons rice vinegar
1	tablespoon toasted sesame oil
1/8	teaspoon chili garlic sauce (found in Thai section of grocery store) or use a dash of cayenne. Add more if you prefer a spicier taste.
1/2	teaspoon honey
1/4	cup raw cashews
3	tablespoons water

. . . .

1/2	carrot
1/2	red pepper
4	ounces whole-wheat angel hair spaghetti
1/2	cup edamame (shelled), thawed if frozen (or use green peas)
1	teaspoon canola oil or toasted sesame oil
1-1/2	teaspoons sesame seed

1. Make sauce by combining all ingredients in small food processor and blend until smooth. Sauce can be made ahead and refrigerated, if desired.
2. Peel and dice carrot.
3. Remove seed, stem and membrane from bell pepper. Dice pepper.
4. Put large pot of water on stove and bring to boil. Cook pasta according to package directions. Add edamame to cook with pasta. If using green peas, sauté with carrot below.
5. Sauté over medium heat, carrot and red pepper with oil until slightly softened. Mixture may also be combined and microwaved for 1 to 2 minutes.
6. Drain spaghetti. Add 1/2 cup sauce, reserving remainder for another use. Add sautéed vegetables and toss.

OPTIONS

For main dish, add 1 cup of cooked, shredded chicken (Page 400), baked tofu or tempeh, or sautéed shrimp.

HELPFUL HINTS

- To make this small amount of sauce, a small food processor works best.

- The sauce freezes well. Make extra and toss with any pasta or cooked grain for a quick meal.

- Also makes a good sauce for vegetables.

- May use 3 tablespoons cashew butter instead of raw cashews.

Servings: 3

NUTRITION PER SERVING

Serving size	1 cup
Calories	283
Protein	10 g
Carbohydrate*	38 g
(*1 g sugars from honey)	
Fiber	6 g
Soluble fiber	1.5 g
Fat	11 g
Saturated fat	1.5 g
Cholesterol	0 mg
Sodium	299 mg
Potassium	229 mg
Calcium	55 mg
Omega-3 ALA	20 mg

Bonus:

Beta-carotene	(37% DV)
Magnesium	(27% DV)
Vitamin C	(27% DV)
Copper	(24% DV)
Zinc	(13% DV)

Sandwich Ideas

Wrap/Bread Choices

❖ Sprouted, whole-wheat, flourless, English muffins
❖ Sprouted, flourless breads
❖ Pita pockets (100% whole-wheat)
❖ Whole-grain tortilla, low-carbohydrate or sprouted-grain
❖ 100% whole-wheat bread with pieces of grains still visible
❖ Lettuce leaf. For a low-carbohydrate version, any of the things that are normally served between slices of bread can be rolled up in a lettuce leaf and/or eaten with a fork, served along with vegetables cut into sticks (carrot, celery, zucchini, jicama, etc.).

Veggie-Stuffed Pita Pocket

❖ Whole-wheat pita pocket
❖ Hummus (Page 428)
   Spread hummus inside pita pocket. Add any of the following:
   ◆ Roasted red pepper (roast fresh peppers from Page 355 or buy in a jar)
   ◆ Thinly sliced cucumber, red bell pepper, jicama, red onion
   ◆ Finely chopped broccoli florets
   ◆ Thinly sliced tomato
   ◆ Thinly sliced avocado
   ◆ Tahini, thinned with water and drizzled on top

HELPFUL HINT
To thinly slice vegetables, a mandolin works great.

Nut Butter

❖ 2 tablespoons almond butter (or natural peanut butter, sunflower, etc.)
❖ Small carrot, finely grated
❖ Lettuce leaf
   ◆ Mix almond butter and carrot together. Spread on bread, tortilla or pita pocket and add lettuce.
   ◆ May also skip the bread. Spread on red or green, leafy lettuce leaf, then roll up and eat.

NUTRITION NOTE
Spread nut butter on celery sticks or cucumber slices and eat.

Creamy Nut Butter

❖ Spread peanut butter on one side and soy cream cheese on other side
❖ Sprinkle of cinnamon
❖ Chopped dried fruit (craisins, currants, raisins) or very thinly sliced apple or pear

NUTRITION NOTE
Try almond butter, sunflower butter, cashew, soy nut, or any other nut butter you find.

Grilled Nut Butter

NUTRITION PER SERVING

Serving size	1 sandwich
Calories	293
Protein	18 g
Carbohydrate*	29 g
(*no added sugars)	
Fiber	5 g
Soluble fiber	1.2 g
Fat	13 g
Saturated fat	3.3 g
Cholesterol	0 mg
Sodium	575 mg
Potassium	260 mg
Calcium	250 mg
Omega-3 ALA	40 mg

- 2 slices whole-wheat bread
- 1 tablespoon natural peanut butter or almond butter
- 1/4 cup shredded low-fat cheese (*Cabot 75% Reduced-Fat Cheddar Cheese*)

1. Spray two slices of whole-wheat bread with cooking spray or spritz with olive oil. On unsprayed side, spread peanut butter.
2. Top with cheese and second slice of bread.
3. Grill on medium heat. Serve.

Nutty Fruity Salmon

NUTRITION PER SERVING

Serving size	1/4 cup filling
Calories	82
Protein	4 g
Carbohydrate*	2 g
(*no added sugars)	
Fiber	0.5 g
Soluble fiber	0.15 g
Fat	6 g
Saturated fat	0.5 g
Cholesterol	11 mg
Sodium	167 mg
Potassium	106 mg
Calcium	49 mg
Omega-3 ALA	71 mg
EPA+DHA	215mg

Bonus:
Vitamin D	(84 IU)

- 1 (7-ounce) pouch salmon
- 2 carrots, grated using small holes on box grater
- 1 apple, cored and shredded
- 1/4 cup light mayonnaise (Page 285)
- 1 teaspoon honey mustard (*East Shore Sweet and Tangy*)
- 1/4 cup walnuts, toasted and chopped

1. Combine all ingredients in small bowl.
2. Place 1/4 cup of mixture into whole-wheat pita pocket, or on a whole-wheat tortilla or whole-wheat bread, along with lettuce and sprouts. Mixture can also be stuffed in celery sticks.

Cottage Cheese Spread

3/4	cup low-fat cottage cheese (no-salt-added preferred)
1/2	teaspoon lemon juice
1/4	teaspoon garlic powder and onion powder
1/4	cup walnuts, toasted and chopped
3	tablespoons dry oat bran
4	red, leafy lettuce leaves
	thinly sliced veggies

1. Blend cottage cheese, lemon juice, and garlic and onion powder in food processor or with handheld blender until smooth. Stir in walnuts and oat bran.
2. Spread 1/4 cup on sprouted whole-wheat bread (toasted if desired). Add lettuce, tomato, thinly sliced bell pepper and zucchini, roasted peppers or any other vegetables.

NUTRITION NOTES
- Has 230 mg sodium if using regular cottage cheese.
- Has omega-3 from walnuts.
- Serve on cucumber slices instead of bread.

Servings: 4

NUTRITION PER SERVING

Serving size	1/4 cup
Calories	121
Protein	8 g
Carbohydrate*	8 g
(*no added sugars)	
Fiber	1.6 g
Soluble fiber	0.6 g
Fat	7.5 g
Saturated fat	1 g
Cholesterol	0 mg
Sodium**	26 mg
Potassium	81 mg
Calcium	63 mg
Omega-3 ALA	920 mg

Deviled Egg Substitute

1/4	cup liquid egg substitute
2	tablespoons light mayonnaise (Page 285)
1/8	teaspoon white pepper
	finely chopped onion and celery (optional)

1. Using a skillet cook the liquid egg substitute as though you were making an omelet. Slip out of pan onto cutting board, cut into small pieces, and allow to cool.
2. Combine the cooled egg substitute with the mayonnaise, mustard, salt and pepper, adding chopped onion and celery, if desired.

NUTRITION NOTE
Has omega-3 from oil in mayonnaise.

Servings: 1

NUTRITION PER SERVING

Serving size	1/4 cup
Calories	125
Protein	5 g
Carbohydrate*	5 g
(*no added sugars)	
Fiber	0 g
Soluble fiber	0 g
Fat	10 g
Saturated fat	0 g
Cholesterol	10 mg
Sodium	331 mg
Potassium	71 mg
Calcium	45 mg
Omega-3 ALA	1,000 mg

Flavored Spreads
(Use instead of butter or margarine)

Feta Spread

Spread a very thin layer instead of mustard or mayonnaise. Kalamata olives add lots of flavor so you won't need much.

4	Kalamata olives, pitted and chopped
2	teaspoon lemon juice
1/2	teaspoon dried basil
1/4	teaspoon dried oregano
1/16	teaspoon Aleppo pepper (*Penzeys Spices*) or cayenne pepper
2	ounces feta cheese
1	teaspoon extra-virgin olive oil

1. With fork, combine and blend until smooth,
2. Add a teaspoon of lemon juice or water if needed.

NUTRITION NOTE

Olives and feta make this higher in sodium; use sparingly.

Servings: 4

NUTRITION PER SERVING

Serving size	1 tablespoon
Calories	69
Protein	2 g
Carbohydrate*	1 g
(*no added sugars)	
Fiber	0.2 g
Soluble fiber	0 g
Fat	6.5 g
Saturated fat	2.5 g
Cholesterol	13 mg
Sodium	219 mg
Potassium	18 mg
Calcium	76 mg
Omega-3 ALA	76 mg

Seasoned Mayonnaise

Start with 1/4 teaspoon of seasoning per half cup mayonnaise or salad dressing and adjust to taste.

Mayonnaise mixed with wasabi powder

Mayonnaise mixed with chipotle chili powder or Aleppo pepper

Thousand Island Spread

1/2	cup light mayonnaise (Page 285)
2	tablespoons organic ketchup
1/2	teaspoon paprika
2	tablespoons pickle relish
1/4	teaspoon onion powder or dry minced onion

Combine and mix well.

Servings: 12

NUTRITION PER SERVING

Serving size	1 tablespoon
Calories	39
Protein	0 g
Carbohydrate*	3 g
(*no added sugars)	
Fiber	0.08 g
Soluble fiber	0 g
Fat	3.5 g
Saturated fat	0 g
Cholesterol	3 mg
Sodium	102 mg
Potassium	8 mg
Calcium	0 mg
Omega-3 ALA	333 mg

Sandwich Spread

3   ounces leftover, cooked chicken breast (no skin); pork; beef (round or loin); or leftover, cooked fish (about 1/2 cup)
2-3 tablespoons light mayonnaise (Page 285)
1   tablespoon finely chopped green pepper or 1 teaspoon sweet pickle relish
1-2 tablespoons chopped onion
1/2 teaspoon mustard, such as *East Shore Sweet and Tangy*
1/8 teaspoon salt-free lemon pepper (*Penzeys Spices' Sunny Spain*)

1. Place all in small food processor.
2. Pulse until coarsely chopped.

When choosing chicken or pork, check ingredient list and label to select one that has not been marinated or injected with a sodium solution.

NUTRITION NOTE
Omega-3 from mayonnaise.

Servings: 2

NUTRITION PER SERVING

Serving size	1/4 cup
Calories	99
Protein	10 g
Carbohydrate*	2.5 g
(*no added sugars)	
Fiber	0.2 g
Soluble fiber	0.04 g
Fat	5.5 g
Saturated fat	0.1 g
Cholesterol	29 mg
Sodium	124 mg
Potassium	124 mg
Calcium	7 mg
Omega-3 ALA	500 mg

Salmon Spread

1   (7-ounce) can salmon, drained, no-salt-added preferred
2   tablespoons light mayonnaise (Page 285)
1   teaspoon yellow mustard

OPTIONAL ADD-INS
❖   chopped chives
❖   finely minced red onion
❖   chopped bell pepper
❖   pickle relish

1. Break apart salmon, mashing bones with fork (adds calcium).
2. Add remaining ingredients.
3. Stir and serve.

Servings: 2

NUTRITION PER SERVING

Serving size	1/4 cup
Calories	115
Protein	10 g
Carbohydrate*	1 g
(*no added sugars)	
Fiber	0 g
Soluble fiber	0 g
Fat	7.5 g
Saturated fat	1 g
Cholesterol	15 mg
Sodium	125 mg
Potassium	139 mg
Omega-3 ALA	125 mg
EPA + DHA	427mg

Tofu Egg Salad

NUTRITION NOTES
Source of omega-3 is
canola based mayonnaise
and tofu.

Servings: 6

NUTRITION PER SERVING

Serving size	1/4 cup
Calories	71
Protein	7 g
Carbohydrate*	2 g
(*no added sugars)	
Fiber	0 g
Soluble fiber	0 g
Fat	4 g
Saturated fat	0 g
Cholesterol	3 mg
Sodium	245 mg
Potassium	84 mg
Calcium	23 mg
Omega-3 ALA	457 mg

Bonus:
Vitamin E   (7% DV)

1	(12.3-ounce) box silken, firm tofu (*Mori-Nu*)
1	cup egg substitute
1/4	teaspoon turmeric (gives a nice yellow color)
1/4	cup light mayonnaise (Page 285)
1	teaspoon yellow mustard
1/8	teaspoon sea salt
	freshly ground pepper to taste

1. Pour egg substitute in a nonstick pan sprayed with cooking spray.
2. Cover and cook over very low heat for 4 to 5 minutes or until it begins to set.
3. Slide out of pan onto a cutting board.
4. Cut into small pieces.
5. Open box of tofu, discard any liquid.
6. Place block of tofu on cutting board. Dice tofu into small pieces.
7. Combine all ingredients together and stir gently. Chill.
8. Serve with lettuce on toasted whole-wheat bread.

OPTIONAL
❖ May also add chopped celery, onion and red bell pepper. Serve open-face on whole-wheat bread, rolled into a whole-wheat tortilla, or mounded onto celery stalks.

Portobello Mushroom Melts

Servings: 2

NUTRITION PER SERVING

Serving size	1 mushroom
Calories	87
Protein	5 g
Carbohydrate*	7 g
(*no added sugars)	
Fiber	1.5 g
Soluble fiber	0.4 g
Fat	4 g
Saturated fat	0.4 g
Cholesterol	0 mg
Sodium	201 mg
Potassium	427 mg
Calcium	167 mg
Omega-3 ALA	30 mg

Bonus:
Selenium   (20% DV)

1	teaspoon olive oil
2	teaspoons balsamic vinegar
1	clove garlic, minced
1/2	teaspoon dried thyme
1/4	teaspoon dry, cracked rosemary
2	large portobello mushrooms
2	tablespoons shredded mozzarella or Parmesan cheese, *soy or almond cheese*

1. Preheat oven to 400° F.
2. In small bowl, mix oil, vinegar, garlic, thyme and rosemary.
3. Tap mushroom to remove any growing medium. They do not need washing. Use a sharp knife to cut the stem even with the gills.
4. Place mushroom, gill side up, in shallow baking dish and spoon mixture over mushrooms. Bake 15 to 20 minutes.
5. Sprinkle with cheese and bake a few minutes more until cheese starts to melt. Mushrooms may also be broiled 6 minutes per side, instead of baked. Serve hot.

NOTE Cooked mushrooms can be frozen and reheated.

Whole-Wheat Veggie Wrap

4   whole-wheat tortillas
1   cup hummus (Page 428)
2   cups baby spinach
1   cup finely shredded carrots
1   large, thinly sliced, yellow bell pepper

1. Lay out tortillas in front of you. Spread top half of each with 1/4 cup hummus.
2. Add layer of spinach, carrots and red pepper over the whole tortilla, ending 1-1/2 inches from the top.
3. Tightly roll each from the edge near you. Wrap each one in plastic wrap, tuck down ends and twist wrap. Do the other end and chill 30 minutes or longer.
4. Remove plastic, eat as is or slice and serve on lettuce-lined plate.

Choose a whole-wheat tortilla that does not contain partially hydrogenated oils or high fructose corn syrup (see Page 287 for suggestions).

Servings: 4

NUTRITION PER SERVING

Serving size	1 wrap
Calories	202
Protein	7 g
Carbohydrate*	37 g
(*no added sugar)	
Fiber	7 g
Soluble fiber	2.1 g
Fat	6 g
Saturated fat	1 g
Cholesterol	0 mg
Sodium	351 mg
Potassium	360 mg
Calcium	66 mg
Omega-3 ALA	80 mg

Bonus:
Beta-carotene	(137% DV)
Vitamin C	(81% DV)
Folate	(20% DV)
Magnesium	(13% DV)
Vitamin K	(78 mcg)

Pizza Crust

Making healthy pizza is easier than you may think. Start by making a healthier crust with whole-wheat flour. Make the dough in the morning or the night before. Allowing it to rest in the refrigerator will help the gluten relax so it is easier to work with. Bring refrigerated dough to room temperature before you roll it out. You can even make it and freeze, then thaw overnight in refrigerator before using.

Crust: for two 9-inch pizzas or one 15-inch pizza

3/4	cup warm water
1	tablespoon extra-virgin olive oil
1-1/2	cup whole-wheat flour (white whole-wheat if available)
1	teaspoon *SAF Perfect Rise Instant Yeast*
1/2	teaspoon sea salt
1/2	cup all-purpose flour

FOOD PROCESSOR (WITH FEED TUBE METHOD

Combine water and oil in measuring cup. Place remaining dry ingredients into the bowl of a food processor with the plastic blade. Pulse a few times to mix well. Turn on the processor and add the water and oil through the feed tube. Stop the machine. If the dough has not formed into a ball, add flour one tablespoon at a time and pulse until ball forms. Once the dough forms into a ball process 30 seconds longer.

BY HAND

Combine water and oil in mixing bowl. Stir in flours, salt and yeast. Stir until stiff dough forms. Turn out onto counter and knead for 5 minutes. Knead by folding the dough onto itself and pressing with the heel of the hand, making a quarter turn and repeating the process. Add a sprinkle of flour to the surface as needed to keep dough from sticking. Use the least amount of flour to prevent the dough from getting too dry. When dough is smooth, return it to the bowl, oil the top and let it rise. If using immediately, let rise 20 to 30 minutes on the counter. If using the next day or later, put into a resealable plastic bag and refrigerate.

HELPFUL HINT
For quick Pizza Sauce, see Page 388.

MIXER WITH DOUGH HOOK METHOD

Follow "by hand" method and use the mixer with the dough hook to knead dough. If dough is too sticky add flour a tablespoon at a time. If it is too stiff, add water a tablespoon at a time.

SHAPING THE CRUST

If dough has been refrigerated, allow it to come to room temperature before rolling out. If frozen, thaw overnight in refrigerator, and then set on counter to reach room temperature.

THIN CRUST. Flatten ball of dough with hands. Let dough rest for 5 minutes. Starting at the center and working toward the outside edges, use finger tips to press down and toward the outside edges. Take care not to tear dough. Continue until the dough is 1/4 inch thick. Add toppings and bake without letting rise.

THICK CRUST. Follow same procedure as thin, but leave it 1/2-inch thick and let crust rise, covered with a cloth, until puffy before adding toppings and baking.

TOPPINGS

Tomato sauce and a little grated Parmesan cheese are all you need. As an alternative to tomato sauce, use Pesto (Page 390) and spread thinly. Use bottled tomato sauces or make your own. If you wish, add very thinly sliced vegetables (a mandolin works well) before baking. Sliced olives; bell peppers; sun-dried tomatoes; frozen, thawed and chopped broccoli florets; mushrooms; onions or any vegetables you enjoy. Finely sliced fresh arugula or baby spinach added to the pizza as soon as it comes from the oven will wilt from the heat.

BAKING PIZZA

If using a baking sheet, spray the area where the pizza will be with cooking spray and dust with stoneground cornmeal. Do not use insulated pans as they prevent browning. Darker pans will brown the bottom best. Bake pizza at 475°F. When crust is lightly browned, lift up an edge to check.

BAKING STONE

If baking on a pizza stone, dust the paddle with cornmeal or rice flour. Heat the stone in a 500°F oven for 30 minutes before you start cooking. If your stone comes with preheating instructions, follow them. Tiles or stones need time to heat up. Sliding the pizza onto the stone requires a bit of practice. Use a quick, jerking action to slide it off the peel. It is easier if you place a piece of parchment paper on the peel, pizza screen or rimless cookie sheet (if cookie sheet has rims turn over and use the bottom). Shape the pizza dough on the parchment paper. Trim excess paper since it can burn at temperature over 450°F. Slide the pizza with the paper onto the preheated baking stone. Discard the paper afer the pizza is baked.

PREBAKED CRUSTS

Make extra dough and then prebake and freeze crusts. On busy days you can take them out and make pizza quickly. After shaping the crust on parchment paper slide the dough, including the parchment paper, onto the baking stone. Bake about 2 to 3 minutes until just set. Remove from oven, remove parchment paper, and allow to cool on a wire rack until completely cooled. Wrap and store in freezer until needed.

OTHER CRUST IDEAS

- ❖ Prebaked frozen crusts such as *French Meadows* (spelt, sourdough, yeast free).
- ❖ Refrigerated pizza dough sold by some stores and pizza shops.
- ❖ Frozen whole-wheat bread dough, thawed and shaped as desired.
- ❖ Whole-wheat tortilla.
- ❖ Whole-wheat pita pocket (separated for thinner crust).
- ❖ Whole-wheat, sprouted, English muffin.

Pesto Salmon Pita Pizza

NUTRITION NOTE
Try canned smoked salmon.

Servings: 1

NUTRITION PER SERVING

Serving size	2 pita halves
Calories	278
Protein	21 g
Carbohydrate*	31 g
(*no added sugar)	
Fiber	5 g
Soluble fiber	2 g
Fat	9 g
Saturated fat	2 g
Cholesterol	37 mg
Sodium	382 mg
Potassium	640 mg
Calcium	390 mg
Omega-3	
EPA+DHA	810 mg

2	tablespoons tomato sauce (no-salt-added preferred)	
1	teaspoon pesto	
1	tablespoon grated Parmesan	
1/4	cup (2 ounces) salmon, skin and bones removed, flaked	
1	whole-wheat pita pocket	

1. Preheat oven to 450°F.
2. Carefully cut pita around the outside by inserting a knife and working around to open it up into two rounds. Lay on pan.
3. Combine tomato sauce and pesto, spread on pita. Top with salmon then Parmesan.
4. Bake 8 to 10 minutes.

Parmesan Pesto Pizza

1. Preheat oven to 400°F. Spread pesto (buy or make – see Page 390) on pizza crust (see Page 345 for ideas).
2. Sprinkle with freshly grated Parmesan.
3. Bake about 5 to 10 minutes.

Broccoli Salmon Pizza

Servings: 1

NUTRITION PER SERVING

Serving size	1 tortilla
Calories	273
Protein	28 g
Carbohydrate*	27 g
(*no added sugars)	
Fiber	17 g
Soluble fiber	1.5 g
Fat	12 g
Saturated fat	4 g
Cholesterol	49 mg
Sodium	370 mg
Potassium	440 mg
Calcium	390 mg
Omega-3	
EPA+DHA	810 mg
Bonus:	
Selenium	(33% DV)
Beta-carotene	(27% DV)
Folate	(17% DV)
Vitamin K	(91 mcg)

1	whole-wheat tortilla (Page 287 for brands)
1	tablespoon whipped, reduced-fat, cream cheese
1/2	cup frozen broccoli, thawed and chopped
2	ounces salmon, leftover or canned (no-salt-added preferred)
2	tablespoons shredded reduced-fat, reduced-sodium, Swiss cheese

1. Preheat oven to 400°F.
2. Place tortilla on baking sheet, and bake a few minutes to crisp. Spread with cream cheese and top with broccoli, salmon and cheese.
3. Bake 10 to 12 minutes.

OPTIONS
❖ Add other veggies, onion, bell peppers, mushrooms, etc.

Creamy Vegetable Soup

1	pound asparagus (or other vegetables including carrots, butternut squash, broccoli or cauliflower)
1/2	medium onion
1	clove garlic
1	teaspoon olive oil
1	teaspoon bouillon vegetable base (Page 283)
2	cups water
1	(12.3 ounce) box silken tofu (*Mori-Nu*)
1	lemon, zested and juiced (1 tablespoon juice)

1. Hold asparagus spear in one hand, and using the other hand, snap off tough ends of asparagus and discard.
2. Cut off tip of each spear and reserve, cut remaining portion of spears into pieces. Peel and cut onion into chunks. Peel garlic clove and mince.
3. In saucepan, sauté onion and garlic with 1 teaspoon olive oil about 3 minutes over medium-low heat until soft but not browned.
4. Add vegetable base, water, asparagus spears (not tips yet), and bring to a boil. Reduce and let simmer 15 minutes or until tender. Place in a food processor or blender (or use immersion handheld blender) along with tofu, and blend until smooth.
5. Place back in pan and add reserved asparagus tips, 1 tablespoon lemon juice and all of the zest. Simmer about 5 minutes or until asparagus tips are tender.

HELPFUL HINT
If using carrots or butternut squash instead of asparagus, peel and cube, and adjust cooking time.

Servings: 5

NUTRITION PER SERVING

Serving size	1 cup
Calories	73
Protein	8 g
Carbohydrate*	9 g
(*no added sugars)	
Fiber	3 g
Soluble fiber	0.5 g
Fat	1.4 g
Saturated fat	0.2 g
Cholesterol	0 mg
Sodium	102 mg
Potassium	390 mg
Calcium	49 mg
Omega-3 ALA	185 mg

Bonus:
Vitamin C	(21% DV)

Root and Bean Soup

HELPFUL HINTS

- Use 1 tablespoon fresh basil and parsley if available.

- Do not use cooking wine, which is high in sodium.

4	cups of root vegetables – any combination of the following:
	• parsnip
	• carrot
	• turnip
	• rutabaga
1	medium onion
1	clove garlic
1	stalk celery
1	tablespoon canola oil
1	cup low-sodium vegetable or tomato juice
4	cups low-sodium vegetable broth
1/4	cup white wine
2	tablespoons tamari, reduced-sodium or soy sauce
1/2	cup pineapple juice
1	cup frozen, cut green beans
1	(15 ounce) can salad beans (kidney, pinto and garbanzo)
1/2	teaspoon dry basil
1/2	teaspoon dry parsley

1. Peel and dice root vegetables, onion and garlic. Dice celery. Sauté vegetables with oil over medium heat about 4 minutes.
2. Add vegetable juice, broth, wine, tamari, pineapple juice, and green beans. Bring to a boil, lower to simmer, and cook 15 minutes or until desired tenderness.
3. Add drained and rinsed salad beans, basil and parsley, and cook 5 minutes longer and serve.

VARIATIONS

❖ Add other vegetables, such as sweet potato, butternut squash, potato, zucchini, yellow squash, or mixed vegetables.

❖ *Very Veggie Low Sodium* by R.W. Knudsen or *V-8 Low-Sodium 100% Vegetable Juice*

Servings: 8

NUTRITION PER SERVING

Serving size	1 cup
Calories	105
Protein	5 g
Carbohydrate*	18 g
(*no added sugars)	
Fiber	7 g
Soluble fiber	2 g
Fat	2 g
Saturated fat	0 g
Cholesterol	0 mg
Sodium	290 mg
Potassium	325 mg
Calcium	40 mg
Omega-3 ALA	17 mg
Bonus:	
Beta-carotene	(37% DV)
Vitamin C	(23% DV)
Vitamin K	(8 mcg)

Quick Minestrone Soup

1/2   cup whole-wheat shells, rotini spirals or ditali pasta (1 cup cooked)
2   cloves garlic, chopped
3   cups water
2   teaspoons *Organic Better Than Bouillon Chicken Base* (Page 283)
1/2   cup low-sodium vegetable or tomato juice
1   teaspoon dry, cracked rosemary (*Penzeys Spices*)
1   (15-ounce) can diced tomatoes (*Muir Glen Fire-Roasted Diced Tomatoes*)
1   cup frozen mixed vegetables or vegetables for soup
1   (15 ounce) can navy beans, or other white beans, no-salt-added preferred drained, and rinsed
1   cup frozen cut-leaf spinach or frozen turnip greens
1   tablespoon Pesto (Page 390) or purchased variety

1. Cook pasta 3 minutes less than suggested on package directions. When cooked, drain and rinse with cold water and set aside until needed.
2. Peel and chop garlic.
3. Meanwhile, combine water, bouillon base, vegetable juice, garlic, rosemary, tomatoes with the liquid, and frozen mixed vegetables. Bring to a boil, reduce heat and simmer 5 minutes.
4. Add drained beans, spinach, pesto and cooked pasta. Cook 3 minutes or until vegetables are as tender as you like.

Servings: 8

NUTRITION PER SERVING

Serving size	1 cup
Calories	101
Protein	4.5 g
Carbohydrate*	17 g
(*no added sugars)	
Fiber	5 g
Soluble fiber	1 g
Fat	1.5 g
Saturated fat	0.3 g
Cholesterol	1 mg
Sodium	220 mg
Potassium	283 mg
Calcium	93 mg
Omega-3 ALA	30 mg

Bonus:
Beta-carotene	(61% DV)
Vitamin C	(34% DV)
Vitamin K	(111 mcg)

Quick and Easy Broccoli Corn Soup

1   can northern, navy or white cannellini beans, no-salt-added preferred
8   ounces (about 3 cups) frozen broccoli, thawed or microwaved for 3 minutes
1-1/2   cups plain, unsweetened soy milk (or 1% milk)
1/4   teaspoon dry, cracked rosemary
1/2   teaspoon onion powder
1/4   teaspoon sea salt
1/2   cup frozen corn

1. Drain and rinse beans.
2. Thaw, cook or microwave broccoli.
3. Add all ingredients except for corn to blender, and blend to desired texture.
4. Place in bowl or pan and add corn.
5. Heat to serving temperature.

Servings: 4

NUTRITION PER SERVING

Serving size	1 cup
Calories	138
Protein	10 g
Carbohydrate*	21 g
(*no added sugars)	
Fiber	9 g
Soluble fiber	3 g
Fat	2 g
Saturated fat	0.2 g
Cholesterol	0 mg
Sodium*	180 mg
(*if beans are	
canned with salt)	280 mg
Potassium	365 mg
Calcium	112 mg
Omega-3 ALA	140 mg

Bonus:
Vitamin C	(54% DV)
Folate	(33% DV)
Iron	(15% DV)
Beta-carotene	(12% DV)
Zinc	(7% DV)
Vitamin K	(52 mcg)

Black Bean Soup

1	tablespoon extra-virgin olive oil
1/2	medium onion, diced
1	stalk celery, diced
1	carrot, peeled and diced
1/2	jalapeno pepper, seeds and veins removed, diced small
1/2	green bell pepper, diced
1	(15-ounce) can black beans, no-salt-added preferred, drained and rinsed
1	cup water
1/2	teaspoon Organic *Better Than Bouillon Chicken Base*
1/2	teaspoon ground cumin
1	teaspoon unsweetened natural cocoa powder
1/2	cup salsa
2	teaspoon lime juice

1. Prepare vegetables. Sauté onion, celery, carrot, jalapeno and bell pepper in oil for 5 minutes or until softened.
2. Meanwhile, drain and rinse beans. Mash about half with a fork.
3. Add water, chicken base, cumin, cocoa powder, beans (mashed and whole), and salsa to vegetables and simmer for 10 minutes.
4. Add lime juice and serve.
5. (Optional) Serve with a dollop of reduced-fat sour cream and chopped cilantro.

NOTE: Sodium content varies by amount of sodium in canned beans and salsa.

Servings: 4

NUTRITION PER SERVING

Serving size	1 cup
Calories	148
Protein	9 g
Carbohydrate*	24 g
(*no added sugars)	
Fiber	9 g
Soluble fiber	1.3 g
Fat	3.6 g
Saturated fat	0.5 g
Cholesterol	0 mg
Sodium	153 mg
Potassium	480 mg
Calcium	78 mg
Omega-3 ALA	14 mg

Bonus:
Beta-carotene	(17% DV)
Vitamin C	(20% DV)

Vegetables, Fruits and Pesticides

To lower your exposure to pesticides, you may want to choose organic fruits and vegetables whenever possible. If eating only organic is not possible, try to eat organic for those that have been found to be highest in pesticides. *The Environmental Working Group* has found some fruits and vegetables higher in pesticides and publishes a toxic 12 based on studies from 2000 to 2004; however, that list has not been updated and may not reflect the current pesticide levels on foods but it is all that is currently available. For more information, visit their Web site at www.ewg.org.

Highest Pesticide Levels

The highest levels of pesticides have been found in: peaches, apples, sweet bell peppers, celery, nectarines, strawberries, cherries, pears, imported grapes, spinach, lettuce and potatoes.

Lowest Pesticide Levels

The lowest levels of pesticide levels are in: onion, avocado, sweet corn, pineapple, mango, asparagus, sweet peas, kiwi, banana, cabbage, broccoli and papaya.

Tips for eating more vegetables

Breakfast

❖ Serve egg white omelets filled with sautéed veggies. Use leftover vegetables or frozen stir-fry vegetables, bell peppers, etc., to save time.
❖ Top scrambled eggs with salsa. Choose a salsa with the least sodium.
❖ Have a low-sodium tomato or low-sodium vegetable juice.

Snack Ideas

Cut up several day's worth of veggies and put in small baggies for easy-to-grab snacks.

❖ Dip baby carrots and bell pepper strips in hummus.
❖ Chop spinach or bell peppers very finely and stir into vegetable or spinach dip, then serve with more veggies.
❖ Spread nut butter, such as almond butter or natural peanut butter on celery.
❖ Peel broccoli stems with a vegetable peeler, then dip in natural almond butter (choose a natural brand which is thin enough to dip when at room temperature). This tip is from Irene Wheeler who named it "broccoli stumps" when she served it to her grandson.
❖ Add freeze-dried veggies to trail mix.
❖ Wash and eat cherry tomatoes.

HELPFUL HINT
First make sure you eat enough vegetables before you worry about other issues such as organic or pesticides

WHAT IS A SERVING OF VEGETABLES?
• 1/2 cup cooked
• 1 cup raw
• 1-1/2 cups raw, green, leafy vegetables

WHAT IS A SERVING OF FRUIT?
• 1 medium piece fruit
• 1/2 cup canned fruit

Lunch

For sandwich ideas, try to cut back on the amount of meat or cheese while super-sizing the veggies.

❖ Try hummus or bean spread made by mashing beans to use as a sandwich spread. (See recipes on Pages 428 to 429).

❖ Stuff leftover grilled veggies, thinly sliced (mandolin works good) fresh bell pepper, or sliced cucumber into a whole-wheat pita pocket or roll up in a whole-wheat tortilla.

❖ Add sprouts, spinach or romaine (the darker green, the better) to any sandwich.

❖ Stir grated carrots into tuna or salmon salad.

❖ Add thinly sliced jicama or daikon to your sandwich for a crunchy texture.

❖ Choose a vegetable or bean-based soup. If using canned soup, add extra frozen veggies such as mixed vegetables, chopped broccoli, peas, or any leftover cooked veggies. For each serving, add a tablespoon or two of black beans, kidney beans, lentils, etc.

❖ If eating out, order a side salad with your sandwich and take half the sandwich home for the next day.

❖ If you're eating lunch out, pack raw veggies to eat when you return to work or for an afternoon snack.

❖ Order sandwiches with half the meat and cheese and double the amount of vegetables.

Dinner

❖ At your main meal of the day, plan to have 1-1/2 cups of cooked vegetables, which is three servings.

❖ Have a tossed salad daily. Make enough for the next day, and put in bowls to take for lunch the next day. Add sliced veggies, such as bell peppers, cucumber, cauliflower, grated carrot, etc., but add dressing or tomatoes right before serving.

❖ Offer two different vegetables, even if there is a vegetable in one of the items prepared, such as a casserole, soup or main dish. We tend to eat more when more choices are provided, which is a good thing if the extra options are vegetables. Try a medley of vegetables lightly sautéed or stir-fried.

❖ Each week, try a new vegetable from the produce area, perhaps kale or rapini, to discover some new favorites. You may have to prepare it in several different ways to see which way you prefer.

❖ Cook familiar vegetables or ones you think you don't like in a new way. For example, try roasted brussel sprouts instead of the steamed version, which will taste very different. Keep them slightly crunchy to avoid the strong flavors that develop if overcooked.

❖ To a frozen pizza, add extra veggies, such as chopped spinach; thawed, frozen chopped broccoli, or thinly sliced bell peppers. Add them before you bake.

❖ If you order pizza for take out or delivery, ask for half of the usual amount of cheese and double the vegetables. Then, have a salad before the pizza arrives so less pizza will satisfy you.

- Add frozen stir-fry veggies to casseroles in addition to the onions, celery, etc., already in them.
- Grate carrots, mash northern beans, or shred zucchini and add to meatloaf or meatballs.
- Turn brown rice or whole-wheat couscous into a pilaf by adding grated carrots; finely chopped celery; onion; mushrooms; bell peppers; frozen, chopped spinach; and frozen, chopped broccoli.
- When grilling out, include sliced zucchini, eggplant, fennel and bell peppers, lightly brushed with some olive oil. These taste great at room temperature, hot or cold. Make extras to put in a sandwich the next day.
- Add vegetables to a jar of pasta sauce, such as finely sliced spinach or frozen leaf spinach, kale, or shredded carrots.
- Add cooked red lentils to pasta sauce.
- Add chopped, cooked kale to mashed potatoes or mashed sweet potatoes.
- Serve your entrée, such as grilled fish or chicken, on top of seasoned, dark greens, such as spinach, kale, collards or chard.

BOTTOM LINE

No single vegetable will provide all the nutrients needed. Choose a wide variety of vegetables in many colors. Green, leafy vegetables are especially important in reducing the risk of heart disease. Aim for six or more servings of vegetables. Frozen vegetables without any added sauces are fine and often a convenient way to add them when time is short. It is best not to drink fruits and vegetables as juice; instead eat them whole. Juice does have some nutrients but can't compare to solid pieces of fruit and vegetables. Some antioxidants and fiber found in skins and peels are not in juices.

Vegetables rich in beta-carotene:

Green, leafy (collard, spinach, kale, Swiss chard, romaine)

Red pepper	Carrots	Brussel sprouts
Sweet potato	Broccoli	Winter squash
Pumpkin	Okra	Green peppers

Cruciferous Vegetables

Eating more of these vegetables has been linked to lower levels of inflammation.

Arugula	Cauliflower	Kohlrabi
Bok choy	Collard greens	Mustard greens
Broccoli	Daikon	Radish
Broccoflower	Horseradish	Rapini
Brussel sprouts	Kale	Rutabaga
Cabbage (red, green, savoy, napa)		Turnip

Indole-3-carbinol is derived from the breakdown of glucobrassicin found in cruciferous vegetables. It acts as an antioxidant protecting against cancer.

Roasted Vegetables

Roasted vegetables are great as is and can be served hot or cold. They can be stuffed into pita pockets or added to pasta or grain salads.

To prepare vegetables for roasting, the following suggestions may be helpful:
❖ Zucchini – cut in thirds lengthwise.
❖ Yellow squash – cut in thirds lengthwise.
❖ Eggplant – leave on skin, remove one long lengthwise strip to make it easier to eat. Slice across into inch-thick slices, and spray with oil as it will darken if left standing.
❖ Red, – yellow or green bell pepper – cut in half, and discard seeds and remove inside veins. Cut into smaller sections or flatten.
❖ Fresh asparagus – snap off ends and discard. Cut remaining stalk in half or thirds.
❖ Onions (sweet, red, or yellow) – Peel and cut into wedges or slices.
❖ Roma tomatoes – cut in half.
❖ Fennel – remove tops and slice.

1. Preheat oven to 400°F. Rub vegetables with canola or olive oil.
2. Grind some fresh black pepper over them, to taste.
3. A tiny pinch of sea salt or seasoning such as Herbes de Provence; lemon pepper; *Penzeys Spices' Sunny Spain, Mural of Flavor, Tuscan Sunset, Shallot Pepper, Greek Seasoning*, etc.
4. Lay in a single layer on heavy-duty rimmed baking sheets. Dark baking sheets such as French black steel work best to brown vegetables.
5. Roast or grill.

To Oven Roast

1. Prepare the vegetables as specified above.
2. Roast at 450°F for about 20 minutes. Sprinkle with balsamic vinegar, if desired, when done.
3. Time varies for different vegetables and the size of the pieces being roasted

To Grill (Gas or Charcoal)

Place directly on preheated grill or use skewers or vegetable grilling baskets to hold several pieces of small items, such as garlic or tomato.

Cast-Iron Stove-Top Grill Pan With Ridges

1. Heat pan on top of stove until it is quite hot. Grill both sides of vegetables, such as zucchini, yellow squash, eggplant and asparagus, until they begin to soften and have grill marks.
2. Grilling generally takes a total of 6 to 8 minutes.

Roasted Garlic

Bake the whole heads slowly so they become soft and mild or roast them at a higher temperature for a caramelized version. Use as a spread on bread instead of butter or margarine, or freeze in ice cube trays and use whenever you need a mild garlic flavor.

HELPFUL HINT
This can be frozen for later use or refrigerated for up to one week.

> Several heads garlic (as many as desired)
> Olive oil cooking spray

1. Preheat oven to 375°F. Cut about a half inch off top of garlic head (not root end). Rub to remove any loose, papery skin. Peel the pieces that have been cut off for use in another recipe. Place in baking dish, cut side up. Spray with cooking spray or olive oil and add a little water. Cover and bake for one hour or until soft enough to use as a spread.
2. If you want caramelized garlic, bake uncovered at 400°F for about 30 to 40 minutes.
3. To serve, use a small knife to scoop out of the skin or squeeze the root end until the cloves will slip out.

Garlic. The compound allicin is believed to be responsible for the blood cholesterol and blood pressure reducing effects seen from eating garlic. When the clove is crushed, an enzyme is activated to convert allin to allicin. Cooking destroys some of the benefits. For the full benefit, chop clove, allow to stand, mix with a little olive oil, and stir into a prepared dish that is finished cooking.

Roasted Beets

Scrub, remove tops, wrap in foil, and roast at 450°F for 45 to 60 minutes or until a toothpick inserts easily. Allow to cool. Rub off skin and discard. If cooking different colors, wrap them separately to preserve their individual colors.

Roasted Bell Peppers

HELPFUL HINT
When bell peppers are in season, roast and freeze for use in the winter.
Place a piece of waxed or parchment paper between each piece for easy removal when needed. You can buy these in jars, but the flavor is not as wonderful as when you prepare them since they are packed in water and salt.

1. When you roast peppers over high heat, their skins blacken and blister. After you peel off the skin, you will have tender flesh with a roasted taste.
2. Roast on BBQ grill or under an oven broiler. You can also place directly into the flame of a gas burner, holding them with a long-handled tongs or fork if your kitchen is well-ventilated.
   Steps:
   a. If using a grill or broiler, cut the pepper in half, and remove and discard stem, membranes and seeds. Flatten by pressing down.
   b. Place on grill or under broiler in single layer with skin side toward heat until skin blackens.
   c. Remove and stack them on a plate, and cover with a bowl turned upside down. Allow to steam about 15 minutes, making it easier to remove the peel.
   d. Peel off skin. Do not rinse with water as this will remove the flavor. If small bits of charred skin remain, that is fine they add to the smoky taste.

Crumb-Topped, Oven-Roasted Vegetables

2 cups (8 ounces) brussel sprouts
2 cups cauliflower florets
1 medium carrot (1 cup)
1 sweet potato or 1/2 butternut squash (1 cup)
1 tablespoon olive oil
1/4 teaspoon sea salt
1/8 teaspoon freshly ground black pepper
1/4 teaspoon dry, cracked rosemary

Topping: (This will make 4 tablespoons – freeze extra for another time.)
1 tablespoon whole-wheat bread crumbs
1 tablespoon walnuts or hazelnuts, toasted and chopped
1 tablespoon ground or milled flaxseed
1 tablespoon Parmesan cheese, freshly grated

1. Preheat oven to 425°F.
2. Prepare vegetables. Trim off bottom of brussel sprouts and cut in half. Break cauliflower into florets and cut each in half, if large. Peel and slice carrot on the diagonal. Peel and cube sweet potato or butternut squash. As you prepare each vegetable, place on a baking sheet.
3. Drizzle with oil, and sprinkle with salt, pepper and rosemary. Toss to coat and spread out in a single layer on pan. If they are too close to each other, they will steam instead of roasting.
4. Place pan with vegetables on the lowest rack in oven. Bake for 30 minutes, stirring after 15 minutes. Ovens vary, so watch to see if they are browning too fast and reduce time. If they are taking too long, increase heat.
5. Meanwhile, combine bread crumbs, nuts, flaxseed and Parmesan. When vegetables are roasted, sprinkle with 1 tablespoon of the topping mixture and serve immediately.

HELPFUL HINT
Use 1/2 teaspoon fresh rosemary if available.

Servings: 4

NUTRITION PER SERVING

Serving size	1 cup
Calories	127
Protein	5 g
Carbohydrate*	19 g
(*no added sugars)	
Fiber	6 g
Soluble fiber	2.2 g
Fat	4.7 g
Saturated fat	0.7 g
Cholesterol	1 mg
Sodium	198 mg
Potassium	600 mg
Calcium	65 mg
Omega-3 ALA	340 mg

Bonus:
Beta-carotene	(239% DV)
Vitamin C	(137% DV)
Vitamin K	(113 mcg)

Ginger-Roasted Carrots

1   pound carrots
1   teaspoon ground cumin seed
1   teaspoon fresh-grated ginger
1   teaspoon brown sugar
2   teaspoons olive oil

1. Preheat oven to 375°F.
2. Peel carrots and slice into circles or slice on the diagonal. Place on a dark cookie
    sheet.
3. Add the cumin, ginger, brown sugar and oil. Toss to coat carrots and spread
    carrots in single layer.
4. Roast on a rack in lower portion of the oven until browned (about 15 minutes).
    Time may vary depending upon your oven.

*Carrots. Carrots contain calcium pectate, a pectin fiber that lowers cholesterol. It may be the
reason why in one study, participants who ate a cup of carrots a day had an average 11%
drop in their cholesterol after three weeks. Carrots are also a good source of the antioxidant
beta-carotene. Forget the advice to avoid carrots that some fad diets promote. They have a
low glycemic load.*

Servings: 4

NUTRITION PER SERVING

Serving size	1/2 cup
Calories	79
Protein	1.5 g
Carbohydrate*	13 g
(*1 gram added sugars)	
Fiber	4 g
Soluble fiber	1.3 g
Fat	3 g
Saturated fat	0.5 g
Cholesterol	0 mg
Sodium	82 mg
Potassium	369 mg
Calcium	51 mg
Omega-3 ALA	20 mg

Bonus:
Beta-carotene	(381% DV)
Vitamin C	(11% DV)

Sage Green Beans With Walnuts

3/4   pound fresh or frozen green beans
2   tablespoons toasted walnuts
1   teaspoon walnut oil
1   clove garlic
2   teaspoons chopped, fresh sage leaves

1. Thaw or steam green beans.
2. Toast walnuts in dry pan (Page 285) over medium heat until slightly golden.
3. Chop garlic and sage.
4. Over medium-low heat, sauté garlic in walnut oil for a minute, but do not brown.
5. Add green beans, walnuts and sage. Toss and cook several minutes until beans are
        warmed.

HELPFUL HINTS
• Use canola oil if walnut
  oil is not available.
• Use 1/2 teaspoon dried,
  rubbed sage to replace
  fresh.

Servings: 3

NUTRITION PER SERVING

Serving size	3/4 cup
Calories	82
Protein	2 g
Carbohydrate*	8 g
(*no added sugars)	
Fiber	3 g
Soluble fiber	1.7 g
Fat	4.8 g
Saturated fat	0.4 g
Cholesterol	0 mg
Sodium	130 mg
Potassium	26 mg
Calcium	61 mg
Omega-3 ALA	610 mg

Bonus:
Beta-carotene	(11% DV)
Vitamin C	(14% DV)

Confetti Veggies With Dill

1/2	small head cauliflower (4 cup florets)
1	carrot
1/2	bunch kale (2 cups leaves)
2	tablespoons diced red bell pepper
1	green onion
1/2	cup reduced-sodium chicken or vegetable broth
2	teaspoons arrowroot or cornstarch
1/4	teaspoon dry dill weed
1/8	teaspoon black pepper, or to taste

1. Break cauliflower into florets, cut if large, discard stem area and leaves.
2. Peel and dice carrots.
3. Remove kale from tough stems, discard stems, and tear leaves into pieces.
4. Dice bell pepper and green onion. Set aside.
5. Steam cauliflower and diced carrots, covered, for 4 minutes or until crisp tender; add kale and steam 2 minutes more. Set into bowl to keep warm.
6. Combine chicken stock and cornstarch in measuring cup; pour into a medium nonstick skillet and heat over medium to high heat. Mixture may be heated to boiling in microwave if preferred.
7. Add bell pepper, green onion, dill weed, pepper and cook for 1 minute.
8. Pour over the cauliflower, carrots and kale and toss all together.

HELPFUL HINTS:
- If kale stalks are thin, such as those found on Lacinato kale, do not discard.

- Add a couple tablespoons of black beans if desired.

Servings: 4

NUTRITION PER SERVING

Serving size	1 cup
Calories	54
Protein	3.5 g
Carbohydrate*	11 g
(*no added sugars)	
Fiber	4 g
Soluble fiber	1.86 g
Fat	0 g
Saturated fat	0 g
Cholesterol	0 mg
Sodium	149 mg
Potassium	495 mg
Calcium	41 mg
Omega-3 ALA	10 mg

Bonus:

Vitamin C	(197% DV)
Beta-carotene	(71% DV)
Vitamin K	(276 mcg)

Easy Italian Vegetables

1/2   bunch broccoli
1   cup sliced carrots (about 2 medium)
1   yellow or red bell pepper
2   tablespoons vinaigrette dressing (Page 371)
1/2   can (or 1 cup) stewed tomatoes, no-salt-added preferred
1/2   teaspoon of dry Italian seasoning or *Penzeys Spices' Tuscan Sunset*

1. Wash broccoli, break into small florets, peel stems and slice diagonally.
2. Peel carrots and slice on the diagonal.
3. Wash bell pepper, cut in half, remove stem and seeds, and slice into strips or cut in chunks.
4. Combine broccoli and carrots, and place in collapsible vegetable steamer set in pan with 1/4 cup water. Bring to boil and cook about 3 minutes.
5. Add bell pepper and cook 1 minute more.
6. Toss the vegetables, dressing, stewed tomatoes and seasoning together.
7. Serve warm, room temperature or chilled.

HELPFUL HINT
Cut carrots with a vegetable crinkle cutter for a special look.

Servings: 6

NUTRITION PER SERVING

Serving size	1 cup
Calories	61
Protein	2.5 g
Carbohydrate*	11 g
(*no added sugars)	
Fiber	3.5 g
Soluble fiber	1.4 g
Fat	1.3 g
Saturated fat	0.1 g
Cholesterol	0 mg
Sodium	48 mg
Potassium	333 mg
Calcium	54 mg
Omega-3 ALA	180 mg
Bonus:	
Beta-carotene	(135% DV)
Vitamin C	(130% DV)

Summer Vegetable Medley

NUTRITION HINT
By adding a can of beans, this becomes a complete, meatless meal.

2	tablespoons extra-virgin olive oil
1	large onion
3	carrots
2	stalks celery
3	small new potatoes, scrubbed
8	ounces (about 1 cup) green beans, fresh or frozen
6	Roma tomatoes or 1 (28-ounce) can diced tomatoes, with liquid
2	cloves garlic (more if desired)
1/3	cup organic ketchup (no high fructose corn syrup)
1/2	teaspoon sea salt

1	small eggplant
1	green bell pepper
1	red bell pepper
1	yellow squash
1	zucchini
1	teaspoon dry basil or 1 tablespoon fresh
1/2	teaspoon dry oregano or 1/2 tablespoon fresh
1/2	teaspoon dry parsley or 1 tablespoon fresh

1. To begin, prepare the first group of vegetables because they take longer to cook. Peel and cut onion into 1-inch chunks. Peel carrots. Slice carrots and celery on the diagonal. Cube potatoes. Cut green beans into 1-inch pieces. Dice tomatoes if using fresh. Mince garlic.
2. In stockpot, add oil, onion, carrots, celery, potatoes, green beans, tomatoes, garlic, ketchup, and salt. Bring to a boil, then reduce heat to slow simmer, cover and cook 1 hour.
3. Meanwhile, prepare remaining vegetables. Cut unpeeled eggplant into one-inch cubes, and cut bell pepper in half. Remove stem, white membrane and seeds from bell peppers and cut peppers into cubes. Remove ends and cut yellow squash and zucchini in half lengthwise and then across into slices.
4. Add remaining vegetables to stockpot with dry herbs and continue to cook, covered, for 30 minutes longer at a slow simmer until desired tenderness. If using fresh herbs, stir in at the end of cooking.

Servings: 12

NUTRITION PER SERVING

Serving size	1 cup
Calories	74
Protein	2 g
Carbohydrate*	12 g
(*no added sugars)	
Fiber	4 g
Soluble fiber	1 g
Fat	2.6 g
Saturated Fat	0.4 g
Cholesterol	0 mg
Sodium	208 mg
Potassium	440 mg
Calcium	33 mg
Omega-3 ALA	50 mg

Bonus:	
Beta-carotene	(67% DV)
Copper	(12% DV)
Vitamin K	(11 mcg)

Baked Vegetable Medley With Flaxseed Topping

1	bunch (2 cups) kale
1/2	red onion or sweet onion
1	yellow squash, sliced
1	zucchini, sliced
1	red bell pepper
1	(14-ounce) can diced tomatoes, no-salt-added preferred

Topping:

2	tablespoons flaxseed, ground
2	tablespoons oat bran
1/4	cup freshly grated Parmesan cheese
	oil (pump spray or cooking spray)

1. Preheat oven to 350°F.
2. Strip off leaves from kale stems and discard thick stems.
3. Peel onion and slice in wedges.
4. Remove ends from yellow squash and zucchini. Cut in half lengthwise and then into slices crosswise.
5. Remove stem and seeds from bell pepper. Cut into cubes.
6. Combine vegetables and diced tomatoes with liquid in 3-quart baking dish.
7. In small dish, combine flaxseed, oat bran and Parmesan. Sprinkle over top. Spray top with oil.
8. Bake, uncovered, in preheated oven for 20 to 25 minutes. If desired, broil after baking to brown the top.

Servings: 4

NUTRITION PER SERVING

Serving size	1 cup
Calories	115
Protein	7 g
Carbohydrate*	17 g
(*no added sugars)	
Fiber	5 g
Soluble fiber	1.5 g
Fat	3.5 g
Saturated fat	1 g
Cholesterol	1 mg
Sodium	108 mg
Potassium	316 mg
Calcium	148 mg
Omega-3 ALA	990 mg

Bonus:

Beta-carotene	(133% DV)
Vitamin C	(127% DV)
Vitamin K	(276 mcg)

Kale. *Among vegetables, the ORAC (antioxidant score) is highest for this leafy green in the studies when it was included as one of the vegetables tested. Two carotenoids important for eye health, lutein and zeaxanthin, are found in kale. Lutein-rich foods are heart protective since they help prevent cholesterol from invading artery walls. For a mere 36 calories, a cooked cup provides 89% of a days' requirement for vitamin C, 5% of vitamin E, 1,3285% vitamin K, 10% copper, 2.6 grams of fiber, and 1.2 grams soluble fiber. It is in the cruciferous family of cancer-fighting vegetables. It tastes like a mild cabbage, works great in stir-fries and soups, diced into pasta sauce, or on its own.*

Green and Gold Vegetable Bake

1	pound butternut squash (2 cups diced) or sweet potato
1	parsnip, grated (1 cup)
1	carrot, grated (1 cup)
2	cups packed, finely chopped, kale
1/2	red bell pepper, diced (1/2 cup)
2	cups fresh or frozen broccoli florets
1	tablespoon canola oil
2	tablespoons maple syrup
1/16	teaspoon fresh pepper
1/8	teaspoon sea salt
1/2	teaspoon ground cinnamon

1. Preheat oven to 350°F. Peel squash with vegetable peeler. Dice into 1-inch chunks.
2. Steam squash using a collapsible steamer set in a pot above 1/4 inch of water until crisp tender, not soft since it will continue to cook in the recipe. If using sweet potato, microwave 6 minutes. Cool, peel and dice.
3. Meanwhile, peel and grate parsnips and carrots. Strip kale from stalks (discard stalks) and chop leaves. Dice bell pepper. Chop broccoli into small pieces.
4. Place prepared vegetables and all remaining ingredients in baking dish. Stir to combine.
5. Cover with foil and bake for 30 to 35 minutes.

Servings: 8

NUTRITION PER SERVING

Serving size	1/2 cup
Calories	128
Protein	3 g
Carbohydrate*	25 g
(*3 g added sugars)	
Fiber	5 g
Soluble fiber	1.5 g
Fat	2 g
Saturated fat	0.2 g
Cholesterol	0 mg
Sodium	76 mg
Potassium	390 mg
Calcium	51 mg
Omega-3 ALA	27 mg

Bonus:	
Beta-carotene	(80% DV)
Vitamin C	(61% DV)
Folate	(11% DV)
Iron	(12% DV)
Vitamin K	(198 mcg)

Butternut squash. It is the superstar of the squash family with almost twice the amount of beta-carotene as other winter squashes. Beta-carotene is converted to vitamin A as the body needs it. One cup provides a daily value of 457% for vitamin A. You can serve it as a vegetable or make it into a wonderful creamy soup or sauce, as well as add it to a stir-fry of other vegetables.

Basic Cooking Method For Sautéed Greens

1	large bunch greens (kale, Swiss chard, collards or other greens)
1/2	medium onion
2	teaspoons olive or canola oil
2	cloves garlic, minced

1. Wash greens and cut off leaves. Cook stems (if thin) and leaves separately. Note that some stems, such as that on lacinato kale, are thin enough that they can be cooked with the leaves. The stems of chard are never too tough to eat.
2. Make 2 separate stacks, one of stems and one of leaves. Slice stems into 2-inch pieces. Chop leaves.
3. Chop onion and garlic.
4. Sauté onion in olive oil a few minutes over medium-low heat. Add garlic and stems, if using them. Cook about 1 minute for chard stems, longer for other greens, until almost as tender as you like them.
5. Add leaves, tossing until wilted, about 1 to 3 minutes.
6. Remove from heat and serve immediately.

NOTE: *1 bunch of greens serves 2 to 4 people.*

VARIATIONS

❖ Add chopped, toasted nuts such as walnuts, almonds or hazelnuts.
❖ Grind fresh black pepper over greens.
❖ Squeeze some lemon juice over cooked greens.
❖ Sprinkle with balsamic vinegar.

SUGGESTIONS – ADD LEFTOVER COOKED GREENS TO:

❖ Scrambled eggs and omelets
❖ Soups
❖ Stews
❖ Chili
❖ Pizza, taco, burritos
❖ Pasta sauce
❖ Stir-fry
❖ Cooked grains
❖ Hamburger, meatloaf
❖ Casseroles
❖ Mixed vegetable

Spinach Parmesan

HELPFUL HINT
Use a 10-ounce bag of
cut-leaf frozen spinach.

1   tablespoon dry roasted, unsalted, sunflower seeds
9   ounces baby spinach (or remove tough stems if not baby)
1   tablespoon Parmesan cheese (fresh grated)

1. Toast sunflower seeds in dry pan over medium heat until golden. Set aside.
2. Grate Parmesan cheese.
3. Wash and drain spinach, place in bowl, and microwave for 2 to 3 minutes until wilted.
4. Immediately top with Parmesan cheese and sunflower seeds, and cover to allow the heat from the spinach to melt the Parmesan.

Servings: 2

NUTRITION PER SERVING

Serving size	1/2 cup
Calories	92
Protein	5 g
Carbohydrate*	16 g
(*no added sugars)	
Fiber	7 g
Soluble fiber	0.7 g
Fat	3 g
Saturated fat	1 g
Cholesterol	0.5 mg
Sodium	255 mg
Potassium	34 mg
Calcium	134 mg
Omega-3 ALA	177 mg

Bonus:
Beta-carotene	(100% DV)
Vitamin C	(33% DV)
Iron	(26% DV)
Vitamin K	(616 mcg)

Garlic Spinach Sauté

2   teaspoons olive oil
2   garlic cloves, chopped
1   pound fresh spinach, preferably organic, washed and drained

1. Heat oil and garlic in skillet over medium-low heat for a minute.
2. Add spinach.
3. Toss and cook until wilted.

Servings: 3

NUTRITION PER SERVING

Serving size	1/2 cup
Calories	92
Protein	3.5 g
Carbohydrate*	17 g
(*no added sugars)	
Fiber	7 g
Soluble fiber	0.6 g
Fat	3 g
Saturated fat	0.5 g
Cholesterol	0 mg
Sodium	240 mg
Potassium	38 mg
Calcium	110 mg
Omega-3 ALA	230 mg

Bonus:
Beta-carotene	(107% DV)
Vitamin C	(37% DV)
Iron	(27% DV)
Vitamin K	(730 mcg)

Emerald Mashed Sweet Potatoes

1	pound sweet potatoes
3	cups finely shredded kale or spinach
1	tablespoon fresh chives or green onion, finely sliced
1/4	cup plain soy milk or skim milk
1	teaspoon walnut or canola oil
1/8	teaspoon sea salt (optional)
1/16	teaspoon freshly ground pepper

1. Bake or microwave potatoes. Cool to touch, then cut in half, remove pulp and place in bowl.
2. Strip leaves from the stems of the kale; wash well. Discard stems. Slice leaves into thin strips. Chop chives.
3. Meanwhile, in saucepan, combine soy milk, walnut oil, chives and kale. Bring to a boil, reduce heat to low, and simmer 2 minutes. Remove from heat.
4. Mash potatoes, adding milk mixture, salt (if using) and freshly ground pepper.

Kale is at the top of the list of healthy foods you can eat. It is high in calcium and vitamin K, which are important for bones. Rich in lutein and beta-carotene, it is good for your eyes and heart, as well.

HELPFUL HINT
Use half white and half sweet potatoes.

Servings: 4

NUTRITION PER SERVING

Serving size	1/2 cup
Calories	163
Protein	3.5 g
Carbohydrate*	34 g
(*no added sugars)	
Fiber	4.5 g
Soluble fiber	1.8 g
Fat	1.5 g
Saturated fat	0 g
Cholesterol	0 mg
Sodium	66 mg
Potassium	526 mg
Calcium	105 mg
Omega-3 ALA	210 mg

Bonus:
Beta-carotene	(539% DV)
Vitamin C	(127% DV)
Vitamin K	(413 mcg)

Garlic Rosemary Sweet Potatoes

8	ounces sweet potato (works with Yukon Gold or red potatoes)
1	clove garlic, minced
1/2	teaspoon dry, cracked rosemary*
1/8	teaspoon sea salt
2	teaspoons extra-virgin olive oil

1. Peel and cube potatoes. Mince garlic.
2. Combine all ingredients in glass dish and cover.
3. Microwave, covered, on high for 5 minutes. Let stand 5 minutes. Potato will continue to cook.
4. Check to see if tender. If not, cook another minute and retest.

Cracked rosemary is available from Penzeys Spices, or use a mortar and pestle to break dried rosemary into smaller pieces.

Servings: 3

NUTRITION PER SERVING

Serving size	1/3 cup
Calories	112
Protein	1.5 g
Carbohydrate*	20 g
(*no added sugars)	
Fiber	2.5 g
Soluble fiber	1.2 g
Fat	3 g
Saturated Fat	0.5 g
Cholesterol	0 mg
Sodium	124 mg
Potassium	210 mg
Calcium	20 mg
Omega-3 ALA	30 mg

Bonus:
Beta-carotene	(256% DV)
Vitamin C	(19% DV)

Sweet Potato Fries

1   large sweet potato (8 ounces)
1   tablespoon olive oil
1/8   teaspoon sea salt

1. Preheat the oven to 425°F.
2. Peel sweet potato and cut into sticks. Toss with oil.
3. Place potato sticks on pan and bake. Time varies with oven and thickness of potatoes. Watch so they don't burn.
4. For a different taste, try adding 1/4 teaspoon ground cinnamon and 1/8 teaspoon ground, dry ginger to potatoes before baking.

Servings: 3

NUTRITION PER SERVING

Serving size	1/3 of sticks
Calories	80
Protein	0.5 g
Carbohydrate*	9 g
(*no added sugars)	
Fiber	2.5 g
Soluble fiber	1.2 g
Fat	4.7 g
Saturated Fat	0.5 g
Cholesterol	0 mg
Sodium	110 mg
Potassium	116 mg
Calcium	13 mg
Omega-3 ALA	30 mg

Bonus:
Beta-carotene	(256% DV)
Vitamin C	(11% DV)

HELPFUL HINTS
• If you can't find cardamom, use cinnamon.
• Use amaretto almond liqueur or almond extract and toasted sliced almonds.

Honey Rum Sweet Potatoes

1-1/2   pounds sweet potatoes (about 2 to 3)
1   teaspoon butter
1   teaspoon canola oil
2   tablespoons plain soy milk or evaporated skim milk
1   tablespoon honey
1   teaspoon rum flavoring or 1 tablespoon rum or bourbon
1/4   teaspoon cardamom spice
1   tablespoon chopped walnuts or pecans

1. Preheat oven to 400°F.
2. Wash potatoes, prick a few times. Place in a microwave dish and cook on high power for 5 minutes. Test for doneness. A toothpick should go in with only slight resistance. Cool to touch.
3. Remove pulp from shell. Place in mixing bowl. Add remaining ingredients, except nuts, and mash until smooth.
4. Place in dish, top with walnuts, and bake for 15 minutes.

Servings: 5

NUTRITION PER SERVING

Serving size	1/2 cup
Calories	126
Protein	2.5 g
Carbohydrate*	25 g
(*5 g added sugars)	
Fiber	3 g
Soluble fiber	0.7 g
Fat	2.4 g
Saturated fat	0.8 g
Cholesterol	0 mg
Sodium	45 mg
Potassium	415 mg
Calcium	42 mg
Omega-3 ALA	136 mg

Bonus:
Beta-carotene	(398% DV)
Vitamin C	(34% DV)
Copper	(10%DV)

Sweet Potato is rich in beta-carotene and has a lower glycemic index and glycemic load than a white potato.

Butternut Orange Sauce Over Spaghetti Squash

1	butternut squash (1-1/2 cup cooked)
1	spaghetti squash
1	tablespoon shallots, minced
1/2	cup white wine (not cooking wine)
1	cup orange juice
1/8	teaspoon sea salt
1	tablespoon chopped flat-leaf parsley

1. To cook squash in microwave, cut in half and remove seeds. Place in microwave with cut side down, and cook 10 to 12 minutes or until soft. Let cool slightly before scooping out flesh with a spoon. Save leftover butternut squash to serve at another time or freeze.
2. Keep the spaghetti squash warm until sauce is made.
3. Peel shallots and mince. Combine shallots, wine and orange juice. Bring to a rapid boil, and cook uncovered until reduced to 3/4 cup.
4. In blender, combine cooked butternut squash, salt and wine mixture. Purée until smooth. Heat sauce until warm.
5. Using a fork, rake the pulp of the spaghetti squash into strands. Serve warm sauce over cooked spaghetti squash, and top with chopped fresh parsley.

Servings: 9

NUTRITION PER SERVING

Serving size	1/4 cup
Calories	48
Protein	1 g
Carbohydrate*	8 g
(*no added sugars)	
Fiber	1 g
Soluble fiber	0.2 g
Fat	0 g
Saturated fat	0 g
Cholesterol	0 mg
Sodium	32 mg
Potassium	135 mg
Calcium	16 mg
Omega-3	none

Bonus:
| Beta-carotene | (24% DV) |
| Vitamin C | (39% DV) |

Creamy Butternut Squash Sauce

1	butternut squash (1 cup cooked pulp)
1	cup plain, unsweetened soy milk
1/2	cup reduced-sodium chicken stock (1/2 teaspoon *Organic Better Than Bouillon Chicken Base* plus 1/2 cup water)
1	clove garlic, minced
1/2	cup chopped onion
2	teaspoons canola oil

1. Cut squash in half and microwave or bake. Place onion, garlic and oil in glass dish and microwave for 1-1/2 minutes.
2. Combine all ingredients in food processor and blend.

VARIATION
❖ Thai curry squash sauce. Replace soy milk with coconut milk, and add 1/4 teaspoon red curry paste (*Thai Kitchen* or other brand), and juice from 1/2 lime.

Quick Meal Suggestion: Serve sauce over cooked frozen ravioli or cooked grains.

NOTE: *Spaghetti squash can be topped with butternut sauce or pasta sauce. It can also be tossed with olive oil and grated Parmesan cheese or pesto sauce.*

Servings: 6

NUTRITION PER SERVING

Serving size	1/2 cup
Calories	55
Protein	2 g
Carbohydrate*	7 g
(*no added sugars)	
Fiber	1.3 g
Soluble fiber	0.2 g
Fat	2.4 g
Saturated fat	0.2 g
Cholesterol	0 mg
Sodium	20 mg
Potassium	190 mg
Calcium	69 mg
Omega-3 ALA	35 mg

Bonus:
| Beta-carotene | (19% DV) |

Wild Rice Stuffed Squash

3	small festival, carnival or sweet dumpling squash
1/4	cup walnuts, toasted (Page 285)
2	tablespoons canola oil
1	medium onion, chopped
1	stalk celery, minced
1/4	teaspoon sea salt
	few grinds freshly ground pepper
1/4	cup craisins or dried cherries
1/4	cup dried apricots, chopped
2	cups cooked *Lundberg Wild Blend* or cooked brown and wild rice

1. Preheat oven to 350°F.
2. Cook rice if you do not have leftover. Use 3/4 cup rice and 1-1/2 cups water.
3. Cut squash in half and remove the seeds.
4. Place cut side down on pan and bake for about 45 minutes to 1 hour until soft but not mushy. This can be done a few days ahead of time if you want.
5. Prepare the filling for the squash. Toast nuts and chop onion, celery and apricots.
6. Sauté onion and celery in oil, until softened, over medium heat.
7. Remove pan from heat and add toasted, chopped nuts, salt, pepper, craisins, apricots and cooked rice.
8. Fill the cavity of the squash with the mixture. Place on pan, cover with foil, and bake for 20 minutes or until heated through. If desired, make ahead and refrigerate until ready to bake.

Servings: 6

NUTRITION PER SERVING

Serving size	1 filled squash half
Calories	197
Protein	3.5 g
Carbohydrate*	28 g
(*no added sugars)	
Fiber	3 g
Soluble fiber	1.3 g
Fat	8.5 g
Saturated fat	1 g
Cholesterol	0 mg
Sodium	112 mg
Potassium	216 mg
Calcium	35 mg
Omega-3 ALA	900 mg

Bonus:
Beta-carotene	(45% DV)
Vitamin C	(12% DV)
Magnesium	(10% DV)
Vitamin E	(6% DV)

Garden Salad

This is not a recipe but a general guideline to create your own. By making different choices, your salad can change every time. Make up a couple day's worth of salad, and then add dressing when ready to eat.

3 cups mixture of leafy greens: or a bag of store purchased mixed greens
- ❖ 2 cups romaine lettuce or red leafy, green leafy, mesculin/spring mix, baby spinach, butter lettuce, or mache (also called lamb's lettuce).
- ❖ 1/2 cup of kale (green, curly or decorative) or cabbage, finely sliced.
- ❖ 1/2 cup of assertive greens cut in strips, such as watercress, escarole, arugula, frissee (a type of chicory), endive, or mustard greens.
- ❖ 2 tablespoons, fresh herbs, such as basil, thyme, dill or parsley.

1 cup colorful vegetables: the more colors you pick, the more phytonutrients are in your salad
- ❖ Jicama, daikon, thinly sliced fennel, cauliflower
- ❖ Yellow bell pepper, yellow squash, shredded carrots, golden beets
- ❖ Red bell pepper, red onion, radishes, roasted red beets
- ❖ Flower petals (chive flowers, nasturtium, pansy)
- ❖ Sprouts, cucumber, kohlrabi, green onions, olives

2 tablespoons nuts, seeds and cheese:
- ❖ 1 tablespoon of one of the following: pumpkin seeds, sunflower seed, walnuts, pine nuts, black sesame seeds
- ❖ 1 tablespoon of an assertive cheese, such as crumbled gorgonzola, feta or shaved Parmesan

2 tablespoon for a touch of sweetness:
- ❖ Chopped, dried apricots, craisins or cherries
- ❖ Orange zest
- ❖ Diced cantaloupe, orange sections or sliced strawberries, thinly sliced pear, diced mango

Dressing (see Page 371)

1. Wash greens and dry with a salad spinner. Dressing will stick to the leaves better when dry.
2. Toss leafy greens with the colorful vegetables in large bowl along with 1 tablespoon dressing for each 2 to 3 cups of greens. Add freshly ground pepper, if desired.
3. Place in salad bowls, adding nuts and seeds and the touch of sweetness.

Servings: 3

NUTRITION PER SERVING

Serving size	2 cups without dressing
Calories	74
Protein	4 g
Carbohydrate*	12 g
(*no added sugars)	
Fiber	5 g
Soluble fiber	0.6 g
Fat	2.5 g
Saturated fat	0.2 g
Cholesterol	0 mg
Sodium	32 mg
Potassium	547 mg
Calcium	116 mg
Omega-3 ALA	220 mg

Bonus:	
Vitamin C	(192% DV)
Folate	(46% DV)
Copper	(12% DV)
Magnesium	(11% DV)
Vitamin E	(4 % DV)
Vitamin K	(502 mcg)

For extra flavor, try one of these ideas:

❖ For best taste, make your own dressing and omit the salt. If desired, add 1 pinch of salt to your salad. A pinch is the amount you can hold between two fingers, which adds 72 mg of sodium. This adds more flavor and less sodium than using purchased, bottled dressing, as most are usually high in sodium.

❖ Adding 1 tablespoon of feta to a salad adds 25 calories, 2 grams of fat, 1.5 grams saturated fat, and 105 mg of sodium.

❖ Tip to take the bite out of onions – slice thinly and marinate covered with fresh lime juice or vinegar before using.

For added protein and soluble fiber, add cooked legumes/beans to salads:

❖ Use any bean you have available.

❖ Small red beans are high in disease-fighting antioxidants. A half cup cooked contains an antioxidant capacity of 4,575, compared to a half cup of wild blueberries which has 6,713, or a half cup of cultivated blueberries which have 4,509.

❖ Adzuki (ah-ZOO-kee) are small red beans, with a distinctive white ridge along one side. They have a slightly sweet flavor and are less "gassy" compared to most beans, making them easier to digest. Japanese use them to make sweet red bean paste. If preparing from dry, they cook faster than most dry beans. If soaked, they will be done in 45 minutes.

Other protein choices you can add to the salad to make a complete meal:

❖ Grilled salmon, Ginger Soy Grilled Salmon (Page 417), Poached Salmon (Page 414).

❖ Grilled chicken, Berry Chicken (Page 402).

❖ Marinated Tempeh (Page 397).

Crispy Tempeh Croutons
("bacon-like" bits to toss on salads)

1　teaspoon canola oil
4　ounces soy tempeh
1　teaspoon *Bragg Liquid Aminos All-Purpose Seasoning*

1. Grate tempeh using large holes on box grater, or chop very small.
2. In medium skillet, heat oil over medium low heat. Add tempeh. Cook, stirring until the tempeh is browned and crisp, about 10 minutes.
3. Add *Bragg* and stir.
4. Store in refrigerator or freezer.

NOTE: These will soften when stored. Recrisp by heating in a sauté pan (cast-iron works great).

NUTRITION NOTE
Antioxidant capacity is the measure of the antioxidant potency of foods.

The most accepted and accurate method is the ORAC method which measures how well a food absorbs oxygen free radicals.

Salad Dressing

Make your own dressing to avoid all the unhealthy ingredients found in most bottled dressings. You will save money, and your salads will taste better. Made with healthy oils, they are a good source of vitamin E and monounsaturated fats.

A simple formula is to toss your salad with a teaspoon or two of extra-virgin olive oil, along with a squeeze of lemon or lime juice, a few drops or tiny drizzle of vinegar (red wine, balsamic, sherry, etc.), a pinch of sea salt, and a few grinds of pepper.

Basic Vinaigrette

1	tablespoon minced shallots
1/4	cup balsamic vinegar
1	teaspoon Dijon mustard
1/4	cup canola, walnut or extra-virgin olive oil
1/8	teaspoon sea salt

1. Combine all ingredients in small jar with tight-fitting lid.
2. Shake well before using.

VARIATIONS

❖ Replace oil with liquid fish oil.

❖ **Raspberry Vinaigrette:** Use raspberry vinegar instead of balsamic vinegar. Canola oil is best, as it does not compete with the raspberry flavor.

❖ **Creamy Dressing:** Add 1 tablespoon light mayonnaise to Basic Vinaigrette

Servings: 8

NUTRITION PER SERVING

Serving size	1 tablespoon
Calories	62
Protein	0 g
Carbohydrate*	1.5 g
(*no added sugars)	
Fiber	0 g
Soluble fiber	0 g
Fat	6 g
Saturated fat	0.4 g
Cholesterol	0 mg
Sodium	76 mg
Potassium	12 mg
Calcium	5 mg
Omega-3 ALA	580 mg

Bonus:
Vitamin E   (5% DV)

Ranch Dressing

2	tablespoons Basic Vinaigrette dressing
2	tablespoons light mayonnaise (Page 285)
2	tablespoons low-fat buttermilk
1	teaspoon chopped flat-leaf parsley
1	clove garlic, chopped

1. Combine all ingredients in small jar with tight-fitting lid.
2. Shake well before using.

Servings: 6

NUTRITION PER SERVING

Serving size	1 tablespoon
Calories	44
Protein	0 g
Carbohydrate*	1.5 g
(*no added sugars)	
Fiber	0 g
Soluble fiber	0 g
Fat	4.3 g
Saturated fat	0.2 g
Cholesterol	2 mg
Sodium	77 mg
Potassium	13 mg
Calcium	8 mg
Omega-3 ALA	360 mg

Bonus:
Vitamin E   (5% DV)

Maple Vinaigrette Dressing

Servings: 8

NUTRITION PER SERVING

Serving size	1 tablespoon
Calories	74
Protein	0 g
Carbohydrate*	3.5 g
(*3 g added sugars from maple syrup)	
Fiber	0 g
Soluble fiber	0 g
Fat	6.8 g
Saturated fat	0.5 g
Cholesterol	0 mg
Sodium	81 mg
Potassium	14 mg
Calcium	4 mg
Omega-3 ALA	710 mg
Bonus:	
Vitamin E	(8% DV)

1/4	cup canola or walnut oil
2	tablespoons cider vinegar
2	tablespoons maple syrup
1/2	teaspoon lemon juice
1	teaspoon Dijon mustard
1	tablespoon chives or any other fresh herb (or 1-1/2 teaspoon dry)
1/8	teaspoon sea salt

1. Combine all ingredients in small jar with tight-fitting lid.
2. Shake well before using.

Honey French Dressing

Servings: 4

NUTRITION PER SERVING

Serving size	1 tablespoon
Calories	17
Protein	0 g
Carbohydrate*	4 g
(*4 g added sugars from honey)	
Fiber	0 g
Soluble fiber	0 g
Fat	0 g
Saturated fat	0 g
Cholesterol	0 mg
Sodium	99 mg
Potassium	7 mg
Calcium	<1 mg
Omega-3	none

1/4	cup organic ketchup
2	tablespoons cider or sherry vinegar
1	tablespoon honey
1	tablespoon water
1/2	teaspoon Worcestershire (*Annie's Natuals*) or *Braggs Liquid Aminos*

1. Combine all ingredients in small jar with tight-fitting lid.
2. Shake well before using.

French dressings have added sugars or are made with artificial sugar substitutes. Avoid those with high fructose corn syrup, those high in carbohydrates from any sweeteners, and artificially sweetened dressings. Make your own for a lower-sugar option.

Creamy Parmesan Dressing

Servings: 12

NUTRITION PER SERVING

Serving size	1 tablespoon
Calories	19
Protein	2 g
Carbohydrate*	1.5 g
(*no added sugars)	
Fiber	0 g
Soluble fiber	0 g
Fat	1 g
Saturated fat	0 g
Cholesterol	0 mg
Sodium	64 mg
Potassium	19 mg
Calcium	42 mg
Omega-3 ALA	30 mg

1/2	cup (or 4 ounces) silken tofu (*Mori-Nu*)
2	tablespoons grated Parmesan
1	tablespoon lemon juice
1	garlic clove, minced
1	tablespoon unsweetened soy milk, skim milk or water
1	tablespoon balsamic vinegar
2	teaspoons Dijon mustard
1/8	teaspoon black pepper

1. Combine all ingredients in food processor.
2. Blend until smooth.

Dark Green/Deep Orange Super Salad With Vinaigrette

1	cup diced cantaloupe
1/4	cup diced red onion
1/2	red bell pepper, diced
1/2	yellow bell pepper, diced
1/2	cup diced jicama
1	tablespoon chopped fresh herbs, parsley, basil, tarragon or any you enjoy
2	tablespoons Vinaigrette (Page 371)
4	cups leafy mesclun greens (spring mix, romaine, red leafy, etc.)

1. Dice cantaloupe and red onion place in bowl.
2. Cut bell pepper in half, and remove and discard top stems, inside white veins and seeds. Dice half, reserving other half for another use. Add to bowl.
3. Peel and cube jicama and add it to the bowl. Chop herbs and add.
4. Make dressing.
5. Just before serving, add 2 tablespoons dressing, along with leafy greens, to bowl with other diced ingredients. Toss and serve.

Mesclun is a French word meaning "mixture." Originally, young, wild field greens were picked in the spring. Now the mix is cultivated. It is a blend of mild, peppery and bitter. It may include a variety of greens, such as red and green oak leaf with sharply indented leaves, dandelion, sorrel, cress, chervil, arugula and delicate mache.

Jicama (pronounced "hick ah mah") is a sweet, nutty, crunchy tuber that has a thin, brown skin. It is available in the produce section of large supermarkets. Do not buy those that have wet or soft spots, which indicates rot and interiors that are starting to get brown. Medium sized have better flavor than the very large ones. They should be kept refrigerated and peeled only when ready to use. Jicama are a fair source of vitamin C and potassium.

Servings: 2

NUTRITION PER SERVING

Serving size	2 cups
Calories	156
Protein	3 g
Carbohydrate*	22 g
(*no added sugars)	
Fiber	6 g
Soluble fiber	2.3 g
Fat	0.5 g
Saturated fat	0.75 g
Cholesterol	0 mg
Sodium	106 mg
Potassium	710 mg
Calcium	60 mg
Omega-3 ALA	910 mg

Bonus:	
Vitamin C	(295% DV)
Beta-carotene	(222% DV)
Vitamin K	(121 mcg)
Folate	(47% DV)
Vitamin E	(7% DV)
Zinc	(6% DV)

Wild Rice Spinach Salad

This recipe is from Irene Wheeler, who assisted at many cooking classes. Irene is an art teacher, which explains the variety of warm colors. The sprinkles of oranges and browns, with flecks of black, against the cool background of spinach, make it both beautiful and nutrient dense. Irene recommends the use of California apricots, such as Trader Joe's slab apricots, which have a deeper orange color and more intense sweet/tart flavor than Turkish or Mediterranean types.

3-1/2	cups water
1	cup uncooked wild rice (or *Lundberg Wild Rice Blend*) or use half of each
1	(10-ounce) package fresh spinach, washed well
1/4	cup chopped flat-leaf parsley
1/3	cup sliced green onions (3 medium) or fresh chives or chopped red onion
1/2	cup dried California apricots
1/2	cup slivered almonds

Dressing:

3	tablespoons canola oil or walnut oil
2	tablespoons rice vinegar
1	tablespoon reduced-sodium soy or Tamari sauce
1/2	teaspoon sugar
1/4	teaspoon sea salt
	freshly ground black pepper

1. Place rice and water in rice cooker to cook. If using stove top, cook covered on for 50 minutes. While rice is cooking, prepare other ingredients.
2. Stack spinach and cut across into thin strips. Place in bowl. Remove thick stems from parsley and chop. Add to spinach mixture.
3. Slice onion (green and white part), adding to the bowl with spinach.
4. Slice apricots into strips and set aside in separate dish.
5. Toast almonds (see Page 285).
6. Mix dressing ingredients in a large bowl. Add rice to bowl while still warm. Let this mixture cool to room temperature.
7. Add the spinach, onion and parsley mixture to rice mixture.
8. Cover and refrigerate 1 to 2 hours. Add almonds and apricots right before serving.

NOTE: *If you will not use the salad within a couple days, the spinach will get very soft. The rice mixture lasts longer if you do not add the spinach until the day you plan to serve it. Add half the spinach to half the rice mixture. Then, when ready for more salad, add the remaining spinach to the remaining rice mixture.*

Servings: 9

NUTRITION PER SERVING

Serving size	1 cup
Calories	186
Protein	5 g
Carbohydrate*	30 g
(*less than 1/2 gram added sugars)	
Fiber	3 g
Soluble fiber	0.4 g
Fat	5 g
Saturated fat	0.5 g
Cholesterol	0 mg
Sodium	99 mg
Potassium	398 mg
Calcium	47 mg
Omega-3 ALA	550 mg

Bonus:
Vitamin E	(85% DV)
Beta-carotene	(64% DV)
Vitamin C	(22% DV)
Folate	(21% DV)
Magnesium	(16% DV)
Vitamin K	(186 mcg)

Kale Salad

4   cups raw kale, stems removed (about 1/2 bunch)
1/2   yellow bell pepper, chopped
1   carrot, peeled and grated
1/4   teaspoon sea salt
1   tablespoon extra-virgin olive oil
1/2   teaspoon brown rice syrup or honey
1   tablespoon fresh lemon juice
1/8   teaspoon (or to taste) freshly grated pepper
1   tablespoon raw sunflower seed, toasted
2   tablespoons dried craisins or dried apricots, chopped

1. Wash kale, remove thick stems, stack leaves and cut across into thin strips. Place in bowl.
2. Chop bell pepper, peel and grate carrot, and add to bowl with kale.
3. Add salt, oil, brown rice syrup and pepper. Toss and refrigerate several hours or overnight to allow kale to soften and wilt slightly.
4. When ready to serve, toast sunflower seeds or do the day before and store refrigerated until needed.
5. Sprinkle with sunflower seeds and craisins and serve.

Servings: 4

NUTRITION PER SERVING

Serving size	3/4 cup
Calories	102
Protein	3 g
Carbohydrate*	14 g
(*0.7 g added sugars)	
Fiber	2.4 g
Soluble fiber	1 g
Fat	4.7 g
Saturated fat	0.7 g
Cholesterol	0 mg
Sodium	190 mg
Potassium	405 mg
Calcium	101 mg
Omega-3 ALA	12 mg

Bonus:
Vitamin K	(550 mcg)
Beta-carotene	(254% DV)

Salmon, Wheat Berry Salad

2   cups cooked wheat berries or cooked, hulled barley or cooked, whole oat groats
2   tablespoons extra-virgin olive oil
2   tablespoons sherry vinegar or balsamic vinegar
1/2   tablespoon Dijon mustard
2   stalks celery, diced
1/2   small red onion, diced
1   carrot, peeled and diced
1/2   red bell pepper, diced
1/2   yellow bell pepper, diced
1/4   cup grape tomatoes
1/2   cup frozen peas, thawed
1   (7-ounce) can salmon, drained and chunked
6   cups mixed salad greens

1. Cook 1 cup dry wheat berries with 3 cups water for 60 minutes (see Page 325). Drain and add oil, vinegar and mustard.
2. Dice celery, onion, carrot, bell pepper, and cut tomatoes in half. Place in bowl along with peas and salmon.
3. Add wheat berries to bowl with vegetables and toss.
4. To serve, place 1 cup greens on plate and top with 1/2 cup wheat berry mixture.

Servings: 6

NUTRITION PER SERVING

Serving size	1 cup salad greens with 1/2 cup wheat berry mixture
Calories	135
Protein	9 g
Carbohydrate*	12 g
(*no added sugars)	
Fiber	2.5 g
Soluble fiber	0.7 g
Fat	6 g
Saturated fat	0.9 g
Cholesterol	15 mg
Sodium	258 mg
Potassium	337 mg
Calcium	100 mg
Omega-3 ALA	380 mg
DHA+EPA	410 mg

Bonus:
Vitamin C	(72% DV)
Beta-carotene	(60% DV)
Selenium	(23% DV)
Vitamin D	(74 IU)

Apple and Spelt Berry Salad with Raspberry Vinaigrette

1	cup spelt berries (2-1/2 cups cooked)
3	cups water

2	tablespoons walnut oil
2	tablespoons raspberry vinegar
1/2	tablespoon Dijon mustard
1	teaspoon honey
1/8	teaspoon sea salt

1/3	cup slivered almonds
1/4	small red onion, diced
1/3	cup dried craisins
1/3	dried cherries
1/3	cup dried currants or blueberries
1	apple, such as gala or honey crisp

1. Bring 3 cups water to a boil. Add 1 cup dry spelt berries, reduce to simmer, cover and cook for 60 minutes. Drain and add oil, vinegar, mustard, honey and salt to warm spelt. Let stand while preparing remaining ingredients.
2. Toast almonds according to Page 285. Set aside.
3. Dice onion, adding with dried fruit to bowl of cooked spelt.
4. Cut apple in half, remove core, and dice into small cubes.
5. Add apple and almonds to bowl, tossing all.
6. Serve at room temperature or chilled.

HELPFUL HINT
May use rye berries, hulled barley or oat groats instead of spelt.

Servings: 10

NUTRITION PER SERVING

Serving size	1/2 cup
Calories	102
Protein	2 g
Carbohydrate*	15 g
(*0.5 g added sugars)	
Fiber	2.4 g
Soluble fiber	0.4 g
Fat	5 g
Saturated fat	0.4 g
Cholesterol	0 mg
Sodium	49 mg
Potassium	120 mg
Calcium	19 mg
Omega-3 ALA	300 mg

Bonus:
Magnesium	(6% DV)
Selenium	(6% DV)

Green Salad With Salmon and Vinaigrette Dressing

2	small red potatoes
1	tablespoon cider vinegar
1	cup frozen green beans, thawed (or cooked fresh and chilled)
1/2	cup grape tomatoes
1/4	cup black olives, sliced
1/4	red bell pepper, sliced thinly
1/4	yellow bell pepper, sliced thinly
1/2	avocado, sliced
1/2	cup canned *Beluga Lentils* (or black beans, garbanzo, etc.)
1/4	cup frozen corn, thawed
1	(7-ounce) filet of broiled or poached sockeye salmon, chunked
4	cups or 1 bag mixed, leafy greens
2	tablespoons raw pumpkin seeds
2	tablespoons craisins

1. Prepare all ingredients.
2. Microwave potatoes, cut in cubes and toss with 1 tablespoon cider vinegar. Set aside to cool.
3. Thaw beans; slice tomatoes if large; and slice olives, bell peppers and avocado.
4. Drain lentils and rinse. Thaw corn.
5. Prepare salmon and break into chunks.
6. When ready to serve, place mixed greens in a bowl.
7. Toss greens with 2 tablespoons of vinaigrette dressing (Page 371), divide onto two plates.
8. Arrange all ingredients on top.

VARIATION

❖ Boiled shrimp or canned tuna instead of salmon.
❖ 7-ounce can or pouch of salmon, broken into chunks

Servings: 2

NUTRITION PER SERVING

Serving size	1 salad with 3-1/2 ounces salmon
Calories	468
Protein	28 g
Carbohydrate*	32 g
(*no added sugars)	
Fiber	10 g
Soluble fiber	4.75 g
Fat	14 g
Saturated fat	3.5 g
Cholesterol	55 mg
Sodium	257 mg
Potassium	1,474 mg
Calcium	120 mg
Omega-3 ALA	2,640 mg
EPA+DHA	1,430 mg

Bonus:	
Beta-carotene	(214% DV)
Vitamin C	(173% DV)
Folate	(58% DV)
Selenium	(54% DV)
Magnesium	(31% DV)
Copper	(30% DV)
Iron	(28% DV)
Vitamin E	(13% DV)
Vitamin D	(589 IU)
Vitamin K	(142 mcg)

Black Bean Salad

2	tablespoons salsa (mild or hot according to your taste preference)
1	tablespoon fresh lime juice
2	tablespoons balsamic or red wine vinegar
2	tablespoons canola oil
1	teaspoon Dijon mustard
1/4	teaspoon sea salt (omit if desired)
1	15-ounce can black beans, no-salt-added preferred
1	bell pepper (orange, yellow, green, red or purple)
1	stalk celery
1/4	cup red onion
3	Roma tomatoes
1	ear corn or 1/2 cup frozen, thawed
1/4	cup fresh flat-leaf parsley, chopped

1. In bowl, combine salsa, lime juice, vinegar, oil, mustard and salt. Whisk and set aside. Drain black beans and rinse. Add to bowl.
2. Chop bell pepper, onion, celery and tomatoes in pieces about the same size, and add to bowl with beans. Cut corn off the cob if using fresh (does not need cooking).
3. Mince parsley and add to bowl.
4. When all ingredients have been added, toss to coat well. Cover and refrigerate for 30 minutes.

SERVING TIP
- Serve on top of bowl of leafy greens.

HELPFUL HINTS
- Red wine vinegar is more tangy than balsamic.

- If you want it spicier, add a minced jalapeno, *Penzeys Spices' Aleppo Pepper* or dash of cayenne.

- Good with pinto beans.

- Substitute cilantro for parsley.

- If preparing dry beans that have been soaked and cooked, use 1-1/2 cups cooked beans.

Servings: 8

NUTRITION PER SERVING

Serving size	1/2 cup
Calories	94
Protein	3.5 g
Carbohydrates*	12 g
(*no added sugars)	
Fiber	3.7 g
Soluble fiber	0.9 g
Fat	3.8 g
Saturated fat	0.3 g
Cholesterol	0 mg
Sodium	106 mg
Potassium	253 mg
Calcium	17 mg
Omega-3 ALA	360 mg

Bonus:	
Vitamin C	(25% DV)
Folate	(15% DV)
Copper	(12% DV)
Iron	(14% DV)
Vitamin K	(36 mcg)

Warm Lentil Salad

1-1/2 cups green lentils, rinsed and picked over
1 bay leaf
1/2 teaspoon dried thyme or a couple sprigs fresh
3 cups reduced-sodium chicken broth (or 2 teaspoons *Organic Better Than Bouillon chicken base* plus 3 cups water)

1. In covered saucepan, combine lentils, bay leaf, thyme and broth.
2. Bring to boil, reduce heat, and simmer 40 to 45 minutes until soft but not mushy.
3. Drain. Add 1/4 cup Basic Vinaigrette Dressing (Page 371).
4. Serve warm or cold as a side dish, or serve over a bed of arugula or leafy greens garnished with tomato wedges.

VARIATION
❖ Add finely chopped parsley, onions, celery, bell peppers and diced carrots to cooked lentils.

Lentils are quick to cook. They come in several varieties, including green, brown and red. The green hold their shape best, but brown can also be used if not overcooked, since they then become mushy. The red ones cook quickly and become mushy, so they are not recommended for this recipe.

Servings: 8

NUTRITION PER SERVING

Serving size	1/2 cup
Calories	144
Protein	11 g
Carbohydrate*	25 g
(*no added sugars)	
Fiber	5 g
Soluble fiber	1 g
Fat	1 g
Saturated fat	0 g
Cholesterol	0 mg
Sodium	150 mg
Potassium	365 mg
Calcium	19 mg
Omega-3 ALA	120 mg
Bonus:	
Iron	(24% DV)

Tempeh Salad

8 ounces tempeh
2 tablespoons toasted sunflower seeds (unsalted) (see Page 285 for information on how to toast)
1/2 stalk celery, minced
1/4 cup finely chopped red onion
1/4 red bell pepper, diced
2 tablespoons chopped fresh chives
2 teaspoons lime juice
1/3 cup *Ojai Cook Lemonaise Light* or light mayonnaise (Page 285)
1/4 teaspoon dry dill weed

1. Cut tempeh into small cubes.
2. Steam for 10 minutes. To steam, place a collapsible vegetable steamer in pan with an inch of water. Place tempeh on steamer.
3. Bring to boil, reduce heat, cover and let steam. Discard water.
4. Toast sunflower seeds.
5. Prepare celery, red onion, bell pepper and chives, adding them to a bowl.
6. Add all ingredients, along with tempeh, to bowl. Stir to mix.
7. Refrigerate for 30 minutes or longer.

SERVING TIP
Serve on a bed of lettuce with sliced tomatoes or sliced roasted beets if desired.

Servings: 4

NUTRITION PER SERVING

Serving size	1/2 cup
Calories	135
Protein	12 g
Carbohydrate*	6.5 g
(*no added sugars)	
Fiber	4 g
Soluble fiber	1.4 g
Fat	7 g
Saturated fat	1 g
Cholesterol	0 mg
Sodium	116 mg
Potassium	45 mg
Calcium	92 mg
Omega-3 ALA	157 mg
Bonus:	
Vitamin C	(33% DV)
Iron	(10% DV)

Zucchini Julienne With Lemon and Chive

Servings: 3

NUTRITION PER SERVING

Serving size	1/4 cup
Calories	32
Protein	2 g
Carbohydrate*	5 g
(*no added sugars)	
Fiber	1.2 g
Soluble fiber	0.2 g
Fat	1 g
Saturated fat	0.5 g
Cholesterol	3 mg
Sodium	161 mg
Potassium	287 mg
Calcium	27 mg
Omega-3 ALA	70 mg

Bonus:
Vitamin C	(23% DV)
Copper	(7% DV)
Vitamin K	(6 mcg)

1	medium zucchini
1	tablespoon plain *Silk Soy Creamer*
1	tablespoon half-and-half
2	teaspoons freshly squeezed lemon juice (or more to taste)
1/2	tablespoon minced fresh chives
1/8	teaspoon sea salt

1. Cut ends off zucchini. Using a mandolin vegetable slicer, cut zucchini into julienne strips.
2. Add remaining ingredients and refrigerate 30 minutes before serving.
3. Serve on a lettuce leaf garnished with chives.

NOTES:
❖ *Great way to use fresh zucchini without heating up your kitchen.*
❖ *You can omit the half-and-half, using only the soy creamer, but it adds only a small amount of saturated fat and a lot of flavor that nothing else seems to match.*

Broccoli Cauliflower Salad

Servings: 6

NUTRITION PER SERVING

Serving	1 cup
Calories	160
Protein	2.5 g
Carbohydrate*	23 g
(*2 g added sugars from honey)	
Fiber	2.5 g
Soluble fiber	1 g
Fat	8.5 g
Saturated fat	0.5 g
Cholesterol	7 mg
Sodium	185 mg
Potassium	345 mg
Calcium 3	1 mg
Omega-3 ALA	666 mg

Bonus:
Vitamin C	(68% DV)
Vitamin E	(20% DV)
Beta-carotene	(15% DV)
Vitamin K	(39 mcg)

2	cups fresh broccoli florets (about 1/2 pound)
2	cups cauliflower (about 1/2 head)
1/4	cup minced red onion
2	cups red or black grapes, cut in half if large
1	tablespoon sunflower or pumpkin seeds
1/4	cup raisins, dried cherries or currants
1/2	cup light mayonnaise (Page 285)
1	tablespoon red wine, balsamic or raspberry vinegar
2	teaspoons honey

1. Break broccoli into small florets, save stems for another use. Break cauliflower into small pieces.
2. Wash broccoli and cauliflower. Peel onion and mince. Wash grapes and cut in half.
3. In large bowl, combine all ingredients, tossing to coat. Make up to 24 hours in advance.

OPTIONAL
❖ Top with soy bacon bits.
❖ Blanch broccoli before using in salad.

Italian Pasta Salad

2	cups (8 ounces) uncooked whole-wheat rotini pasta or brown rice pasta

· ·

1	(6-ounce) jar roasted red peppers, drained
1	tablespoon balsamic vinegar
2	tablespoons canola oil
1	teaspoon Dijon mustard
1/4	cup fresh basil leaves

· ·

11	ounces artichoke hearts, water-packed, drained
1	(15-ounce) can black beans (no-salt-added preferred)
1	ounce part-skim mozzarella cheese
1	cup grape tomatoes
1/4	cup sliced black or Kalamata olives
6-12	cups of mixed salad greens torn into bite-size pieces

1. Cook pasta according to package directions, omitting salt or fat; drain and rinse under cold water immediately. Place drained pasta in a large serving bowl.
2. While pasta is cooking, place roasted peppers, vinegar, oil, mustard and basil in blender and process until almost smooth. Add to pasta and toss.
3. Chop artichokes.
4. Drain and rinse beans.
5. Cube mozzarella.
6. Cut tomatoes in half.
7. Slice olives.
8. Add all ingredients except salad greens to bowl with pasta. Toss.
9. Serve 1 to 2 cups salad greens on plate, topping with 1/2 cup pasta mixture.

VARIATION

❖ Use cooked, green soybeans instead of black beans.
One 15-ounce can of beans equals about 1-1/2 cups cooked beans.

Servings: 6

NUTRITION PER SERVING

Serving size   1 cup salad greens, 1/2 cup pasta mixture

Calories	287
Protein	13 g
Carbohydrate*	48 g
(*no added sugars)	
Fiber	9 g
Soluble fiber	3.5 g
Fat	5 g
Saturated fat	1 g
Cholesterol	2.5 mg
Sodium	191 mg
Potassium	325 mg
Calcium	89 mg
Omega-3 ALA	320 mg

Bonus:	
Folate	(27% DV)
Vitamin C	(22% DV)
Iron	(20% DV)
Vitamin E	(4% DV)

Potato Salad

6	medium red potatoes (about 6 cups cooked)

Dressing:

1/4	cup vinegar
1/4	cup water
1/4	cup sugar
1/4	teaspoon sea salt (optional)
2	tablespoons yellow mustard
2	eggs (omega-3 enriched)
1	cup light mayonnaise (Page 285)
1/2	teaspoon celery seed
1/4	teaspoon black pepper

1. Scrub potatoes. Place in saucepan, cover with water and bring to boil. Reduce heat and cook about 20 minutes or until a toothpick can be inserted into center without too much resistance. Drain and let cool 10 minutes. Peel if desired and slice into a bowl.
2. Meanwhile, make dressing. Combine vinegar, water, sugar and salt in a saucepan. Bring to a boil. Stir together mustard and egg. Add a little of the hot mixture to egg mixture, then transfer egg mixture to saucepan and cook until it bubbles and thickens. Remove from heat and stir in mayonnaise, celery seed and black pepper.
3. Pour dressing over potato mixture and stir. Chill and serve.

OPTIONAL

❖ To cooked potatoes in bowl, add 2 tablespoons chopped green onion, 1 cup finely chopped celery, 1/2 cup chopped red onion, 1 shredded carrot, as desired.

Alternate Potato Salad Dressing

Prepare potatoes as above using the following dressing.

1/2	(0.7 ounce) package dry Italian salad dressing mix
1	(12.3-ounce) box silken tofu (*Organic Silken Mori-Nu*)
1/4	cup light mayonnaise (Page 285)
1	tablespoon canola oil
1-1/2	teaspoons prepared yellow mustard
1/8	teaspoon pepper
1	tablespoon sugar

1. Carefully divide dressing on a plate to evenly distribute seasonings, saving half for another use.
2. Place everything in a food processor, and blend until creamy. Scrape sides and blend again.

NOTE: *Omega-3 is less if mayonnaise with soybean oil is used (228 mg), since canola oil has more omega-3 ALA than soybean oil.*

Servings: 8

NUTRITION PER SERVING

Serving size	1/2 cup
Calories	247
Protein	4 g
Carbohydrate*	34 g
(*6 grams added sugars)	
Fiber	2 g
Soluble fiber	0.5 g
Fat	11.5 g
Saturated fat	0.2 g
Cholesterol	55 mg
Sodium*	392 mg
(*without salt)	299 mg
Potassium	450 mg
Calcium	12 mg
Omega-3 ALA	1,025 mg

Bonus:
Vitamin E	(27% DV)
Vitamin C	(26% DV)

Servings: 8

NUTRITION PER SERVING

Serving size	1/2 cup
Calories	226
Protein	6 g
Carbohydrate*	31 g
(*2.5 g added sugar)	
Fiber	3 g
Soluble fiber	1.5 g
Fat	9 g
Saturated fat	0.5 g
Cholesterol	4 mg
Sodium	292 mg
Potassium	839 mg
Calcium	49 mg
Omega-3 ALA	428 mg

Bonus:
Vitamin C	(48% DV)
Copper	(17% DV)
Magnesium	(14% DV)
Vitamin E	(4% DV)

Vegetarian Chili

1	medium onion, chopped
1	green pepper, chopped
1	stalk celery, chopped
1	medium zucchini with peel, diced
2	medium carrots, peeled and diced
2	cloves garlic, minced or crushed
1	jalapeno, seeds removed and finely diced (optional)
2	teaspoons canola oil

1	(28-ounce) can crushed tomatoes, no-salt-added preferred, or *Muir Glen Chunky Tomato Sauce*
1	(8-ounce) can *Health Valley No-Salt-Added Tomato Soup* or no-salt-added tomato sauce
1	(15-ounce) can tomato sauce, no-salt-added preferred
1	(15-ounce) can chili beans, mild or hot, not drained
1	(15-ounce) can pinto or red beans, no-salt-added preferred
1	(15 ounce) can garbanzo or black beans, no-salt-added preferred
1	tablespoon chili powder
3/4	teaspoon ground cumin
1	tablespoon cocoa (powdered, unsweetened)
1	(12-ounce) package soy meat-like crumbles (*Yves Veggie Ground Round* or *Morningstar Farms Meal Starters Recipe Crumbles*)
2	cups water or low-sodium vegetable juice (*Very Veggie by RW Knudsen*) or water to thin chili if too thick.

1. Prepare vegetables. Chop onion, green pepper, celery, zucchini, carrot, garlic and jalapeno. Drain and rinse pinto and garbanzo beans.
2. In dutch oven, over medium heat, sauté the vegetables with the oil until softened.
3. Add remaining ingredients. Bring to a boil, reduce to simmer, and cook covered for 30 minutes or until vegetables are as soft as you like. May also be cooked in a crockpot on low for 6 to 8 hours.
4. Make ahead and reheat if you have time, since flavors get better after standing.

Servings: 15

NUTRITION PER SERVING

Serving size	1 cup
Calories	145
Protein	11 g
Carbohydrate*	24 g
(*no added sugars)	
Fiber	7.6 g
Soluble fiber	1.7 g
Fat	1 g
Saturated fat	0 g
Cholesterol	0 mg
Sodium*	260 mg
(*if beans and tomato	
with salt)	509 mg
Potassium	488 mg
Calcium	67 mg
Omega-3 ALA	90 mg

Bonus:	
Copper	(359% DV)
Iron	(15% DV)
Vitamin C	(37% DV)
Beta-carotene	(60% DV)
Vitamin K	(4 mcg)

Lentil Taco Filling

HELPFUL HINTS
- Leftovers freeze well.

- *Penzeys Spices' Aleppo Pepper* is a Turkish crushed chili with an ancho-like flavor that has a little more heat and tartness than black pepper.

1	medium onion, finely chopped
1	garlic clove, minced
1/2	green bell pepper, diced
1	carrot, peeled and shredded
1	teaspoon canola oil
1	cup dry, brown lentils
2	teaspoons chili powder
1/2	teaspoon Aleppo pepper, chipotle chili powder or black pepper
1	teaspoon ground cumin
1	teaspoon dried oregano
2-1/2	cups reduced sodium broth (or 2-1/2 cups water plus 2 teaspoons *Organic Better Than Bouillon Chicken Base*)
1	cup salsa

1. Chop onion, mince garlic, dice bell pepper, and shred carrot on box grater.
2. In heavy-bottom saucepan over medium heat, sauté onion, garlic, green pepper and carrot with the oil until they begin to soften.
3. Add remaining ingredients (except salsa) and bring to boil. Reduce and simmer, covered, until lentils are very tender. About 30 minutes
4. Mash lentils with potato masher. If too thin, continue to cook uncovered to thicken mixture.
5. Stir in salsa.
6. Serve in taco shells without trans fat, such as *Bearitos* brand, or roll up in high-fiber whole-wheat tortilla, or use to make a taco salad. Add chopped romaine; shredded, reduced-fat cheese (*Cabot* 50% Reduced-Fat Jalapeno Cheddar); diced grape tomatoes; and Greek-style yogurt, if desired.

Servings: 16

NUTRITION PER SERVING

Serving size	1/4 cup
Calories	61
Protein	5 g
Carbohydrate*	12 g
(*no added sugars)	
Fiber	5 g
Soluble fiber	0.6 g
Fat	0.3 g
Saturated fat	0 g
Cholesterol	0 mg
Sodium	102 mg
Potassium	165 mg
Calcium	28 mg
Omega-3 ALA	20 mg
Bonus:	
Folate	(15% DV)
Beta-carotene	(25% DV)

Spaghetti Squash Casserole

Layer One:
- 1   pound spaghetti squash

. . . .

Layer Two: (Combine the following in a bowl)
- 1/2   package (about 5 ounces) frozen cut-leaf spinach, thaw & squeeze out water
- 1/2   cup 1% cottage cheese, no-salt-added preferred
- 1   egg (omega-3 enriched)
- 1/2   teaspoon dried Italian seasoning
- 2   ounces (1/2 cup) shredded, part-skim mozzarella cheese

. . . .

Layer Three:
- 1   (14-ounce) can *Muir Glen Fire-Roasted Crushed Tomatoes* or pasta sauce
- 1   ounce (1/4 cup) shredded, part-skim mozzarella cheese
- 1   tablespoon freshly grated Parmesan cheese

1. Preheat oven to 350°F. Spray 9 x 9-inch glass pan with cooking spray.
2. Cut squash in half and remove seeds. If squash is large, use only half for this recipe and use the other half for a meal later in the week.
3. Lay squash cut side down on glass dish or tray (not covered) and microwave until tender, about 10 to 15 minutes (about 5 minutes per pound). Let stand 5 minutes.
4. Turn squash cut side up, and using fork, rake across to remove strands of squash from the shell. If too difficult to remove, it is not done. Cook a couple minutes longer. If overcooked, will get mushy instead of being in strands.
5. Meanwhile, combine Layer Two ingredients in a bowl.
6. Arrange squash on the bottom of the 9-inch glass pan.
7. Top with spinach ricotta mixture (Layer Two).
8. Top with Layer Three ingredients.
9. Bake uncovered for 30 minutes.

HELPFUL HINT
Italian seasoning: Use 1/4 teaspoon each basil, marjoram and oregano.

Servings: 4

NUTRITION PER SERVING

Serving size	2-1/4 inch square piece
Calories	190
Protein	14 g
Carbohydrate*	14 g
(*no added sugars)	
Fiber	4 g
Soluble fiber	0.8 g
Fat	9.5 g
Saturated fat	5 g
Cholesterol	83 mg
Sodium	390 mg
Potassium	460 mg
Calcium	321 mg
Omega-3 DHA	12 mg

Bonus:
Beta-carotene	(131% DV)
Vitamin C	(57% DV)
Folate	(19% DV)
Magnesium	(14% DV)
Vitamin K	(179 mcg)

Tomato Rosemary Polenta Bake

Basic Polenta: (or purchase ready-to-use polenta)

1/2	cup dry corn grits polenta (not degerminated which is refined, choose one that is whole grain)
1-1/2	cups water
1/4	teaspoon dry, cracked rosemary
1	teaspoon *Organic Better Than Bouillon Vegetable or Chicken Base*

1	carrot, peeled and shredded
1/4	red bell pepper, diced
2	cups kale or spinach, torn into pieces
1	cup Pasta Sauce (recipe Page 388) or purchased
1	cup low-fat ricotta cheese
1	large egg (omega-3 enriched)
1/4	cup Parmesan cheese, divided

To make polenta: Bring water, vegetable base and rosemary to a boil. Add the cornmeal mixture slowly (to avoid lumps), whisking constantly. Then reduce heat and gently simmer for 20 to 30 minutes or until mixture thickens and pulls away from sides of pan. At this point, whisk about every 5 minutes, and change from a whisk to a wooden spoon as it thickens. Be careful as mixture will bubble and pop as it cooks. Spread into 9 X 9 pan. Smooth the top with a spoon.

If using the prepared polenta: Slice and lay in pan, slightly overlapping.

1. Preheat oven to 350°F. Spray 9-inch square pan with cooking spray.
2. While polenta is cooking, place carrot, red pepper and kale in glass bowl with 1 tablespoon water, and microwave about 2 to 3 minutes or until crisp tender. Add pasta sauce. Set aside.
3. Combine ricotta cheese, egg, and half of the Parmesan in bowl.
4. Drop ricotta mixture over polenta, then spoon pasta sauce mixture evenly over ricotta cheese.
5. Sprinkle with remaining grated Parmesan cheese.
6. Cover with foil; bake for 30 minutes.
7. Let stand 5 minutes before serving.

Servings: 4

NUTRITION PER SERVING

Serving size	2-1/4 inch square
Calories	160
Protein	9 g
Carbohydrate*	25 g
(*no added sugars)	
Fiber	4.5 g
Soluble fiber	1.3 g
Fat	3 g
Saturated fat	1 g
Cholesterol	49 mg
Sodium	289 mg
Potassium	386 mg
Calcium	118 mg
Omega-3 DHA	13-37 mg

Bonus:	
Beta-carotene	(181% DV)
Vitamin C	(94% DV)
Vitamin K	(273 mcg)

Flavorful Vegetable Stew

8	whole cloves
1	tablespoon cumin seeds
1/2	teaspoon whole coriander spice

1/4	teaspoon saffron
1/4	teaspoon ground nutmeg
1-1/2	teaspoon turmeric
1	bay leaf

Bowl One:

2	small red potatoes (8 ounces) with peel scrubbed and cut into chunks
1/2	pound yellow turnip, cut into pieces
2	carrots, peeled and cut into diagonal slices
1/2	teaspoon grated fresh ginger
2	cloves garlic, chopped

Bowl Two:

1	sweet potato or 1 cup of cubed butternut squash

Bowl Three:

1	green pepper, remove seeds and membranes and cut into cubes
1	small zucchini, cut in half lengthwise and then crosswise
1	yellow squash, cut in half lengthwise and then crosswise

1	tablespoon olive oil
1	medium yellow onion, diced

1	tablespoon chicken or vegetable base and 5 cups water or 5 cups reduced-sodium chicken broth
1	(15-ounce) can chick peas, no-salt-added preferred, drained
1	(15-ounce) can diced tomatoes, no-salt-added preferred, with liquid
2	tablespoons canned *Harissa Paste* (more or less according to your preference)
1	teaspoon *Aleppo Pepper* (*Penzeys Spices*) or 1/2 teaspoon black pepper
1/4	teaspoon sea salt

2	teaspoons arrowroot or corn starch mixed with 1 tablespoon cold water

1. Place cloves, cumin seeds and coriander in dry stainless steel pan over medium heat, and toast until fragrant and a shade or two darker. Remove and grind with mortar and pestle or in coffee mill. Set aside adding saffron, nutmeg, turmeric and bay leaf.
2. Prepare vegetables. Separate them into three bowls which will be added at different times based on how long they take to cook. In **Bowl One**, place potatoes, turnips, carrots, ginger and garlic. In **Bowl Two**, place sweet potato or butternut squash. In **Bowl Three**, add the bell pepper, zucchini and yellow squash.
3. Chop onion and sauté with oil in large dutch oven or stockpot. Add spices, chicken base, water and vegetables in Bowl One; simmer 10 minutes. Add sweet potatoes and simmer 5 minutes. Add Bowl Three vegetables, chick peas, diced tomato and Harrisa paste, pepper and salt. Simmer 5 minutes longer or until desired tenderness of all vegetables.
4. Stir together arrowroot and water. Add to stew and stir. Makes 12 cups stew. Serve alone or over any cooked grain desired.

Harissa paste is a fiery hot, spicy sauce made from chili pepper and garlic. Look for it in the ethnic food section of the store or a Middle Eastern food store.

Make this when you have some extra time it is well worth the effort. It makes a large amount which you can freeze for a later meal.

Servings: 8

NUTRITION PER SERVING

Serving size	1-1/4 cup
Calories	147
Protein	5 g
Carbohydrate*	26 g
(*no added sugars)	
Fiber	5.4 g
Soluble fiber	1.9 g
Fat	2.5 g
Saturated fat	0 g
Cholesterol	0 mg
Sodium	331 mg
Potassium	537 mg
Calcium	71 mg
Omega-3 ALA	190 mg

Bonus:

Copper	(537% DV)
Vitamin C	(102% DV)
Iron	(12% DV)

Pasta Sauce

A typical store-bought pasta sauce has 70 to 120 calories and 2 teaspoons of added sugars per half cup. Make your own with this simple recipe.

HELPFUL HINT
Do not use cooking-type wines; they are high in sodium.

2	teaspoons olive oil
3	cloves garlic, crushed
1-1/2	teaspoons dry basil (1/4 cup fresh)
2	tablespoons chopped fresh flat-leaf parsley (or 2 teaspoons dry)
2	teaspoons dry oregano
2	teaspoons balsamic vinegar
1/8	teaspoon sea salt
	few grinds freshly ground pepper
1	(28-ounce) can *Muir Glen Fire-Roasted Tomatoes* with juice
1	(28-ounce) can *Dei Fratelli Crushed Tomatoes No-Salt-Added with Basil and Herbs*
1	tablespoons red wine (optional)

1. Sauté olive oil and garlic over medium to low heat for 1 minute. Do not brown garlic.
2. Add remaining ingredients. Bring to boil, reduce and simmer 15 minutes.

VARIATION
❖ Add 1/2 to 3/4 cup dry, textured vegetable soy protein (TVP), reconstituted with equal amount of boiling water
❖ Pasta Primavera: Add a 1-pound bag of frozen stir-fry vegetables or broccoli, cauliflower, carrots or mixed vegetables.
❖ Cook 1 cup red lentils for 5 minutes, then add dry pasta and cook together for 10 minutes longer. Drain and combine with pasta sauce.

QUICK TIP
❖ Add a 28-ounce can crushed, no-salt-added tomatoes to any jar of pasta sauce to reduce sodium by half.

QUICK SAUCE
❖ To a 28-ounce can of crushed tomatoes, add 1 to 2 cloves of chopped garlic and a tablespoon of extra-virgin olive oil. Add fresh, chopped basil if you have it.

QUICK PIZZA SAUCE
❖ Line a mesh strainer with a paper coffee filter. Add can of crushed tomatoes and let some of the liquid drain to thicken sauce.

Servings: 14

NUTRITION PER SERVING

Serving size	1/2 cup
Calories	41
Protein	1.5 g
Carbohydrate*	8 g
(*no added sugars)	
Fiber	1.5 g
Soluble fiber	0.6 g
Fat	0.5 g
Saturated fat	0 g
Cholesterol	0 mg
Sodium	193 mg
Potassium	10 mg
Calcium	12 mg
Omega-3 ALA	10 mg

Bonus:
Vitamin C	(37% DV)
Beta-carotene	(18% DV)

Spinach and Basil Pasta

1/4	cup sun-dried tomatoes, diced
1	carrot, peeled and shredded
2	cloves garlic
1	(10-ounce) package fresh baby spinach
1/2	cup tightly packed basil
1	tablespoon sliced almonds
1/4	teaspoon sea salt
1/3	cup grated Parmesan cheese
1	tablespoon extra-virgin olive oil

. . . .

8	ounces whole-wheat angel hair pasta or brown rice pasta

1. Bring pot of water to boil to cook pasta.
2. If sun-dried tomatoes are hard, soften by covering slightly with boiling water. Let stand for 15 minutes. Omit soaking step if soft. Dice tomatoes.
3. Peel and shred carrot using small holes on box grater; set carrots aside for later.
4. Chop garlic in food processor. Add spinach, basil, almonds, salt, Parmesan and oil. Blend thoroughly.
5. Cook and drain pasta. Immediately add spinach mixture to cooked pasta, along with sun-dried tomatoes and carrots. Toss and serve.

HELPFUL HINT
To reduce sodium to 171 mg, omit salt.

Servings: 4

NUTRITION PER SERVING

Serving size	1 cup
Calories	175
Protein	8 g
Carbohydrate*	22 g
(*no added sugars)	
Fiber	4.5 g
Soluble fiber	0.95 g
Fat	6.5 g
Saturated fat	1.7 g
Cholesterol	6 mg
Sodium	314 mg
Potassium	248 mg
Calcium	173 mg
Omega-3 ALA	70 mg

Bonus:
Vitamin C	(40% DV)
Selenium	(23% DV)
Vitamin K	(363 mcg)

Pesto

Make this when basil is in season and available at the farmers' market, or grow it yourself in the summer. Freeze in the amounts you use.

2	cloves garlic, peeled (use only fresh)
2	cups lightly packed, fresh basil leaves (1 ounce), wash and dry (a salad spinner works great)
3	tablespoons pine nuts (walnuts or almonds also work well)
1/4	teaspoon sea salt
1/2	cup freshly grated Parmesan cheese (1 ounce)
1/4	cup extra-virgin olive oil

1. Wash basil. Remove leaves and discard thick stems.
2. Place garlic cloves in food processor and pulse into small pieces.
3. When garlic is minced, add basil, nuts, parmesan and salt. Pulse again until chopped.
4. Add oil, process, and scrape sides as needed.
5. Toss with cooked whole-wheat pasta (8 ounces dry)

HELPFUL HINTS
- Makes 1/2 cup, enough to coat 8 ounces of cooked pasta.
- Use only fresh basil. This is one recipe where dried won't work.
- Use only extra-virgin olive oil.

Servings: 8

NUTRITION PER SERVING

Servings size	1 tablespoon
Calories	77
Protein	1.5 g
Carbohydrate*	0.5 g
(*no added sugars)	
Fiber	0.2 g
Soluble	0 mg
Fat	8 g
Saturated fat	1.5 g
Cholesterol	3 mg
Sodium	127 mg
Potassium	24 mg
Calcium	46 mg
Omega-3 ALA	70 mg

Bonus:	
Beta-carotene	(4 % DV)
Vitamin K	(15 mcg)

Servings: 4

NUTRITION PER SERVING

Serving size	1 cup pasta with pesto
Calories	287
Protein	8.5 g
Carbohydrate*	43 g
(*no added sugars)	
Fiber	7 g
Soluble fiber	0.9 g
Fat	9 g
Saturated fat	1.5 g
Cholesterol	3 mg
Sodium	137 mg
Potassium	92 mg
Calcium	69 mg
Omega-3 ALA	390 mg

WHOLE-WHEAT PASTA: 2 ounces of dry pasta, when cooked, provides copper (29% DV), iron (21% DV), magnesium (11% DV), selenium (73% DV), zinc (11% DV)

PARMESAN CHEESE. No Parmesan can compare to *Parmigiano Reggiano,* which is made partly from skimmed, unpasteurized cow's milk. No chemical preservatives or artificial additives are used in its preparation. The cheese is encased with a yellowish rind on which the brand name *Parmigiano Reggiano* is stenciled in small dots. It is produced in Italy in a zone limited to the Provinces of Parma, Reggio-Emilia and Modena, and parts of the Provinces of Mantua and Bolgona in the Italian region of Emlia-Romagna. Grate it as needed since freshly grated is best.

USING FROZEN PESTO
If using the pesto frozen, it is ideal to thaw it overnight in refrigerator. If you don't have time, microwave 10 seconds, stir, and repeat if needed until just slightly soft. Be careful because if it is heated too much, it will clump and not coat the pasta strands.

Roasted Bell Peppers and Basil Sauce

1	large red bell pepper, roasted
1	large yellow bell pepper, roasted
1/4	cup sun-dried tomatoes (Page 287)
1/2	teaspoon fennel seeds, crushed with mortar and pestle or in coffee grinder
1	tablespoon olive oil
1	medium sweet onion, cut in thin wedges
1	clove garlic, minced
1	(15-ounce) can stewed tomatoes, no-salt-added
1/8	teaspoon *Penzeys* Spices' *Aleppo Pepper* (may also use cayenne or diced jalapeno)
1/8	teaspoon sea salt
1/4	cup fresh basil, sliced
1/4	cup freshly grated Parmesan cheese

Serve over cooked whole-wheat penne pasta, spaghetti squash, Multi-Grain Mix (Page 327), or cooked oat groats.

1. Roast bell peppers (Page 355), or purchase them in jars, see note below.
2. Soften tomatoes if needed, cut in strips.
3. Crush fennel seed. Chop onion and mince garlic.
4. In sauté pan over medium heat, sauté onion, fennel seed and oil. Cover and cook 5 minutes; stir occasionally. Onions should be soft but not browned.
5. Add garlic, canned tomatoes, diced sun-dried tomatoes (include the liquid if they needed soaking), and bring to a boil. Reduce heat and simmer uncovered for 20 minutes.
6. Meanwhile, remove skin from roasted bell peppers. Cut peppers in strips. Add any liquid that collects while standing to the recipe.
7. Add Aleppo pepper, salt, basil and roasted peppers to tomato mixture. Cover and cook 5 minutes. Serve 1/2 cup over desired grain, and sprinkle with Parmesan cheese.

Note: *May purchase roasted bell pepper. If canned, drain the salty brine and discard. If using canned, the skin is already removed.*

Servings: 5

NUTRITION PER SERVING

Serving size	1/2 cup
	(sauce only)
Calories	92
Protein	3 g
Carbohydrate	13 g
(*no added sugar)	
Fiber	3 g
Soluble fiber	0.54 g
Fat	3.5 g
Saturated fat	0.8 g
Cholesterol	2 mg
Sodium	185 mg
Potassium	216 mg
Calcium	58 mg
Omega-3 ALA	40 mg

Bonus:	
Vitamin C	(146% DV)
Beta-carotene	(39% DV)
Vitamin K	(32 mcg)

Broccoli Pesto Penne

1	tablespoon pine nuts, toasted
1/2	teaspoon fresh garlic, minced (1 clove)
1/4	cup fresh basil (leaves only) (do not use dry basil as a substitute in this recipe)
1/2	cup frozen broccoli florets, thawed
1/4	cup fat-free ricotta cheese or no-salt-added cottage cheese
1-1/2	teaspoons extra-virgin olive oil
1/2	cup water
1/4	teaspoon *Organic Better Than Bouillon Vegetable Base*
1/8	teaspoon sea salt
2	tablespoons freshly grated Parmesan cheese
	freshly grated black pepper to taste

3	ounces uncooked whole-wheat penne, rotini, bow tie or any other shape (3 cups cooked)

1. In dry pan over medium heat, toast nuts, stirring until toasted to a slightly golden color. Watch carefully so they don't burn. Remove from heat and set aside.
2. Place nuts, garlic, basil, broccoli, ricotta, olive oil, water, vegetable base and salt in small food processor and blend thoroughly. Add Parmesan and pulse a few times to blend.
3. Cook pasta as directed on package to desired doneness; omit salt and oil if package directions include them. Drain pasta. Immediately add sauce to pasta, toss and serve.

- Make extra sauce as it freezes well. For a quick meal, thaw and toss with any cooked pasta or cooked grain, such as couscous, millet or multi-grain mix, (Page 327).

- A good way to sneak in broccoli.

Servings: 6

NUTRITION PER SERVING

Serving size	1/2 cup
Calories	140
Protein	6 g
Carbohydrate*	23 g
(*no added sugars)	
Fiber	1.5 g
Soluble fiber	0.24 g
Fat	3 g
Saturated fat	0.6 g
Cholesterol	3 mg
Sodium	119 mg
Potassium	74 mg
Calcium	55 mg
Omega-3 ALA	10 mg

Bonus:

Folate	(16% DV)
Vitamin C	(10% DV)

Baked Pasta and Cheese Florentine

Topping:
1	tablespoon whole-wheat dry bread crumbs (Page 284) (or *Ian's Panko Whole-Wheat Bread Crumbs*)
1	tablespoon ground flaxseed
1	teaspoon dry parsley
1	tablespoon very finely chopped walnuts
1	tablespoon grated Parmesan cheese

· ·

2	cups (4-ounces) uncooked whole-wheat rotini pasta (or brown rice pasta)
1/4	cup fat-free sour cream or low-fat yogurt
1/2	cup 1%, no-salt-added cottage cheese
4	ounces *Cabot 75% Light Cheddar* or similar reduced-fat cheddar

· ·

3/4	cup plain, unsweetened soy milk
2	tablespoons whole-wheat flour
1/8	teaspoon sea salt
1/4	teaspoon dry mustard
1/4	teaspoon onion powder

· ·

2	cups frozen cut-leaf spinach, thawed; or 1-1/2 cups frozen broccoli florets, thawed and chopped; or frozen mixed or stir-fry vegetables, thawed

1. Combine topping ingredients (first five ingredients) and set aside.
2. Preheat oven to 350° F.
3. Cook pasta 3 minutes less than package directs. Drain and combine with yogurt and cottage cheese.
4. Shred cheese.
5. In glass bowl or 4-cup measuring cup, combine soy milk, flour, salt, mustard and onion powder. Microwave and stir every minute with whisk until mixture bubbles. Add, along with cheddar cheese, to the pasta mixture. Stir.
6. Spread half the mixture in a glass (1-1/2 quart) baking dish. Top with spinach. Add remaining pasta mixture. Sprinkle with topping and bake uncovered for 20 to 25 minutes.

NOTE: *Casserole-type dishes such as this should be served with a salad or a side of vegetables, since they contain some vegetables but not enough.*

Servings: 5

NUTRITION PER SERVING

Serving size	1 cup
Calories	174
Protein	17 g
Carbohydrate*	18 g
(*no added sugars)	
Fiber	2 g
Soluble fiber	1.5 g
Fat	4 g
Saturated fat	1.8 g
Cholesterol	2 mg
Sodium	350 mg
Potassium	160 mg
Calcium	321 mg
Omega-3 ALA	320 mg

Fettuccini With Tofu Alfredo

Servings: 5

NUTRITION PER SERVING

Serving size	3/4 cup
Calories	271
Protein	14 g
Carbohydrate*	45 g
(*no added sugars)	
Fiber	7 g
Soluble fiber	1.7 g
Fat	5 g
Saturated fat	1 g
Cholesterol	3 mg
Sodium	156 mg
Potassium	270 mg
Calcium	94 mg
Omega-3 ALA	50 mg

Bonus:
Selenium   (60% DV)

1	clove garlic
1	tablespoon extra-virgin olive oil
1/3	cup freshly grated Parmesan cheese
1/2	cup plain soy milk or skim milk
1/4	teaspoon sea salt
1	(12.3-ounce) box silken tofu (*Mori-Nu*)
12	ounces whole-wheat fettuccini pasta

1. Combine all ingredients except fettuccini in food processor, and blend until smooth.
2. Cook fettuccini pasta according to package directions.
3. Drain pasta and toss sauce with cooked pasta.

White Bean and Tofu Stuffed Shells

Servings: 6

NUTRITION PER SERVING

Serving size	3 filled shells
Calories	216
Protein	13 g
Carbohydrate*	35 g
(*no added sugars)	
Fiber	4.5 g
Soluble fiber	1.5 g
Fat	3 g
Saturated fat	0.7 g
Cholesterol	3 mg
Sodium	151 mg
Potassium	219 mg
Calcium	86 mg
Omega-3 ALA	124 mg

Bonus:
Folate   (16% DV)
Magnesium   (12% DV)
Iron   (12% DV)

18	jumbo macaroni shells, cooked (6 ounces dry)
5	halves or 2 tablespoons sun-dried tomatoes, chopped (Page 287)
1	clove fresh garlic
1	(12.3-ounce) box firm silken tofu (*Mori-Nu*)
1	(15-ounce) can cannellini or other white beans, rinsed and drained
2	tablespoons chopped fresh basil, or 1/2 teaspoon dried basil
1/2	teaspoon dried Italian seasoning*
1-1/2	cups pasta sauce (Page 388)
1/2	cup part-skim shredded mozzarella
1	tablespoon grated Parmesan cheese

1. Preheat oven to 350°F.
2. Cook pasta shells according to package directions.
3. Pulse garlic in food processor until finely chopped.
4. Add tofu; process until smooth.
5. Add beans, basil and Italian seasoning; pulse until beans are coarsely chopped. Add chopped sun-dried tomatoes; pulse only until blended.
6. Spread 1/2 cup pasta sauce on bottom of a 9 x 13-inch baking dish.
7. Spoon 1/4 cup tofu mixture into each shell. Arrange shells in dish.
8. Spoon remaining pasta sauce over shells, covering only part of each shell; sprinkle with mozzarella and Parmesan cheese.
9. Bake covered for 30 minutes.

Italian Seasoning: Place 1 tablespoon of each dried herb in coffee mill and pulse several times: basil, oregano, rosemary, marjoram, sage, savory and thyme. Store in tightly covered jar. Or try Tuscan Sunset or Mural of Flavor by Penzeys Spices.

Tofu With Fire-Roasted Tomatoes

1   package (1 pound) firm tofu (not silken style)
2   teaspoons canola oil
1   (14.5 ounce) can *Muir Glen Fire-Roasted Diced Tomatoes*

1. Prepare tofu as stated below. Heat heavy skillet 4 minutes on medium heat. Add 2 teaspoons canola oil and tofu in a single layer. Allow to cook undisturbed for 4 to 5 minutes or until golden. Turn pieces and brown other side.
2. Add tomatoes and simmer until some of the liquid has evaporated.

Basic preparation of Tofu:
1. Do this the night before you plan to cook. The additional time allows tofu to become firmer.
2. Remove tofu from packaging, drain water and wrap in several layers of cotton towel. Then, place inside plastic bag and refrigerate 30 minutes to 24 hours. This will allow the water to be absorbed, making the tofu firmer.
3. When ready to prepare unwrap tofu and cut into slices, then cube or break into irregular shapes.

For this recipe use a tofu that maintains its shape. Choose firm or extra firm. Do not use silken. Note that all Mori-Nu tofu is silken style. Silken tofu works best when you want to blend it into a smooth, creamy texture.

Servings: 4

NUTRITION PER SERVING

| Serving size | 1 cup |
| | (4 ounces tofu) |

Calories	149
Protein	12 g
Carbohydrate*	7 g
(*no added sugars)	
Fiber	1.3 g
Soluble fiber	1 g
Fat	9 g
Saturated fat	1 g
Cholesterol	0 mg
Sodium	304 mg
Potassium	156 mg
Calcium	217 mg
Omega-3 ALA	650 mg

Bonus:	
Vitamin C	(39% DV)
Selenium	(21% DV)
Iron	(15% DV)
Magnesium	(15% DV)

Ginger Soy Marinated Tofu and Rice

1	cup brown rice or *Lundberg Wild Rice Blend* or Multi-Grain Mix (Page 327)
1	pound firm tofu (not silken type)
2	teaspoons canola oil for browning tofu

Marinade:

2	tablespoons canola oil
3	tablespoons reduced-sodium soy sauce
2	cloves garlic, minced
1-1/2	teaspoons grated, fresh ginger root
1	teaspoon honey

1	teaspoon canola oil
1	carrot, peeled and diced
1/2	small red onion, diced
1	stalk celery, diced
1/2	red or yellow bell pepper, diced
1	cup frozen peas
1	cup frozen corn

1. Prepare tofu as described on Page 395.
2. Cook rice with 2 cups water in rice cooker. Rice may also be cooked on stove top (Page 325).
3. While rice is cooking, prepare marinade by combining oil, soy sauce, garlic, ginger and honey in bowl.
4. Peel and dice carrot and onion. Dice celery. Set aside in bowl.
5. Dice bell pepper. Place in another bowl, along with frozen peas and corn.
6. Heat heavy skillet 4 minutes on medium heat. Add 2 teaspoons canola oil and tofu. Allow to cook undisturbed for 4 to 5 minutes or until golden. Turn pieces and brown other side. Remove from pan and add tofu to bowl with marinade. Let marinade soak into tofu while sautéing vegetables.
7. Sauté celery, carrot and onion in oil for 1 minute. Add peas, corn and bell pepper and cook 1 minute longer. Keep the vegetables crispy.
8. Add vegetables and cooked rice to tofu/marinade mixture. Toss and serve warm, room temperature or chilled.

Servings: 7

NUTRITION PER SERVING

Serving size	1 cup
Calories	252
Protein	12 g
Carbohydrate*	35 g
(*0.6 g added sugars from honey)	
Fiber	5 g
Soluble fiber	1.2 g
Fat	8 g
Saturated fat	0.5 g
Cholesterol	0 mg
Sodium	272 mg
Potassium	214 mg
Calcium	53 mg
Omega-3 ALA	400 mg

Bonus:

Beta-carotene	(50% DV)
Vitamin C	(38% DV)
Selenium	(14% DV)
Magnesium	(13% DV)
Iron	(11% DV)
Zinc	(6% DV)
Vitamin K	(14 mcg)

Lemon-Baked Tempeh

1/4	cup freshly squeezed lemon juice
1	teaspoon lemon zest
1/3	cup water
1	teaspoon onion powder
1	teaspoon garlic powder
2	teaspoons reduced-sodium tamari or soy sauce
1	tablespoon canola oil
1	(8-ounce) package tempeh

1. Remove zest from lemon and squeeze out juice.
2. Combine all ingredients, except tempeh, in 8-inch glass loaf pan.
3. Cut tempeh into 2 pieces and add to dish with marinade. Cover and refrigerate for 24 hours.
4. Preheat oven to 350°F.
5. Remove dish and bake uncovered with marinade for 15 minutes. Turn and bake 10 minutes longer. Serve hot or cold.

Look for tempeh in the refrigerated or frozen food area of a grocery store's health section or a natural foods store. Tempeh has a firm, not crunchy, but toothy texture.

Servings: 2

NUTRITION PER SERVING

Serving size	4 ounces
Calories	160
Protein	8 g
Carbohydrate*	9 g
(*no added sugars)	
Fiber	3.5 g
Soluble fiber	4 g
Fat	11 g
Saturated fat	1.5 g
Cholesterol	0 mg
Sodium	238 mg
Potassium	60 mg
Calcium	25 mg
Omega-3 ALA	255 mg

Bonus:
Vitamin C	(29% DV)
Iron	(18% DV)

Pan-Grilled Marinated Tempeh Slices

1	(8-ounce) package tempeh

Marinade:

1/4	cup reduced-sodium soy sauce or tamari
2	tablespoons lemon juice
3/4	cup water
1	teaspoon grated fresh ginger
1	teaspoon minced garlic
2	teaspoons toasted sesame oil

1. Combine marinade ingredients in 9-inch square glass pan.
2. Slice tempeh into thin, 1/4-inch strips adding to marinade. Cover. Refrigerate 20 minutes or overnight if you have time.
3. Remove from marinade and brown tempeh slices in pan sprayed with cooking spray. Serve as is or use tempeh for sandwiches. Good warm or cold.

Servings: 2

NUTRITION PER SERVING**

Serving size:	4 ounces tempeh
Calories	202
Protein	25 g
Carbohydrate*	11 g
(*no added sugars)	
Fiber	7 g
Soluble fiber	2.6 g
Fat	7 g
Saturated fat	2 g
Cholesterol	0 mg
Sodium	207 mg
Potassium	57 mg
Calcium	178 mg
Omega-3 ALA	250 mg

Bonus:
Iron	(19% DV)

** Analysis based on 1/4 of marinade being absorbed.

Fire-Roasted Tomatoes, Lentils and Pasta

1	medium onion, chopped
1	stalk celery, diced
1	carrot, peeled and diced
2	teaspoons extra-virgin olive oil
1/2	cup lentils
1	clove garlic, minced
1	(28-ounce) can *Muir Glen Fire-Roasted Crushed Tomatoes*
1 1/2	cup water
1/2	teaspoon *Organic Better Than Bouillon Chicken Base*
1	cup tiny tube pasta (ditali) or whole-wheat shell pasta
1/4	cup freshly grated Parmesan cheese

1. Peel and chop onion and carrot. Dice celery. Chop garlic. Measure out other ingredients and set aside.
2. Add oil to saucepan and sauté onion, celery, carrot and lentils for 4 minutes.
3. Meanwhile, cook pasta in pot of boiling water for 6 minutes until tender but still firm (al dente).
4. Add garlic, tomatoes, water and chicken base to the saucepan with onion mixture and bring to a boil. Reduce to simmer and cook covered, 30 to 40 minutes, or until lentils have softened. If it becomes too thick, add additional water.
5. Add cooked pasta and Parmesan cheese. Stir and serve.

NOTE: *Use crushed no-salt-added tomatoes to reduce sodium to 107 mg.*

OPTIONAL: *Serve with cooked kale or spinach*

Servings: 6

NUTRITION PER SERVING

Serving size	1 cup
Calories	145
Protein	9 g
Carbohydrate*	25 g
(*no added sugars)	
Fiber	3.8 g
Soluble fiber	1.5 g
Fat	1 g
Saturated fat	0.5 g
Cholesterol	3 mg
Sodium	386 mg
Potassium	615 mg
Calcium	74 mg
Omega-3 ALA	1 mg

Bonus:
Vitamin C	(15% DV)

Chicken Pesto Pasta

1	carrot, peeled and diced
1/2	small onion, chopped
1	clove garlic, minced
1/2	bell pepper (any color), diced
1/4	cup diced sun-dried tomato (soak if needed)
1	teaspoon canola oil
1	cup frozen cut-leaf spinach, thawed, or cooked kale

4	ounces (2 cups) dry whole-wheat rotini, penne pasta or brown rice pasta
2	cup shredded or cubed cooked chicken (Page 400) or see below for meatless options
1/4	cup pesto (buy or make see Page 390)

1. Peel and dice carrot and onion. Mince garlic. Dice bell pepper and sun-dried tomato. Place in bowl with oil. Set aside.
2. Thaw spinach. Thaw chicken if using frozen.
3. Cook pasta according to package directions. About 1 minute before pasta is done, add the cubed chicken so it will warm through. Drain pasta and chicken. If using frozen *Quorn,* add it to the boiling pasta when it is about 2 minutes from being done to allow it to thaw and heat through.
4. Meanwhile, microwave carrot, onion, bell pepper, garlic and oil for 2 minutes. Stir in spinach and cook one minute longer.
5. Toss together the pasta, chicken, vegetables, sun-dried tomatoes and pesto. Serve.

MEATLESS OPTIONS AS SUBSTITUTES FOR CHICKEN

❖ *Quorn* **chick'n tenders** are meat free and soy free. Use one 12-ounce bag in this recipe. The main ingredient in all *Quorn* products is mycoprotein ("myco" is Greek for "fungi"). The mycoprotein comes from Fusarium venenatum, which was originally discovered growing in a field in England. It is a nutritious protein source. Since some individuals may be sensitive or allergic to *Quorn,* it should be treated as any new food ingredient that has the potential for reactions in some individuals, such as shell fish or peanuts.

❖ *Morningstar Farms Chicken Meal Starters Chick'n Strips.* Found in the freezer section. Made from soy.

❖ *Veat's Chick'n-Free Nuggets.* Found in the frozen food section of health food stores. Made from textured soy protein.

Servings: 6

NUTRITION PER SERVING

Serving size	1 cup
Calories	184
Protein	14 g
Carbohydrate*	15 g
(*no added sugars)	
Fiber	3 g
Soluble fiber	0.7 g
Fat	8 g
Saturated fat	1.7 g
Cholesterol	22 mg
Sodium	225 mg
Potassium	227 mg
Calcium	70 mg
Omega-3 ALA	120 mg

Bonus:	
Vitamin C	(30% DV)
Folate	(14% DV)
Magnesium	(10% DV)
Selenium	(13% DV)
Vitamin K	(94 mcg)

Chicken Rice Primavera

1-1/2	cups frozen vegetables (mixed, stir-fry, etc.), thawed
1	clove garlic, minced (or 1/4 teaspoon garlic powder)
1/4	cup finely minced onion
2	cups reduced-sodium chicken broth (2 cups water plus 1-1/2 teaspoons *Organic Better Than Bouillon Chicken Base*
1	cup instant brown rice
1	cup (5 ounces) cooked, shredded chicken (see below)

1. Thaw vegetables.
2. Peel and chop garlic and onion. Add, with broth, to saucepan. Bring to a boil.
3. Add rice, vegetables and chicken. Cover and simmer for 10 minutes or until liquid is absorbed.

MEATLESS OPTIONS
❖ See Page 399 for substitutes for chicken.
❖ Substitute a can of drained and rinsed black beans for chicken.

READY-TO-USE CHICKEN
❖ To make quick and easy dishes, prepare chicken in advance and freeze in 1 cup portions.
❖ Place chicken breasts in crock pot and cover with water. Add a bay leaf, a teaspoon of bouillon chicken base, and a sprinkle of thyme. Cook on high for 2 hours. Let cool for an hour in the broth. Remove and shred with 2 forks into strips or cut in cubes. Save the broth and use to replace water when making soup, rice or other recipes.

Servings: 4

NUTRITION PER SERVING

Serving size	1 cup
Calories	229
Protein	5 g
Carbohydrate*	39 g
(*no added sugars)	
Fiber	5 g
Soluble fiber	2.2 g
Fat	1.7 g
Saturated fat	0.2 g
Cholesterol	24 mg
Sodium	281 mg
Potassium	384 mg
Calcium	43 mg
Omega-3 ALA	10 mg

Chicken Rolls

2 boneless, skinless chicken breasts
1 slice reduced-fat, reduced-sodium Swiss cheese, such as *Sargento,* or 1/4 cup shredded reduced-fat cheese such as *Cabot 50% Reduced-Fat Jalapeño Cheddar*
1/2 cup frozen cut-leaf spinach, thawed or (1 cup fresh baby spinach or kale)
1/4 teaspoon garlic powder or 1 clove fresh garlic, minced
1 cup Pasta Sauce (Page 388) or canned, crushed, no-salt-added tomatoes
1 tablespoon grated Parmesan cheese

1. Preheat oven to 350°F.
2. Remove any fat from chicken. Place chicken between two sheets of waxed paper. Using a rubber mallet, lightly pound from center toward edges until flattened.
3. Place cheese then spinach on flattened chicken and roll up.
4. Put half of pasta sauce in glass loaf pan or other baking dish. Place chicken, seam side down, in pan. Top with remaining sauce. Sprinkle on Parmesan.
5. Cover and bake for 40 minutes. Meat thermometer should read 170°F when done.

KITCHEN HELPER
A rubber mallet, found in the tool department, works great for all sorts of kitchen chores. It can be used to pound chicken or meat into thin pieces.

Servings: 2

NUTRITION PER SERVING

Serving size	1 chicken breast
Calories	274
Protein	42 g
Carbohydrate*	14 g
(*no added sugars)	
Fiber	5 g
Soluble fiber	0.25 g
Fat	4.5 g
Saturated fat	2.3 g
Cholesterol	68 mg
Sodium	395 mg
Potassium	292 mg
Calcium	279 mg
Omega-3 ALA	40 mg

Bonus:
Selenium	(16% DV)
Vitamin K	(222 mcg)

Tuscan Chicken

1 can white kidney or northern beans, no-salt-added preferred, drained and rinsed
1 can diced, no-salt-added tomatoes (not drained)
2 tablespoon Pesto (Page 390) or purchased pesto
2 chicken breasts (4 ounces each)
2 teaspoons grated Parmesan cheese

1. Preheat oven to 350°F.
2. Place beans, tomatoes and pesto in glass baking dish. Stir to blend.
3. Top with chicken; sprinkle with Parmesan.
4. Cover and bake for 20 minutes.

HELPFUL HINTS
Use cannellini (white kidney beans), great northern or navy beans. If using canned beans and tomatoes with salt instead of no-salt-added beans and tomatoes, a serving has 553 mg sodium.

Servings: 8

NUTRITION PER SERVING

Serving size	4 ounces
	chicken and 3/4 cup beans
Calories	422
Protein	43 g
Carbohydrate*	37 g
(*no added sugars)	
Fiber	12 g
Soluble fiber	3.3 g
Fat	10.5 g
Saturated fat	2.5 g
Cholesterol	72 mg
Sodium	259 mg
Potassium	746 mg
Calcium	237 mg
Omega-3 ALA	110 mg

Bonus:
Magnesium	(39% DV)
Vitamin C	(29% DV)
Selenium	(29% DV)
Iron	(26% DV)
Zinc	(25% DV)

Berry Chicken

2   chicken breasts (4 ounces each)

Sauce:
1   clove garlic
1   tablespoon canola oil
1   tablespoon raspberry vinegar
2/3 cup frozen mixed berries, thawed (or fresh)

1. To cook chicken, rub with a little oil and place in countertop grill, sauté pan, grill pan or under broiler. Cook to an internal temperature of 170°F.
2. To make sauce, add garlic to food processor while machine is running. Turn off. when garlic is minced. Add remaining sauce ingredients to processor and process until blended.
3. When ready to serve, heat sauce until only warm.

Servings: 2

NUTRITION PER SERVING

Serving size	4 ounces chicken + 1/4 cup sauce
Calories	222
Protein	27 g
Carbohydrate*	8 g
(*no added sugars)	
Fiber	1.5 g
Soluble fiber	0.5 g
Fat	8.5 g
Saturated fat	0.8 g
Cholesterol	66 mg
Sodium	176 mg
Potassium	297 mg
Calcium	21 mg
Omega-3 ALA	690 mg

Bonus:
Selenium	(29% DV)
Vitamin C	(20% DV)

Asian Chicken

2   chicken breasts (4 ounces each)

Sauce:
1   clove garlic, minced fine or 1/4 teaspoon garlic powder
1-1/2   tablespoons reduced-sodium soy sauce
2   teaspoons rice wine vinegar
2   teaspoons toasted sesame oil
1/2   teaspoon honey
2   tablespoons natural peanut butter
2   tablespoons hot water
1   teaspoon fresh grated ginger
1/4   teaspoon red chili pepper flakes, cayenne or *Thai Chili Garlic Sauce*, use more or less depending upon spiciness you desire.

1. Preheat oven to 350°F.
2. Make sauce. Place all ingredients in a jar with tight-fitting lid and shake vigorously. This can also be made with a handheld blender or small food processor.
3. Place chicken in baking dish, top with sauce, and sprinkle with sesame seeds.
4. Cover and bake 20 minutes.

Servings: 2

NUTRITION PER SERVING

Serving size	4 ounces
Calories	275
Protein	31 g
Carbohydrate*	6 g
(*1-1/2 g sugars from honey)	
Fiber	1 g
Soluble fiber	0.3 g
Fat	14 g
Saturated fat	2.5 g
Cholesterol	66 mg
Sodium	369 mg
Potassium	404 mg
Calcium	22 mg
Omega-3 ALA	50 mg

Bonus:
Selenium	(30% DV)
Magnesium	(14% DV)

Chicken Broccoli Stir-Fry

2	boneless, skinless chicken breasts (4 ounces each)
2	teaspoons canola or olive oil
1	stalk broccoli (about 2 cups broccoli florets)
1	yellow squash
1/2	small red onion
1/4	cup Balsamic Vinaigrette Dressing (Page 371)

HELPFUL HINT
Serve with Oat Groat Pilaf (Page 329), brown rice pasta, whole-wheat rotini, or over a bed of leafy greens.

1. Remove any fat from chicken. Cut into strips.
2. Prepare vegetables and set aside in separate piles.
   ❖ Remove florets from broccoli stalk, saving stems for another use or peel and cut stem into slices.
   ❖ Remove stem end from squash and cut into slices.
   ❖ Remove peel from onion. Cut onion into wedges.

3. Heat skillet over medium heat for 4 minutes. Toss 1 teaspoon oil with half of chicken strips. Add to skillet and stir-fry about 2 minutes, then set aside and keep covered.
4. Repeat with another teaspoon of oil and the remaining half of chicken strips. Set aside with first batch of chicken.
5. Add vegetables to pan and sauté about 1 minute. Add chicken back into pan along with dressing. If you prefer softer vegetables, cover and cook until vegetables are crisp tender.

BROWNING CHICKEN

Browning chicken strips in two batches will prevent crowding, enabling better browning. If chicken strips are too close, they will steam instead of browning. Flavor is improved when chicken is browned.

Servings: 2

NUTRITION PER SERVING

Serving size   4 ounces chicken, 1-1/2 cups vegetables

Calories	269
Protein	30 g
Carbohydrate*	17 g
(*no added sugars)	
Fiber	4.5 g
Soluble fiber	0.4 g
Fat	10 g
Saturated fat	1 g
Cholesterol	66 mg
Sodium	134 mg
Potassium	571 mg
Calcium	74 mg
Omega-3 ALA	910 mg

Bonus:

Vitamin C	(120% DV)
Selenium	(32% DV)
Folate	(15% DV)
Vitamin K	(90 mcg)

Oven-Fried Parmesan Chicken Nuggets

HELPFUL HINT
To make whole-wheat bread crumbs, see Page 284.

2	boneless, skinless chicken breasts (6 ounces each)
1	egg or 2 egg whites (or plain, nonfat yogurt)
2	tablespoons ground flaxseed or flaxseed meal
2	tablespoons dry oat bran
3/4	cup whole-wheat bread crumbs or *Ian's Whole-Wheat Panko Bread Crumbs*
1/4	cup grated Parmesan cheese
1/8	teaspoon black pepper
1	teaspoon dried parsley flakes
1/2	teaspoon garlic powder
1/4	teaspoon sea salt (or use 1/2 teaspoon salt-free lemon pepper)
	cooking spray

1. Preheat oven or toaster oven to 400°F.
2. Remove all fat from chicken. Cut chicken into bite size pieces.
3. Place egg in a small bowl and whisk with fork.
4. In another bowl, combine flaxseed, oat bran, bread crumbs, Parmesan, pepper, parsley, garlic and salt.
5. Dip chicken pieces into egg then crumb mixture, turning to coat.
6. Place chicken on a large, dark baking sheet (not air bake types, since it will not brown as well). Make sure pieces do not touch, or they will steam and not brown.
7. Spray lightly with cooking spray.
8. Bake for 10 minutes; turn chicken pieces and bake 10 minutes longer.
9. Serve with dipping sauce, if desired

Servings: 3

NUTRITION PER SERVING

Serving size	4 ounces
Calories	227
Protein	37 g
Carbohydrate*	23 g
(*no added sugars)	
Fiber	2 g
Soluble fiber	0.5 g
Fat	6.5 g
Saturated fat	1.5 g
Cholesterol	70 mg
Sodium	331 mg
Potassium	385 mg
Calcium	82 mg
Omega-3 ALA	980

Bonus:	
Zinc	(59% DV)
Selenium	(38% DV)

DIPPING SAUCE: 3 VARIATIONS

❖ **Ginger mustard:** Combine 2 tablespoons mustard, 1 tablespoon honey and 1/4 teaspoon freshly grated ginger.

❖ **Pasta Sauce** (Page 388): Heat and serve.

❖ **Honey Dijon:** Combine 1/4 package (about 3 ounces or 1/4 cup) *Organic Silken Mori-Nu Tofu*, 1 tablespoon honey and 1 tablespoon Dijon mustard in small food processor. Blend until smooth.

Stuffed Pork Tenderloin

Stuffing:

1/4	cup diced red bell pepper
1/4	cup minced onion
1	clove garlic, minced
1	teaspoon extra-virgin olive oil
1	cup frozen cut-leaf spinach, thawed
1/4	cup slivered almonds, toasted and chopped
1/4	cup grated Parmesan cheese
1/4	teaspoon sea salt
1/4	teaspoon black pepper

. . . .

1	pork tenderloin (about a pound), trimmed of any fat

Prepare stuffing:

1. Cut bell pepper in half, remove and discard top stems and inside white veins and seeds. Dice about 1/4 of the pepper, reserving the rest for another use. Peel and mince onion and garlic.
2. Toast almonds (see Page 285).
3. Sauté bell pepper, onion and garlic in oil over medium heat until softened.
4. Turn off heat and stir in spinach, almonds, Parmesan, salt and pepper. Set aside until needed.
5. Preheat oven to 375°F.

Butterfly the pork tenderloin (see below) or ask the butcher to double butterfly it for you.

1. Spread filling on flattened pork and roll up. Secure with toothpicks or tie with heavy cotton string or butcher's twine. Space the ties about three fingers width apart.
2. Rub outside with a little olive oil. At this point, you can refrigerate it if you are making it ahead of time.
3. When ready to cook, heat a large frying pan over medium-high heat, and sear tenderloin on all sides until evenly browned. Do not add oil to the pan; the oil rubbed on the pork is enough to brown the meat.
4. Remove browned tenderloin and place in a shallow roasting pan. Place in preheated oven for 20 minutes. Use a meat thermometer inserted into center and cook to 145°F.
5. Remove and let stand, covered with foil, for 3 to 5 minutes before slicing. You can spoon any juices that accumulate in the roaster over the pork.

How to butterfly a pork tenderloin:

1. Place the tenderloin on a cutting board. Hold your knife parallel to the board, with the blade facing the side of the meat, in the middle of the tenderloin.
2. Make a lengthwise cut into the center of the tenderloin until you are almost at the opposite edge. **Do not cut all the way through.** You want the meat to remain attached so you can open and fold the meat back. It is like a book that you open with the spine holding it together.
3. Lay a piece of plastic or waxed paper on the opened tenderloin. Tap meat gently to desired thickness, using a rubber mallet or rolling pin, working from middle toward the edges. Wash mallet or rolling pin with warm soapy water when done.

Servings: 4

NUTRITION PER SERVING

Serving size	4 ounces
Calories	112
Protein	34 g
Carbohydrate*	4 g
(*no added sugars)	
Fiber	2.3 g
Soluble fiber	0.2 g
Fat	9.4 g
Saturated fat	1.7 g
Cholesterol	106 mg
Sodium	251 mg
Potassium	215 mg
Calcium	125 mg
Omega-3 ALA	170 mg
Bonus:	
Selenium	(61% DV)
Copper	(23% DV)
Vitamin D	(687 IU)
Vitamin K	(50 mcg)

Ground Beef Burger Variations

If you eat red meat, see Page 75 for discussion on 100% grass-fed beef. Below are some ways to reduce the saturated fat in ground beef.

Turkey Beef Burgers
❖ Combine extra lean ground beef with equal amounts of ground turkey or chicken white meat or breast.

Soy and Beef Burgers
❖ Combine 1 pound of extra lean ground beef with 1/2 cup of textured vegetable soy protein (TVP). Look for TVP in the natural food section of the store or the bulk section of a natural/health food store. (Pour 1/4 cup boiling water over soy protein, stir, and then add ground beef.)
❖ Combine 1 pound of extra lean ground beef with about 2 cups of refrigerated soy meat-like substitute, such as *Gimme Lean* or *Yves Ground Round*. In the frozen food section, look for *Morningstar Farms Meal Starters Recipe Crumbles.*

Salmon Beef Burgers
❖ Combine 1 pound lean ground beef (ideally 100% grass-fed beef) with 1 pound of wild salmon, skin removed, and cut into small cubes, then minced with a knife. Small cubes may also be pulsed in food processor a few times.

Beef and Beans
❖ Add 1/4 cup bean flour to a pound of lean ground beef. You can make your own bean flour by grinding dry beans in a hand or electric grain mill. It's also available from www.bobsredmill.com and some health food stores.
❖ Combine 1/2 to 1 can of mashed black beans or kidney beans with a pound of ground beef.

See recipes for making a healthy "burger" on Pages 407 to 408.

Italian Beef and Chicken Patties

2	teaspoons extra-virgin olive oil
1	cup finely chopped onion
1	cup shredded carrots
4	cloves garlic, minced
1	teaspoon Italian herb mix (*Penzeys Spices' Tuscan Sunset*)
1	tablespoon sausage seasoning (*Penzeys Spices' Italian Sausage Seasoning*)
1	pound ground, 100% grass-fed beef or bison
1	pound ground turkey breast
1	cup old-fashioned rolled oats
1/4	cup crushed tomatoes, no-salt-added
1	(15-ounce) can kidney beans, no-salt-added preferred, drained and mashed

1. Heat oil in skillet over medium heat; add onion and carrot and cook 4 minutes. Add garlic and herb mix; cook 1 minute longer. Remove from heat and cool 5 minutes.
2. In a large bowl, mash beans. Add beef, turkey, oats, crush tomatoes, onion mixture; mix well.
3. Shape meat mixture into 22 patties (1/4 cup each). At this point patties may be frozen for later use, if desired.
4. Spray patties with cooking spray, and brown in skillet until internal temperature is 165°F.
5. If desired, serve with *Muir Glen Organic Black Bean and Corn Salsa* or similar brand.

A cooking class favorite.

Servings: 22

NUTRITION PER SERVING

Serving size	1 burger
Calories	109
Protein	11 g
Carbohydrate*	7 g
(*no added sugars)	
Fiber	1.5 g
Soluble fiber	1.1 g
Fat	4 g
Saturated fat	1.5 g
Cholesterol	27 mg
Sodium	108 mg
Potassium	275 mg
Calcium	15 mg
Omega-3 ALA	2 mg

Bonus:
Selenium	(13% DV)

Easy Salmon Burgers

1	(15-ounce) can Alaskan pink or sockeye salmon or 1-1/2 cups leftover cooked salmon
1/4	cup finely chopped red or yellow onion
1/4	cup finely minced green pepper
1	stalk finely minced celery
1/4	cup finely chopped fresh flat-leaf parsley
2	teaspoons extra-virgin olive oil
3/4	cup whole-wheat bread crumbs
1	teaspoon dry dill weed
2	eggs, omega-3 enriched preferred

1. Flake salmon in bowl, removing bone and skin.
2. Chop onion, green pepper, celery and parlsey.
3. Sauté on medium-high heat the onion, green pepper, celery and oil until tender. Add to bowl with salmon
4. Add parsley, bread crumbs, dill weed and egg. Shape into 8 patties (about 1/4 cup each) and chill for 30 minutes or overnight.
5. Spray patties with cooking spray. Heat pan over medium-high heat. Cook until browned on each side, about 4 to 5 minutes.
6. Serve with Salsamole (Page 422).

Servings: 8

NUTRITION PER SERVING

Serving size	1 burger
Calories	123
Protein	9 g
Carbohydrate*	8 g
(*no added sugars)	
Fiber	1 g
Soluble fiber	0.1 g
Fat	6 g
Saturated fat	0.8 g
Cholesterol	57 mg
Sodium	246 mg
Potassium	167 mg
Calcium	89 mg
Omega-3	
EPA + DHA	651 mg

Bonus:
Selenium	(18% DV)
Vitamin D	(63 IU)

Chicken Beany Burgers

HELPFUL HINT
If you prefer spicy, add
Tabasco or minced
jalapeno pepper.

Servings: 8

NUTRITION PER SERVING

Serving size	1 burger
Calories	120
Protein	16 g
Carbohydrate*	11 g
(*no added sugars)	
Fiber	4 g
Soluble fiber	0.8 g
Fat	1.9 g
Saturated fat	0.08 g
Cholesterol	23 mg
Sodium	128 mg
Potassium	145 mg
Calcium	33 mg
Omega-3 DHA	20 mg

1	can northern or navy beans, no-salt-added preferred, drained, rinsed and mashed with fork
1	pound ground chicken (or turkey) breast, all white meat
1/4	cup dry oat bran
1	onion, finely grated
1	clove garlic, minced, or 1/4 teaspoon garlic powder
1/2	teaspoon ground cumin
1	teaspoon Worcestershire (Page 288)
1/4	teaspoon sea salt
	few grinds fresh pepper

1. Place all ingredients in a bowl. Mix together well.
2. Form into 8 patties (1/4 cup each).
3. Spray each patty on both sides with cooking spray or rub with canola oil.
4. Heat sauté pan on medium for 4 minutes. Add patties and cook about 4 minutes. Turn and cook other side.
5. Cook until internal temperature reaches 165°F.

❖ *Look for oat bran in the hot cereal section or the health section of your grocery store.*
❖ *Choose poultry raised without antibiotics.*

Tuscan Turkey Burgers

Servings: 8

NUTRITION PER SERVING

Serving size	1 burger
Calories	129
Protein	19 g
Carbohydrate*	9 g
(*no added sugars)	
Fiber	2.2 g
Soluble fiber	0.2 g
Fat	2.8 g
Saturated fat	0.75 g
Cholesterol	26 mg
Sodium	275 mg
Potassium	98 mg
Calcium	87 mg
Omega-3 DHA	10 mg
Bonus:	
Zinc	(19% DV)
Vitamin K	(150 mcg)

1	teaspoon canola oil
1	medium onion, chopped
1	clove garlic, minced
1/4	cup sun-dried tomatoes, minced (pulsed in food processor)
1	pound ground turkey breast or chicken breast
1	(10-ounce) package frozen cut-leaf spinach, thaw, excess water squeezed out, chopped to ensure small pieces
1	ounce freshly grated Parmesan cheese
1/2	cup whole-wheat bread crumbs or dry oat bran
1/4	teaspoon sea salt
	few grinds black pepper as desired

1. Sauté onion and garlic in a teaspoon of oil until softened.
2. Place onion and garlic in bowl, along with remaining ingredients. Mix well. Form into 8 patties (1/4 cup each).
3. Spray both sides of each patty with cooking spray or rub with canola oil.
4. Heat sauté pan on medium for 4 minutes. Add burgers and cook about 4 minutes. Turn and cook other side.
5. Cook until internal temperature reaches 165°F.

❖ *Onions are sautéed to soften the texture. You can skip this step if you pulse onion in food processor or grate onion on box grater.*
❖ *Make your own whole-wheat bread crumbs (Page 284) or buy Ian's Whole-Wheat Panko Bread Crumbs.*

How Do You Know When Fish Is Done?

One guideline is the 10-Minute Rule or Canadian Cooking Method. Measure the fish where it is the thickest, and plan to turn fish halfway through the cooking process, unless it's very thin. This estimates grilling or broiling time, but baking will often take a little longer generally about 12 minutes per inch. If baking an entire fish or filet even more baking time may be needed.

Testing For Doneness

The best way to gauge doneness is to test fish. If you are new to cooking fish, you may need to test often. After cooking fish a few times, you will know about how long it takes. Check about 2 minutes before it is expected to be done. Use the point of a sharp knife to make a small cut into the flesh, or use a fork to separate the flesh at the thickest part (you cannot separate the fish until it is almost done.) If the flesh flakes and the color has changed from translucent to opaque almost all the way to the center, it is done. Salmon will change from a darker to a lighter shade of red/pink. Remove fish when it reaches 130°F, let it stand covered about 5 minutes. Fish will continue to cook when it is removed from the heat source, so cook it slightly less than what you want it to be (145°F is done). Wild salmon will be dry if overcooked, since it has less fat than farmed salmon.

Baking Fish

The length of time it takes will vary by the temperature of the oven, the thickness of the fish, the size of the filet, and whether it is baking in an open or closed dish. For best results, test for doneness.

Should You Rinse Fish Before Cooking?

There is no scientific evidence that rinsing is helpful in getting rid of bacteria. The USDA says not to rinse fish, chicken or meat since it does little to remove bacteria. Bacteria are killed in cooking. By rinsing you will spread bacteria around your sink, which can then cross-contaminate other foods.

Why Remove Skin?

To minimize exposure to contaminants, remove skin from fish before cooking. An exception is farmed rainbow trout, which is raised in a controlled environment, free of contaminates. Look for local sources and ask how they raise their trout.

How To Remove Skin

Using a knife, gently remove a small portion of the flesh away from the skin to get it started. Place fish skin side down. It is important to hold the knife at the correct angle and to pull on the skin, keeping a steady pressure against the knife, but not sawing or cutting with the knife. Holding the blade too flat will result in a jagged cutting action and probably leave some skin on. Hold it too upright, and you will slice through the skin and make it difficult to restart the procedure. There is no substitute for practice, so give it some trial and error until you find the right angle that works with the blade of your knife.

Walnut-Crusted Salmon

4	ounces wild sockeye salmon filet (see fish substitute suggestions)
1-1/2	teaspoons light mayonnaise (see Page 285)
1-1/2	teaspoons Dijon mustard

. . . .

Topping:

1	tablespoon chopped walnuts
1-1/2	teaspoons plain, dried, whole-wheat bread crumbs or *Ian's Whole-Wheat Panko Bread Crumbs* (or use more walnuts)
1-1/2	teaspoons grated Parmesan cheese
1/4	teaspoon dry parsley

1. Preheat oven to 450°F.
2. In a food processor, make topping. Pulse the walnuts, bread crumbs, Parmesan, and parsley. Do not overprocess or it will become "nut butter."
3. Spray skin side of fish with cooking spray or rub with oil. Place the fish filets in a shallow baking dish with oiled side down.
4. In a small bowl, combine the mayonnaise and mustard. Spread the mayonnaise mixture on the top side of the fish.
5. Sprinkle the topping mixture over the fish, patting it on.
6. Bake until the fish just flakes when tested with a fork, about 10 minute per inch.

VARIATIONS

❖ Add ground cumin, onion powder or garlic powder to mayonnaise
❖ Suggested substitutes: barramundi, catfish, cod, flounder, halibut, pollock
❖ Try other nuts, such as pecan or almonds

HELPFUL HINT
Omit bread crumbs
for lower carbohydrate
version.

Servings: 1

NUTRITION PER SERVING

Serving size	4 ounces
Calories	233
Protein	28 g
Carbohydrate*	3 g
(*no added sugars)	
Fiber	0.3 g
Soluble fiber	0.08 g
Fat	13 g
Saturated fat	2 g
Cholesterol	74 mg
Sodium	195 mg
Potassium	660 mg
Calcium	38 mg
Omega-3 ALA	680 mg
EPA + DHA	1,620 mg

Bonus:	
Selenium	(68% DV)
Copper	(15% DV
Zinc	(11% DV)
Magnesium	(11% DV)
Vitamin D	(687 IU)

Flounder Mexicali

Breading:
1/4	cup dry whole-wheat bread crumbs
3	tablespoons ground or milled flaxseed
1/2	teaspoon cumin
1/4	teaspoon chili powder

. . . .

1	egg (omega-3 enriched), whisked with fork
2	(4-ounce) flounder filets
2	tablespoons salsa
2	tablespoons grated cheese (*Cabot 50% Reduced-Fat* Jalapeno Cheese)

1. Preheat oven to 425°F.
2. Combine bread crumbs, flaxseed, cumin and chili powder. Place in shallow dish.
3. Place egg in another shallow dish.
4. Dip fish in egg, then crumbs.
5. Spray breaded fish with cooking spray, and bake on baking pan for 10 minutes or until fish flakes.
6. Top each fish filet with 1 tablespoon of salsa and 1 tablespoon of cheese.
7. Bake 5 minutes longer or until cheese melts.

VARIATIONS
❖ Substitute catfish, cod, pollock, trout, barramundi or perch
❖ Instead of bread crumbs, use ground nuts, such as almonds, walnuts, pecans, etc.

Servings: 2

NUTRITION PER SERVING

Serving size	4 ounces
Calories	172
Protein	24 g
Carbohydrate*	10 g
(*no added sugars)	
Fiber	2 g
Soluble fiber	1.5 g
Fat	7 g
Saturated fat	1.7 g
Cholesterol	91 mg
Sodium	184 mg
Potassium	314 mg
Calcium	79 mg
Omega-3	
EPA + DHA	199 mg
Bonus:	
Selenium	(53% DV)
Zinc	(20% DV)
Magnesium	(6% DV)

Breading Recipes for Baked "Oven-Fried" Fish

❖ The breading can be made ahead of time and stored in the freezer until needed. Leftover breading can be stored in freezer for next time.

❖ For a low carbohydrate option, use ground nuts instead of bread crumbs.

Parmesan Breading

In shallow bowl or resealable bag combine:

1/4	cup dry, whole-wheat bread crumbs (Page 284) or *Ian's Whole-Wheat Panko Bread Crumbs*
1	tablespoon freshly grated Parmesan cheese
1/2	teaspoon dry parsley
1/8	teaspoon paprika
1/4	teaspoon salt-free lemon pepper (*Penzeys Spices' Sunny Spain*)
1/8	teaspoon each dried oregano and basil

Servings: 1

NUTRITION PER SERVING

Serving size	1 tablespoon breading
Calories	16
Protein	2 g
Carbohydrate*	5 g
(*no added sugars)	
Fiber	0.6 g
Soluble fiber	0 g
Fat	1 g
Saturated fat	0 g
Cholesterol	1 mg
Sodium	17 mg
Potassium	5 mg
Calcium	13 mg
Omega-3	none

Whole-Wheat Graham Cracker Breading

8	squares or 1/2 package of *Midel 100% Whole-Wheat Graham Crackers*
1/4	teaspoon sea salt
1/8	teaspoon salt-free lemon pepper (Penzeys Spices' Sunny Spain)
2	tablespoons chopped pecans (may also use walnuts or almonds)

1. Place all ingredients in a food processor.
2. Pulse until finely ground. Store leftover breading in freezer.

❖ Try other nuts, such as pecan or almonds.

❖ Choose a graham cracker that lists whole-wheat as the first ingredient and does not have any partially hydrogenated fat in ingredients.

Servings: 10

NUTRITION PER SERVING

Serving size	1 tablespoon breading
Calories	62
Protein	1 g
Carbohydrate*	9 g
(*2.5 g sugars from graham cracker)	
Fiber	1 g
Soluble fiber	0.3 g
Fat	2.4 g
Saturated fat	0 g
Cholesterol	0 mg
Sodium	146 mg
Potassium	6 mg
Calcium	1 mg
Omega-3	none

Crispy Baked Fish
With Parmesan Breading

    1   (4-ounce) fish filet per person
    1   tablespoon Parmesan Breading (Page 412) per filet
    1   egg white, whisked with fork

1. Pat fish dry with paper towel.
2. Preheat oven to 425°F.
3. Dip fish in beaten egg white or egg.
4. Dip in breading mixture.
5. Place on baking sheet and spray top of breaded fish with cooking spray.
6. Bake for 10 minutes, turn, and bake 10 to 15 minutes longer.

FISH SUGGESTION

❖   perch, haddock, flounder, catfish, cod, pollock

Servings: 1

NUTRITION PER SERVING

Serving size   3-1/2 ounces
      cooked portion haddock
      with Parmesan breading
Calories   124
Protein   24 g
Carbohydrate*   5 g
(*no added sugars)
Fiber   0.06 g
Soluble fiber   0 g
Fat   2.6 g
Saturated fat   0.8 g
Cholesterol   57 mg
Sodium   76 mg
Potassium   347 mg
Calcium   24 mg
Omega-3
   EPA + DHA   238 mg

Bonus:
Selenium   (53% DV)
Zinc   (20% DV)
Magnesium   (6% DV)

Crispy Baked Fish
With Whole-Wheat Graham Cracker Breading

    1   (4-ounce) fish filet per person
    1   tablespoon Whole-wheat Graham Cracker Breading (Page 412) per filet
    1   egg white, whisked with fork

1. Pat fish dry with paper towel.
2. Preheat oven to 425°F.
3. Dip fish in beaten egg white or egg.
4. Dip in breading mixture.
5. Place on baking sheet and spray top of breaded fish with cooking spray.
6. Bake for 10 minutes, turn, and bake 10 to 15 minutes longer.

Servings: 1

NUTRITION PER SERVING

Serving size   3-1/2 ounces
      cooked portion haddock
      with whole-wheat
      graham breading
Calories   124
Protein   24 g
Carbohydrate*   5 g
(*no added sugars)
Fiber   0.06 g
Soluble fiber   0 g
Fat   2.6 g
Saturated fat   0.8 g
Cholesterol   57 mg
Sodium   76 mg
Potassium   347 mg
Calcium   24 mg
Omega-3
   EPA + DHA   238 mg

Bonus:
Selenium   (53% DV)
Zinc   (20% DV)
Magnesium   (6% DV)

Poached Fish

Poaching refers to the technique of cooking food slowly and gently in a simmering, but not boiling, liquid that covers the fish.

NUTRITION NOTE
Do not use cooking wine. It has salt added.

8 ounces of fish, cut into pieces if desired. (If serving more than 2 people or you want leftovers, increase the number of ounces of fish.)
1 cup dry white wine
6 sprigs fresh parsley
1 small onion, sliced
1 carrot, sliced
1 stalk celery, sliced
2 bay leaves
   juice of half lemon
   reduced-sodium broth or water as needed

1. Place fish in covered sauté or skillet/fry pan. Add remaining ingredients and enough broth to cover fish.
2. Take out fish and bring the ingredients to a boil, then adjust heat to a simmer.
3. Add fish back and gently simmer for 5 minutes; take off heat and let stand, covered, for 10 minutes. This is only a guideline; check, with a knife at the thickest part, to see if it separates and is flaky.
4. Let stand longer if more cooking time is required. (At the proper doneness, finfish is flaky, and seafood is white in the center rather than translucent.)
5. Remove the fish with a slotted spoon. Place fish on plate and keep warm.
6. Boil the ingredients in the pan rapidly, uncovered, until reduced by half.
7. Spoon reduced liquid or sauce over fish, if desired.
8. If desired, make sauce (Page 415).

Fish to Poach:

Poached leftover fish can be used cold on a salad or in any way you would use canned fish. Poaching works well for salmon, cod, catfish, lobster, halibut, perch, sea bass, scallops, shrimp, etc.

Servings: 2

NUTRITION PER SERVING

Serving size	3-1/2 ounces wild sockeye salmon
Calories	216
Protein	27 g
Carbohydrate*	0 g
(*no added sugars)	
Fiber	0 g
Soluble fiber	0 g
Fat	14 g
Saturated fat	1.9 g
Cholesterol	87 mg
Sodium	66 mg
Potassium	555 mg
Calcium	14 mg
Omega-3 EPA +DHA	1,620 mg
Bonus:	
Selenium	(59% DV)
Copper	(14% DV)
Zinc	(11% DV)
Magnesium	(9% DV)
Vitamin D	(687 IU)

Sauces For Poached Fish

Cucumber Sauce

1	cucumber
1	clove garlic
2	teaspoon lemon juice (fresh)
1/4	teaspoon dry dill weed
1/4	teaspoon sea salt and few grinds pepper to taste
1/2	cup Greek yogurt or use plain, low-fat yogurt, drained (see Page 288 for yogurt cheese)

1. Peel, remove and discard seeds from cucumber. Place in a food processor with garlic and puree. Add lemon juice, dill, salt and pepper and pulse several times in processor.
2. Place in dish and stir in yogurt. Chill several hours before serving.

Servings: 8

NUTRITION PER SERVING

Serving size	2 tablespoons
Calories	11
Protein	1 g
Carbohydrate*	1 g
(*no added sugars)	
Fiber	0 g
Soluble fiber	0 g
Fat	0.5 g
Saturated fat	0 g
Cholesterol	1 mg
Sodium	84 mg
Potassium	50 mg
Calcium	30 mg
Omega-3	none

Lemon Herb Sauce

1/3	cup light mayonnaise (see Page 285)
1/3	cup reduced-sodium chicken broth (or the reduced liquid from poaching fish)
1	tablespoon Dijon mustard
1	tablespoon extra-virgin olive oil
1	tablespoon fresh lemon juice
4	teaspoons chopped fresh flat-leaf parsley
2	teaspoons chopped fresh tarragon (leaves not stems) or 1/2 teaspoon dry
2	teaspoons chopped fresh chives
1/16	teaspoon fresh ground black pepper or to taste.

1. Place mayonnaise in small saucepan, gradually add broth, whisking until smooth. Heat over medium to low heat until warm but not bubbling.
2. Remove from heat, stir in mustard, oil, lemon juice and herbs. Serve over fish.

Servings: 13

NUTRITION PER SERVING

Serving size	1 tablespoon
Calories	32
Protein	0 g
Carbohydrate*	1 g
(*no added sugars)	
Fiber	0 g
Soluble fiber	0 g
Fat	3 g
Saturated fat	0.1 g
Cholesterol	2 mg
Sodium	104 mg
Potassium	8 mg
Calcium	3 mg
Omega-3 ALA	203 mg

Sun-Dried Tomato Basil Sauce

1/2	cup water
1/2	cup sun-dried tomatoes
1	teaspoon olive oil
1	medium onion, finely chopped
1	teaspoon garlic, crushed
1	(14-ounce) can diced tomatoes, no-salt-added preferred
1/4	teaspoon fennel seed (grind in mortar and pestle)
1/2	cup packed fresh basil leaves, snipped or chopped
1/8	teaspoon fresh ground black pepper

1. Pour 1/2 cup boiling water over sun-dried tomatoes. (If tomatoes are soft, skip this step.) Let stand 5 minutes, then chop into pieces, saving the liquid.
2. In small sauté pan, sauté onion in 1 teaspoon oil on low heat about 5 minutes. Add garlic, diced tomatoes, sun-dried tomatoes, reserved liquid from sun-dried tomatoes, and fennel.
3. Bring to boil and reduce heat, simmer <u>uncovered</u> for 20 minutes until thickened. Stir in basil and black pepper. Serve over fish.

Servings: 5

NUTRITION PER SERVING

Serving size	1/2 cup
Calories	51
Protein	2 g
Carbohydrate*	8 g
(*no added sugars)	
Fiber	2.5 g
Soluble fiber	0.3 g
Fat	1 g
Saturated fat	0 g
Cholesterol	0 mg
Sodium	136 mg
Potassium	243 mg
Calcium	31 mg
Omega-3 ALA	10 mg

Basic Grilled Fish

1. Do not rinse fish. Pat fish dry with paper towels.
2. Remove skin before cooking (see Page 409).
3. Marinate or brush with a little oil.
4. Measure at thickest part. Rule of thumb: cook 10 minutes per inch.
5. Heat grill. If outdoor grill, use tongs to rub grates with an oil-soaked paper towel.
6. If using basket for delicate fish such as flounder, trout, tilapia and catfish, spray basket with nonstick spray.
7. Lay fish presentation side down (side that did not have skin) toward the heat. The side that had skin removed will be away from the heat. Do not attempt to move the fish until it is ready to flip to the other side. Moving the fish too soon will cause it to stick and tear.
8. When ready to turn fish, use a long-tined fork to lift the fish from between the grates as you slide a spatula under. This helps keep the spatula from tearing the fish.
9. Using spatula, roll fish over onto an open space on the grill and finish cooking.

NOTE: An indoor grill with grates on both sides usually cooks twice as fast as broiling or outdoor grilling since heat is on both sides. However, because heat is not as hot, less browning occurs. There is no need for turning the fish when using this type of grill.

Grilled Salmon with Honey Mustard Dijon Sauce

1	tablespoon honey
1	tablespoon Dijon mustard
2	teaspoons balsamic vinegar
	few grinds fresh ground pepper
1/4	teaspoon garlic powder or 1 clove crushed
8	ounces wild sockeye salmon

1. Combine all ingredients, except salmon, in a small bowl or pan and set aside. This will be used to brush on fish a few minutes before grilling is done. Heat sauce before using.
2. Follow directions for Basic Grilled Fish (see above).
3. Cook fish a few minutes less than suggested time. Spread a thin layer of warm sauce over fish, and turn the sauced side toward the heat to finish grilling and allow it to caramelize. If sauce is added too soon, it may burn before the fish is done. Serve immediately.

MEAL SUGGESTION

❖ Serve salmon over a bed of mixed greens that have been tossed with Raspberry Vinaigrette (Page 371) and top with fresh raspberries.
❖ Substitute catfish, cod, halibut, sablefish, tilapia.

Servings: 2

NUTRITION PER SERVING

Serving size	4 ounces
Calories	208
Protein	23 g
Carbohydrate*	11 g
(*8 1/2 g sugars from honey)	
Fiber	0 g
Soluble fiber	0 g
Fat	8 g
Saturated fat	1 g
Cholesterol	62 mg
Sodium	241 mg
Potassium	579 mg
Calcium	26 mg
Omega-3 EPA + DHA	1,620 mg

Bonus:	
Selenium	(59% DV)
Copper	(15% DV)
Zinc	(11% DV)
Magnesium	(9% DV)
Vitamin D	(687 IU)

Fish - Smart 4 Your Heart

Ginger Soy Grilled Salmon

Use this sauce to serve on any grilled fish for an Oriental flavor.

Sauce: combine in small jar, leftover stores well in refrigerator

2	tablespoons reduced-sodium tamari or soy sauce (see Page 286)
2	tablespoons rice vinegar
2	tablespoons water
1	teaspoon sugar, honey or maple syrup
1	teaspoon grated fresh ginger
3/4	teaspoon toasted sesame oil
1/4	teaspoon red pepper flakes

. . . .

1-1/2   pound wild sockeye salmon or another fish

1. Combine all sauce ingredients, and microwave for a few seconds until sweetener dissolves and sauce is warm.
2. Heat grill. If outdoor grill, use tongs to rub grates with an oil-soaked paper towel.
3. Lay salmon presentation side down (side that did not have skin) toward the heat. The side that had skin removed will be away from the heat. Do not attempt to move the fish until it is ready to flip to the other side. Moving the fish too soon will cause it to stick and tear. Turn after cooking 4 or 5 minutes.
4. When ready to turn salmon, use a long-tined fork to lift the fish from between the grates as you slide a spatula under. This helps keep the spatula from tearing the fish.
5. Using spatula, roll salmon over onto an open space on the grill and finish cooking. Fish is done when there is a small amount of dark pink in the center. It will continue to cook while standing off the heat.
6. Spoon sauce over salmon before serving.

VARIATIONS

❖ Substitute trout, shrimp, catfish, halibut, barramundi

Servings: 6

NUTRITION PER SERVING

Serving size 1 tablespoon
           marinade only

Calories	11
Protein	0 g
Carbohydrate*	1 g
(*0.6 g added sugars)	
Fiber	0 g
Fat	1 g
Saturated fat	0 g
Cholesterol	0 mg
Sodium	152 mg
Potassium	9 mg

NUTRITION PER SERVING

Serving size   3-1/2 ounce
       portion salmon with
       1 tablespoon ginger
       soy marinade

Calories	227
Protein	27 g
Carbohydrate*	1 g
(*0.6 g added sugars)	
Fiber	0 g
Soluble fiber	0 g
Fat	12 g
Saturated fat	1.9 g
Cholesterol	87 mg
Sodium	218 mg
Potassium	555 mg
Calcium	19 mg
Omega-3	
EPA + DHA	1,620 mg

Bonus:	
Selenium	(59% DV)
Copper	(14% DV)
Zinc	(11% DV)
Magnesium	(9% DV)
Vitamin D	(687 IU)

Simply Seasoned Grilled Salmon

| 8 | ounces wild sockeye salmon, skin removed |

Combine the following in a small bowl to make seasoning mixture:

2	tablespoons extra-virgin olive oil
1-1/2	teaspoons lemon pepper (Penzeys Spices' Sunny Spain which is salt free, or another similar brand)
1	teaspoon dill weed
3/4	teaspoon fennel seed, ground in spice grinder
1/4	teaspoon sea salt

1. Wipe salmon with paper towel. Spread seasoning mixture on both sides of salmon. If using an 8-ounce piece, you will have leftover seasoning that you can store refrigerated.
2. Cover and refrigerate salmon 30 minutes to 2 hours.
3. Heat grill. If outdoor grill, use tongs to rub grates with an oil-soaked paper towel.
4. Lay salmon presentation side down (side that did not have skin) toward the heat. The side that had skin removed will be away from the heat. Do not attempt to move the fish until it is ready to flip to the other side. Moving the fish too soon will cause it to stick and tear. Turn after 4 or 5 minutes.
5. When ready to turn salmon, use a long-tined fork to lift the fish from between the grates as you slide a spatula under. This helps keep the spatula from tearing the fish.
6. Using spatula, roll salmon over onto an open space on the grill and finish cooking. Fish is done when there is a small amount of dark pink in the center. It will continue to cook while standing off the heat.

VARIATIONS
❖ Bake at 350°F for about 10 to 15 minutes.
❖ Substitute catfish, cod, halibut, trout, tilapia

NOTE: *If using seasoning on another fish the nutrition data with be different. In the seasoning alone, 1-1/2 teaspoons has 25 calories, 3 g fat, 0.4 g saturated fat, and 116 mg sodium.*

Servings: 2

NUTRITION PER SERVING

Serving size   4 ounce
  piece with 1-1/2
  teaspoon of mixture

Calories	241
Protein	27 g
Carbohydrate*	0 g
(*no added sugars)	
Fiber	0 g
Soluble fiber	0 g
Fat	14 g
Saturated fat	1.9 g
Cholesterol	87 mg
Sodium	184 mg
Potassium	555 mg
Calcium	20 mg
Omega-3	
EPA + DHA	1,620 mg

Bonus:
Selenium	(59% DV)
Copper	(14% DV)
Zinc	(11% DV)
Magnesium	(9% DV)
Vitamin D	(687 IU)

Fish - Smart 4 Your Heart

Pecan-Stuffed Salmon Filet

2	teaspoons organic extra-virgin olive oil
1/4	cup minced red onion
1	clove garlic, minced
3	cups fresh spinach or kale, chopped, or 1 cup frozen cut-leaf spinach, thawed
1/2	cup fresh basil, chopped
1/4	teaspoon sea salt
1/4	teaspoon black pepper

. . . .

2	teaspoons lemon zest
1/4	cup sun-dried tomatoes, diced
1/2	cup pecans, toasted and chopped

. . . .

2	pounds filet of wild sockeye salmon, skin removed

. . . .

1/4	cup reduced-fat cheddar, shredded

1. Preheat oven to 375°F.
2. In large skillet over medium heat, sauté onion in oil until tender but not browned, about 5 minutes. Stir in garlic, spinach, basil, salt and pepper and cook until spinach starts to wilt, about 3 minutes. If using frozen spinach, cook 1 minute. Remove from heat. Stir in lemon zest, sun-dried tomatoes and pecans.
3. After removing skin, cut salmon lengthwise into two thin pieces. Lift off the top piece. Spread spinach mixture evenly over bottom half of salmon and sprinkle with cheese. Lay top half of salmon on top of spinach mixture.
4. Place salmon on a foil or parchment-lined, rimmed baking sheet, and bake about 25 minutes until fish reaches 130°F. (check it after 20 minutes to avoid overcooking). It should be slightly dark pink in the center when you check. It will finish cooking while standing.
5. Transfer fish to a warm platter, cover with foil, and let rest 10 minutes. Cut into serving pieces with an electric knife or sharp, serrated knife.

Servings: 8

NUTRITION PER SERVING

Serving size	4 ounces
Calories	245
Protein	25 g
Carbohydrate*	3 g
(*no added sugars)	
Fiber	1 g
Soluble fiber	0.3 g
Fat	14 g
Saturated fat	2 g
Cholesterol	64 mg
Sodium	290 mg
Potassium	723 mg
Calcium	72 mg
Omega-3	
EPA + DHA	1,620 mg
Bonus:	
Selenium	(61% DV)
Copper	(23% DV)
Vitamin D	(687 IU)
Vitamin K	(50 mcg)

Creamy Lemon Salmon Over Multi-Grains

HELPFUL HINT
May use tuna, shrimp or leftover poached fish.

2	cups cooked Multi-Grain Mix (Page 327) or any other cooked grain, such as brown rice, oat groats, rye or barley

2	tablespoons fresh parsley, minced (or 2 teaspoon dry)
1	carrot, shredded
1/4	cup sun-dried tomatoes, diced
1	cup frozen peas
1/2	cup reduced-sodium chicken or vegetable broth

1	lemon, zested and 3 tablespoons fresh lemon juice (adjust to your preference)
1	(12.3-ounce) box silken tofu (*Organic Silken Mori-Nu*)
1/8	teaspoon salt-free lemon pepper (*Penzeys Spices' Sunny Spain*)

1	(6-ounce) can or pouch, wild salmon

1. Cook grain or rice to serve with recipe.
2. Mince parsley.
3. Peel and shred carrot using large holes of a box grater.
4. If sun-dried tomatoes are not soft, cover with boiling water to soften. Dice tomatoes.
5. Set aside a little of the parsley, carrot and tomato for topping the finished dish.
6. Wash lemon, remove peel using a zester, then squeeze out juice.
7. Drain salmon if canned and remove bones and skin. Pouch-type does not require draining. Break into pieces. If using shrimp, cut into pieces if large.

8. When ready to prepare place carrot, sundried tomatoes, peas and broth in glass bowl, and microwave 2 minutes or cook on stove top.
9. Place tofu, lemon peel and juice, and lemon pepper in blender or food processor, and blend until smooth and creamy. Taste and add more lemon juice if desired. Add to carrot mixture, along with parsley and salmon. Stir and heat for a minute until desired serving temperature.
10. Serve over brown rice or any other cooked grain, such as millet, quinoa or pasta. Garnish with reserved parsley mixture and serve.

FOR BROTH USE: *1/4 teaspoon Organic Better Than Bouillon Base plus 1/2 cup water.*

May use cooked, green soybeans for peas or canned and drained beans, such as black beans or aduki, etc.

May substitute half of a diced red, yellow or green bell pepper, for the sun-dried tomatoes.

Servings: 4

NUTRITION PER SERVING

Serving size	3/4 cup sauce + 1/2 cup rice
Calories	240
Protein	19 g
Carbohydrate*	32 g
(*no added sugars)	
Fiber	4 g
Soluble fiber	0.5 g
Fat	4.5 g
Saturated fat	1 g
Cholesterol	25 mg
Sodium*	430 mg
(*230 mg if no-salt-added canned salmon)	
Potassium	364 mg
Calcium	122 mg
Omega-3	
EPA + DHA	740 mg
Bonus:	
Selenium	(81% DV)
Iron	(17% DV)

Seafood Stew

2   teaspoons olive oil
1   medium onion
2   garlic cloves, chopped
2   stalks celery, sliced
1   small green pepper, cut into small cubes

1   (28-ounce) can *Muir Glen Fire-Roasted Crushed Tomatoes*
3   cups water
2   medium Yukon Gold or red potatoes
1   cup frozen mixed vegetables
1   teaspoon fennel, grind seed for more flavor

1   pound halibut or other firm fish cut into 2-inch pieces
1/2   pound small, peeled shrimp (cut into pieces if larger)
1/3   cup fresh flat-leaf parsley, chopped
    black pepper, to taste

HELPFUL HINT
Use halibut, catfish, perch or tilapia.

1. Prepare vegetables. Peel and cut onion into thin wedges; chop garlic; slice celery; and cube bell pepper after removing stem, seeds and membrane.
2. Scrub potatoes and cut into 2-inch chunks.
3. Measure frozen vegetables.
4. Grind fennel in mortar and pestle.
5. Cut fish and shrimp into pieces.
6. Over medium heat, sauté onion, garlic, celery and green pepper in oil until softened.
7. Add tomatoes, water, potatoes, vegetables and fennel; bring to a boil. Simmer 10 minutes.
8. Add fish and shrimp and simmer 10 minutes or until fish is done.
9. Chop parsley and add to stew, along with black pepper to taste, and serve.

Servings: 10

NUTRITION PER SERVING

Serving size	1 cup
Calories	184
Protein	13 g
Carbohydrate*	15 g
(*no added sugars)	
Fiber	2.5 g
Soluble fiber	0.86 g
Fat	8 g
Saturated fat	1.5 g
Cholesterol	55 mg
Sodium	315 mg
Potassium	454 mg
Calcium	45 mg
Omega-3	
EPA + DHA	530 mg
Bonus:	
Vitamin C	(66% DV)
Selenium	(36% DV)
Vitamin A	(27% DV)
Vitamin D	(74 IU)

Tartar Sauce

1/2   cup light mayonnaise (see Page 285)
2   tablespoons dill pickle relish or chopped dill pickle
1/8   teaspoon onion powder
1/2   teaspoon lemon juice

1. In small bowl, combine all ingredients.
2. Cover; refrigerate at least 30 minutes. Serve with fish.

Salsamole

This is a great topping to serve with fish, chicken or tofu.

1/4   cup finely chopped red onion
1   clove garlic
1/2   jalapeno (more or less to taste)
1   mango or 1 cup pineapple
3   Roma tomatoes
1/4   cup cilantro or flat-leaf parsley, chopped
1   tablespoon cider vinegar
1   tablespoon fresh lime juice
1/8   teaspoon sea salt
1/8   teaspoon ground cumin
1/2   ripe avocado

1. Peel and chop onion and garlic. Finely mince jalapeno after removing seeds and membranes. Dice mango and tomatoes into small cubes. Chop cilantro. Place each in a bowl as you prepare them.
2. Add vinegar, lime juice, salt and cumin to bowl and stir. Chill until ready to serve.
3. When ready to serve, mash avocado with a fork and stir into bowl.

A good snack is one that provides long-lasting energy. Many of the foods we choose for a snack, such as fruit drinks, candy bars, pretzels, crackers and granola bars, are high in refined carbohydrates, which provide a quick burst of energy that quickly disappears when our blood sugars drop. The best snacks are foods that are not processed and packaged with a long list of ingredients. Including some protein and good fat such as that found in raw nuts or hummus, prevents the quick rise and fall of blood sugars. The best choice includes vegetables, since most Americans don't get enough of them and snacking is a great way to get more. A few more ideas are:

ANYTIME SNACKS

NUTRITION NOTE
For snacks the best choice includes vegetables.

❖ Raw vegetables with Rosemary-Roasted Red Pepper and Bean Dip (Page 430).

❖ Frozen or leftover cooked vegetables, such as whole green beans and asparagus spears. These are great to eat cold. If frozen thaw them.

❖ Cucumber slices topped with Cottage Cheese Spread (Page 339).

❖ Vegetables with Spinach Dip (Page 431).

❖ Broccoli stumps: Peel the tough skin from broccoli stems and then dip into creamy almond butter.

❖ Sugar snap peas or snow peas.

❖ Arugula leaves or baby spinach, topped with pickled beets that have been cut into strips. Top with 1 tablespoon crumbled feta cheese (go easy – high sodium).

❖ Edamame in the pods. Cook these immature green soybeans, and use your teeth to get the beans. Discard the pod. These may be available already cooked in the frozen foods section.

❖ 1/4 avocado, sliced and arranged on lettuce leaf with sliced, roasted beets.

❖ Hummus (Page 428) with baby carrots, celery or zucchini sticks, jicama, or other veggies.

❖ Hummus spread on large lettuce leaf and rolled up.

❖ Hummus on cucumber or daikon slices.

1/4 cup raw almonds	1/4 cup of cashews roasted in oil
137 calories	187 calories
11 grams fat	15 g fat
<1 g saturated fat	3 g saturated fat
2.7 g fiber	1 g fiber

SOMETIME SNACK

- ❖ Raw nuts or dry roasted instead of nuts roasted in oil.

- ❖ Small piece of fresh fruit.

- ❖ Heart Fuel Nutty Snack Mix (Page 427).

- ❖ 1 ounce part-skim Swiss cheese or *Cabot 75% Reduced-Fat Cheddar Cheese* and 15 grapes.

- ❖ 1 part-skim mozzarella string cheese stick.

- ❖ Boiled or steamed shrimp. Dip into mixture of 2 tablespoons organic ketchup and 1/2 tablespoon horseradish.

- ❖ Thinly sliced smoked salmon (lox) or turkey slice, wrapped around a piece of cooked asparagus and a roasted red bell pepper strip. Add mustard or horseradish if you like before rolling. Then cut the rolls crosswise to form bite-size pieces.

- ❖ 1 ounce leftover cooked fish or chicken.

- ❖ 1 hard-cooked/boiled egg (omega-3 enriched).

- ❖ Baked, seasoned tofu, purchased ready-to-eat.

- ❖ Lemon-Baked Tempeh (Page 397).

- ❖ Cottage cheese (1%, no-salt-added preferred). Sprinkle with lemon pepper, and top with a teaspoon of sunflower seeds.

- ❖ Cottage cheese (1% no-salt-added), topped with thawed or fresh mixed berries, blueberries or crushed pineapple. You won't miss the salt with the added flavors of the fruit.

- ❖ Sandwich Spread (Page 341) on toasted flourless, sprouted bread

- ❖ Yogurt (plain, low-fat), topped with thawed mixed berries and Chocolate Sauce (Page 437).

VEGETABLES TO
SNACK ON ANYTIME
Asparagus spears,
  cooked
Baby carrots
Beets, roasted
Broccoli florets
Broccolini
Cauliflower florets
Celery
Cherry or grape
  tomatoes
Cucumber slices
Daikon
Edamame
Green beans, whole
  cooked
Green bell peppers
Jicama
Kohlrabi
Mushrooms
Orange bell peppers
Pea pods
Purple bell peppers
Radishes
Red bell peppers
Roasted root
  vegetables
Yellow bell peppers
Zucchini strips

See Page 435
for yogurt
information.

Snacks - Smart 4 Your Heart

- ❖ Smoothie (Pages 304 to 306).

- ❖ Lettuce leaves topped with thinly sliced Asian pear topped and 1 tablespoon crumbled blue cheese.

- ❖ Apples with Pumpkin Dip (Page 431).

- ❖ Apples with nut butter, such as almond, sunflower or natural peanut butter.

- ❖ Frozen grapes, with a couple of unsalted nuts.

- ❖ Apricot bites: Dried apricots with a bit of Greek-style yogurt or Yogurt Cheese (Page 317) or fat-free cream cheese topped with chopped pistachio nuts.

- ❖ 3 cups of popcorn popped in canola oil, sprinkled with a teaspoon of Parmesan cheese or nutritional yeast.

- ❖ A piece of dark chocolate (30 calories). Put it on your tongue and hold it in your mouth until it melts. Resist the temptation to chew, as it will be gone quickly.

- ❖ Apricot dipped in chocolate. Melt dark chocolate and dip one end into chocolate. Let cool until set on waxed paper.

FEWER TIMES SNACK

- ❖ Whole-Wheat Veggie Wrap (Page 343).

- ❖ Quesadilla made with a low-carb or sprouted-grain tortilla and low-fat cheese.

- ❖ *Nairn's Rough Oat Cakes* spread with light cream cheese and thinly sliced radishes, cucumber or jicama. Use a mandolin to slice thinly.

- ❖ *Nairn's Rough Oat Cakes* spread with Greek yogurt or drained yogurt cheese, drizzle of honey and sprinkle of cinnamon.

- ❖ Amaranth graham crackers spread with Greek yogurt or fat-free cream cheese and topped with a drizzle of chocolate sauce.

- ❖ Granola bar that does not include any high fructose corn syrup and has protein or good fat. Make your own with the recipe on Page 426.

Granola Bars

In bowl, combine the following:

4	cups *Kashi 7 Whole Grain Puffs 0g Sugar* or brown rice crisps
1/4	cup chopped walnuts
1/4	cup raw pumpkin seeds
1/4	cup sliced or slivered almonds
1/4	cup raw, unsalted sunflower seeds
1/4	cup ground flaxseed (milled flaxseed or flax meal)
1/4	cup oat bran
1/2	cup whey protein powder (chocolate or vanilla) or soy protein powder

In small sauce pan, combine:

1/3	cup almond butter or natural peanut butter
1/3	cup honey
1/3	cup maple syrup or brown rice syrup
1	teaspoon coconut extract (almond or orange extract work well)

1. Preheat oven 350° F. Place foil or parchment paper in a 9 X 13-inch pan. The bars need to be lifted out for cutting and this will help get them out.
2. Place all dry ingredients in bowl.
3. Bring the mixture in the sauce pan to a boil over medium heat and boil 2 minutes, stirring. Pour over dry ingredients in bowl, mix, then dump into the prepared pan.
4. Press mixture tightly into pan. A small pizza roller works well for this, but you can also use a piece of waxed paper and press with a spoon until firm. If mixture is too loose, it will crumble when you cut it.
5. Bake 15 minutes or until the top is golden. Cool in pan and then remove from pan by pulling up on paper. Turn bars over and remove foil or parchment.
6. Use a long, very sharp serrated knife to cut into 24 pieces. Wrap each in wax wrap, or place each in a baggie, and freeze. They will get stale quickly, since there are no added preservatives as in commercial bars. This also helps with eating them in moderate amounts.

HELPFUL HINTS

- Add 1/4 cup mini chocolate chips to dry ingredients, which will melt and give a chocolate flavor.

- If using whole flaxseed, pulse in coffee mill.

- Look for oat bran in the hot cereal section of grocery store.

Servings: 24

NUTRITION PER SERVING

Serving size	2-1/4" X 2" piece
Calories	123
Protein	6 g
Carbohydrate*	13 g
(*6.5 g sugars from honey and maple syrup)	
Fiber	1.8 g
Soluble fiber	0.4 g
Fat	7 g
Saturated fat	0.7 g
Cholesterol	2 mg
Sodium	6 mg
Potassium	87 mg
Calcium	29 mg
Omega-3 ALA	550 mg

Bonus:

Magnesium	(9% DV)
Vitamin E	(7% DV)
Copper	(7% DV)
Zinc	(5% DV)
Iron	(4% DV)

Snacks - Smart 4 Your Heart

Heart Fuel Nutty Snack Mix

Make your own individual heart healthy snack packs. Set out the number of small resealable snack-size baggies you want to make. Using a measuring spoon, start with one of the ingredients, and place some into each bag. Repeat with each ingredient until you have added all the ingredients to the individual bags. Vary the ingredients as you desire. When done, close the bags and store them in the refrigerator or freezer, taking them out as needed. This keeps everything equally divided, portion controlled and fresh.

For 1 baggie	6-1/2 cups	Ingredients
2 tablespoons	1-1/2 cup	*Nature's Path Optimum Power Blueberry Cereal**
1/2 tablespoon	1/2 cup	Slivered almonds
1/2 tablespoon	1/2 cup	Diced, dried California apricots or golden raisins
1 tablespoon	3/4 cup	Raw sunflower seeds
1 tablespoon	3/4 cup	Raw pepita/pumpkin seeds
1/2 tablespoon	1/2 cup	Pistachio or pecans
1/2 tablespoon	1/2 cup	Walnuts or hazelnuts
1 tablespoon	1 cup	Dry-roasted, unsalted soy nuts
1/2 tablespoon	1/2 cup	*Ghiradelli 60% Coacao Baking Chips* or cocoa nibs

*OTHER CEREALS
❖ Choose those that have large pieces – Kashi's U, *Back to Nature's Heart Basics, Optimum Slim, Health Valley's Organic Oat Bran Flakes, Barbara's Bakery Organic Grain Shop's High Fiber Medley*, or *Nature's Path's Smart Bran*

VARY THE NUTS AND SEEDS
❖ **Pumpkin Seed:** High in magnesium and zinc and a source of omega-3-fats. Pepita, which is the inside heart of the seed, is another name that you may see on these dark green seeds. The ones that are commercially available are from a variety of squash that is grown specifically for its seeds.

❖ **Almonds:** Like all nuts, almonds are high in fat but have nine times more healthy fats than unhealthy fats. They are also the nut that is the richest in vitamin E.

❖ **Walnuts:** Unique among nuts because they have heart healthy omega-3 fats.

❖ **Sunflower Seeds:** Are excellent sources of vitamin E and a good source of cholesterol-lowering phytosterols and magnesium, making them heart protective.

❖ **Pecans:** Are rich in antioxidants and gamma tocopherols, which reduce oxidation of blood lipids. This helps to lower the risk of heart disease.

❖ **Hazelnuts:** For the greatest amount of antioxidants use hazelnuts with the skins intact. There are ten times more antioxidants than without the skins.

Servings: 1 to 13

NUTRITION PER SERVING

Serving size	1/2 cup
Calories	252
Protein	10 g
Carbohydrate*	20 g
(*3.5 g added sugars from cereal and chocolate chips)	
Fiber	4.5 g
Soluble fiber	1.6 g
Fat	18 g
Saturated fat	2.6 g
Cholesterol	0 mg
Sodium	28 mg
Potassium	384 mg
Calcium	71 mg
Omega-3 ALA	460 mg

Bonus:	
Magnesium	(27% DV)
Copper	(25% DV)
Vitamin E	(22% DV)
Iron	(16% DV)
Selenium	(11% DV)
Zinc	(11% DV)

Hummus

HELPFUL HINTS
- For a thinner consistency, add more water.

- Add more or less garlic to taste. Roasted garlic is more mellow.

- The varieties of hummus are endless. Try adding fresh spinach, fresh basil, kalamata olives, sun-dried tomatoes, or jalapeno.

- Vary the spices by using chipotle, Aleppo pepper, dill weed or pesto instead of cumin.

- Try using peanut butter instead of tahini. It's not the true version but still tasty.

- Make with black beans instead of garbanzo beans.

Servings: 16

NUTRITION PER SERVING

Serving size	2 tablespoons
Calories	58
Protein	2 g
Carbohydrate*	6 g
(*no added sugars)	
Fiber	1 g
Soluble fiber	0.3 g
Fat	3 g
Saturated fat	0.4 g
Cholesterol	0 mg
Sodium	44 mg
Potassium	72 mg
Calcium	16 mg
Omega-3 ALA	2 mg

Bonus:
Copper	(269% DV)

1	(15-ounce) can garbanzo beans or chickpeas, drained
1	clove garlic
1/4	cup tahini (sesame seed paste)
2	tablespoons lemon juice
1	tablespoon extra-virgin olive oil
1/4	teaspoon cumin
1/4	teaspoon sea salt
1/4	cup water

1. With food processor running, drop garlic in chute and process until finely chopped. If your processor does not have a chute, place in bowl, cover and process until chopped. Turn off and add remaining ingredients. Process until smooth.
2. Taste and adjust, adding more lemon juice if you want more, or adding water if you want it thinner. It may thicken as it chills and need thinning to get the desired consistency.
3. Refrigerate up to two weeks. Hummus may also be frozen. Thaw in refrigerator overnight to use.

SERVING SUGGESTIONS
❖ Serve with sticks of celery, zucchini, jicama, baby carrots, sliced cucumbers, etc.

HELPFUL HINTS
If you have the time, soak dry chickpeas and cook them because the flavor is fresher. Don't add salt when cooking. They soften better without it.

*The texture will remain somewhat coarse with most food processors. If you have a **Vita-Mix** blender it will blend it into a very smooth consistency. Doubling the recipe provides enough volume to mix well.*

***Tahini** is sesame seed paste and can be found in jars in the ethnic foods section or health food section of the grocery store or a Middle Eastern grocery store. Stir before using. Store in the refrigerator once opened. Try several brands, as they vary in taste from mild to bitter. My favorite is **Ziyad**.*

White Bean Spread

1   (15-ounce) can beans (Northern, navy or cannellini), drained and rinsed
2   tablespoons light mayonnaise (Page 285)
1   tablespoon extra-virgin olive oil
1   clove garlic, minced
1/2   teaspoon lemon zest (outermost portion of the peel, no white pith)
1/8   teaspoon sea salt
1/4   green pepper, minced
1   stalk celery, minced
2   tablespoon finely minced red onion

1. Add beans, mayonnaise, oil, garlic, lemon peel and salt to food processor. Blend until smooth.
2. Mince green pepper, celery and onion. Add to processor and pulse to blend.
3. Thin with water to desired consistency.
4. Serve with cut-up vegetables like celery, carrots, daikon, jicama, broccoli, kohlrabi, pea pods and cauliflower florets.

NUTRITION NOTE
Canola oil in mayonnaise provides omega-3.

Servings: 12

NUTRITION PER SERVING

Serving size	2 tablespoons
Calories	66
Protein	3 g
Carbohydrate*	8 g
(*no added sugars)	
Fiber	3 g
Soluble fiber	0.7 g
Fat	2.5 g
Saturated fat	0.2 g
Cholesterol	0 mg
Sodium	95 mg
Potassium	159 mg
Calcium	26 mg
Omega-3 ALA	125 mg

Green Soybean Guacamole

1   bag (2 cups) shelled green soybeans also called edamame/sweet beans
2   cloves garlic, peeled
1   avocado
2   tablespoons lime juice
1/4   teaspoon sea salt
2   tablespoons light mayonnaise (Page 285)
2   tablespoons fat-free or reduced-fat sour cream
2   tablespoons water or more as needed

1. Cook soybeans according to package directions or microwave with 1 tablespoon water about 4 minutes. Let cool 10 minutes.
2. In food processor, chop garlic and edamame, then add all other ingredients and blend until smooth. Add a little more water if needed.
3. Optional: 1/4 cup fresh cilantro (leaves only) or parsley (leaves and stems). Nice, but not necessary!

Cilantro looks like parsley and is found in the produce section.
Look for edamame in the frozen foods section of grocery and natural food stores.

HELPFUL HINT
May use frozen green peas instead of green soybeans.

Servings: 16

NUTRITION PER SERVING

Serving size	2 tablespoons
Calories	54
Protein	2 g
Carbohydrate*	4 g
(*no added sugars)	
Fiber	1.5 g
Soluble fiber	0.83 g
Fat	3.5 g
Saturated fat	0.4 g
Cholesterol	1 mg
Sodium	57 mg
Potassium	175 mg
Calcium	27 mg
Omega-3 ALA	182 mg

Rosemary-Roasted Red Pepper and Bean Dip

Servings: 12

NUTRITION PER SERVING

Serving size	2 tablespoons
Calories	44
Protein	2 g
Carbohydrate*	7 g
(*no added sugars)	
Fiber	2 g
Soluble fiber	0.63 g
Fat	1 g
Saturated fat	0 g
Cholesterol	0 mg
Sodium	52 mg
Potassium	86 mg
Calcium	26 mg
Omega-3 ALA	10 mg

Bonus:

Vitamin C	(17% DV)
Beta-carotene	(14% DV)
Iron	(5% DV)
Zinc	(2% DV)

1	medium red bell pepper, roasted*
2	cloves garlic, minced
1	(15-ounce) can navy or Northern beans, no-salt-added preferred, drained and rinsed
1	teaspoon dry, cracked rosemary
1	tablespoon fresh lemon juice
2	teaspoons extra-virgin olive oil
1/4	teaspoon sea salt (optional)
1/8	teaspoon freshly ground black pepper

1. See Page 355 (in vegetable section) for roasting instructions for bell pepper.
2. Drop garlic in food processor with motor running. When minced, turn off and add all other ingredients. Puree until smooth.
3. Chill and refrigerate until ready to serve.

May use 6-ounce jar of purchased roasted red bell peppers, drained. Canned have added salt, so sodium increases to 112 mg per 2 tablespoons.

VARIATION – BROCCOLI BEAN DIP

❖ Replace roasted bell pepper with 2 cups (5 ounces) frozen, broccoli florets that have been thawed, 1/4 cup fresh flat-leaf parsley instead of rosemary, and add 1/4 teaspoon dry dill weed and water as needed to thin to desired consistency.

Garden Herbed Dip

NUTRITION NOTES
Parsley and basil provide vitamin C.

Servings: 8

NUTRITION PER SERVING

Serving size	2 tablespoons
Calories	55
Protein	5 g
Carbohydrate*	2 g
(*no added sugars)	
Fiber	0.3 g
Soluble fiber	0.2 g
Fat	3.3 g
Saturated fat	1.7 g
Cholesterol	10 mg
Sodium	157 mg
Potassium	106 mg
Calcium	33 mg
Omega-3 ALA	93 mg

Bonus:

Beta-carotene	(12% DV)
Vitamin C	(11% DV)

1	(12.3-ounce) box silken tofu (*Organic Silken Mori-Nu*)
1	garlic clove
1/2	cup (or 4 ounces) reduced-fat cream cheese
1/2	cup fresh parsley, (flat-leaf preferred)
1/2	teaspoon dry dill weed
1/3	cup snipped chives
1/3	cup fresh basil, chopped
1	teaspoon fresh lemon juice
1/2	teaspoon sea salt
	freshly ground pepper

1. Place a coffee filter or cheesecloth into a mesh strainer set on a bowl. Mash tofu with a fork, and place into a mesh strainer, refrigerating at least one hour to allow it to drain. This will remove some of the liquid, making the dip thicker.
2. With food processor running, drop in garlic. When chopped, add tofu and cream cheese and blend until very smooth.
3. Add remaining ingredients and blend well.
4. Chill 2 hours to blend flavors. Best if it can stand 8 hours.
5. Serve with raw veggies.

Spinach Dip

1/4	cup red bell pepper, chopped
1	clove garlic, crushed, or 1/2 teaspoon garlic powder
2	tablespoons finely chopped or grated onion or 1/2 teaspoon onion powder
1	(10-ounce) package frozen chopped spinach, thawed and well-drained
1-1/2	cups light mayonnaise (3 grams of fat per tablespoon)
1	cup light or reduced-fat sour cream (2.5 grams of fat per tablespoon)
1/2	package dry vegetable soup mix, such as *Fantastic Soup and Dip Recipe Mix*
1/8	teaspoon liquid hot pepper seasoning (optional)

1. Chop bell pepper, garlic and onion finely; add to bowl.
2. Press spinach against the sides of a mesh strainer to remove liquid. Place on cutting board and chop; add to bowl.
3. Add all remaining ingredients into bowl. Mix until well blended.
4. Cover and chill until serving time.
5. Serve as a dip with raw vegetables.

NOTES
If you use regular mayonnaise and regular sour cream dip has 208 calories, 21 g fat, 2.7 g saturated fat, 222 mg sodium, and 2.8 g carbohydrate.

If you use fat-free mayonnaise, dip has 42 calories, 0 g fat, 317 mg sodium, 8.5 g carbohydrate, and no omega-3 or vitamin E since they come from oil.

May substitute sun-dried tomato for bell pepper.
Organic spinach is preferred.

HELPFUL HINT
Divide the dry soup mix on a plate to get an equal amount of veggies and granular mixture.

Servings: 14

NUTRITION PER SERVING

Serving size	2 tablespoons
Calories	54
Protein	2 g
Carbohydrate*	4 g
(*no added sugars)	
Fiber	1.5 g
Soluble fiber	0.83 g
Fat	3.5 g
Saturated fat	0.4 g
Cholesterol	1 mg
Sodium	57 mg
Potassium	175 mg
Calcium	27 mg
Omega-3 ALA	182 mg

Pumpkin Dip

1/3	cup Greek-style yogurt (nonfat)
2	ounces light cream cheese (about 1/4 cup)
1/2	cup mashed butternut squash or canned pumpkin
1/2	teaspoon pumpkin pie spice
1	package stevia herbal sweetener or few drops liquid stevia

1. Combine all mixing until smooth.
2. Serve with apple or pear slices.

HELPFUL HINT
• Add maple flavoring.
• Serve with sliced apples.

Servings: 8

NUTRITION PER SERVING

Serving Size	2 tablespoons
Calories	28
Protein	1.5 g
Carbohydrate*	2.8 g
(*no added sugars)	
Fiber	0.4 g
Soluble fiber	0.04 g
Fat	1.3 g
Saturated fat	0.8 g
Cholesterol	4 mg
Sodium	29 mg
Potassium	57 mg
Calcium	31 mg
Omega-3 ALA	2 mg

Simple Fresh Salsa

2	cups diced Roma or grape tomatoes
1	clove garlic, minced
1/4	cup finely minced sweet or red onion
1/2	jalapeno pepper, diced (more or less to taste)
1/4	cup cilantro, leaves only, chopped
1	tablespoon lime juice
2	teaspoon extra-virgin olive oil
1/4	teaspoon sea salt

1. Chop ingredients and add to a bowl as you prepare each.
2. Combine all ingredients and allow to rest for 30 minutes.
3. If you prefer a less chunky consistency, pulse mixture in a food processor to desired texture. Be careful not to overprocess.

VARIATIONS
- ❖ Tomato Mango Salsa: Add 2 cups diced mango
- ❖ Avocado Salsa: Add 1 avocado, mashed

HELPFUL HINT
Great as a topping on salads, broiled fish, baked chicken or as a dip with vegetables.

Servings: 4

NUTRITION PER SERVING

Serving size	1/2 cup
Calories	41
Protein	1 g
Carbohydrate*	5 g
(*no added sugars)	
Fiber	1.2 g
Soluble fiber	0.3 g
Fat	2.5 g
Saturated fat	0.3 g
Cholesterol	0 mg
Sodium	149 mg
Potassium	240 mg
Calcium	13 mg
Omega-3 ALA	none

Bonus:
Vitamin K	(9 mcg)
Beta-carotene	(17% DV)
Vitamin C	(23% DV)

Quick Dessert Ideas

Choose fresh fruit for dessert most often. Some quick ideas are:

❖ Freeze washed grapes or cherries; eat them while still frozen.

❖ Cut kiwifruit in half, and use a spoon to scoop out.

❖ In a parfait glass, layer yogurt; Granola (Page 316) or toasted, rolled oats or rolled barley; and cut-up fruit, such as kiwi, mandarin oranges and red grapes or strawberries, blueberries and mango.

❖ Grill some fruit for dessert, such as pieces of pineapple, peaches, plums, pears or mango, until barely softened. Serve topped with cocoa nibs or a few shavings of grated dark chocolate and a sprinkle of unsweetened coconut.

❖ Serve berries for dessert. If frozen, let them thaw slightly in the refrigerator while eating the meal and they will be ready to eat in time for dessert. Drizzle on some Chocolate Sauce (Page 437) if desired.

❖ Mix 1/2 teaspoon each balsamic vinegar and sugar, and toss with a cup of sliced strawberries. Let stand 5 minutes and enjoy.

❖ Mix yogurt cheese (drained yogurt, Page 317) or Greek-style yogurt with some fresh lemon juice and a bit of stevia. Serve a dollop over cut-up fruit.

❖ Pina colada parfait: Place plain, low-fat yogurt in dish. Add a bit of rum or coconut extract and stir. Top with crushed pineapple, mandarin oranges and diced kiwi. Sprinkle with a bit of coconut (toasted in the oven) and a few chopped nuts.

❖ Spread yogurt cheese or almond butter on whole-wheat graham crackers or rough oat cakes, and top with a small dollop of mashed fruit, sliced banana or no-sugar-added jam.

❖ Spread yogurt cheese on toasted raisin and cinnamon sprouted-grain bread and drizzle with a bit of chocolate sauce.

❖ Place 1 cup of blueberries in a microwave-safe dish. Top with 1/3 cup granola, and microwave 3 minutes. Top with dollop of Greek-style yogurt and enjoy.

❖ Cut up mango or any other fruit. Place in footed dish, and sprinkle with 1/2 teaspoon kirshwasser or triple sec (orange flavored liqueur) and a squeeze of lime juice.

Simple Desserts That Look Extra Special

The way you present food can make a difference in how much you enjoy eating it.

❖ Use a dish with a footed stem or a glass with a tall stem, such as a champagne glass.

❖ Drizzle a little chocolate or berry sauce in a zig-zag or "Z" shape on a plate, and arrange fruit attractively on the plate so the sauce still shows.

❖ Make a kabob of fruits on wooden skewers, alternating colors and shapes. Arrange them on a tray or stick them into a grapefruit half, cut side down.

Nutrition Notes For Some Fruits

❖ **Cherries** contain anthocyanins which give them their red color. They have anti-inflammatory properties. Cherries may help lower not only heart attack risk, but also risk of stroke. They are also rich in fiber and potassium. Freeze them when in season to enjoy later.

❖ **Kiwifruit** are rich in vitamin C, having twice as much as an orange, and more potassium than a banana. A medium kiwifruit has only 45 calories and 2 grams of fiber. According to one study, eating two or three kiwifruit a day may lower triglycerides by 15%. Kiwifruit should "give" slightly when pressed rather than being rock hard. Like bananas, they ripen at room temperature. When ripe, store in the refrigerator.

HELPFUL HINT
Freeze pomegranate seeds when in season for use at a laer date.

❖ **Pomegranate** – The high antioxidant content of pomegranates appears to have many health benefits, including healthier arteries. Pomegranates stimulate nitric oxide production, which helps relax and open arteries and reduce blood pressure. These antioxidants are the same ones found in red wine, cranberries, blueberries and other dark purple colored foods that benefit arteries and improve blood flow. A small study from Israel with people who had diabetes found a reduced risk of heart disease when study participants drank 6 ounces of juice daily. The 6 ounces of juice daily did not raise blood glucose levels in this study.

❖ **Organic Fruits** – The Environmental Working Group (www.ewg.org) evaluated 46 fruits and vegetables and produced a list of the 12 fruits and vegetables that are the most contaminated. You may wish to use organic for those that are most likely to be contaminated. See Page 351 for the complete list.

Most Pesticides:
- peaches
- strawberries
- apples
- nectarines
- pears
- cherries
- red raspberries
- imported grapes

Lowest Pesticides:
- bananas
- kiwi
- mangos
- papayas
- pineapple

Yogurt For Dessert

Choose fat-free or low-fat yogurt which has less saturated fat. Try Greek yogurt, such as *FAGE Total 0% Greek Yogurt* or *Oikos*. Greek yogurt has been drained and is thick and creamy with a rich flavor. It is lower in carbohydrates and higher in protein than other yogurts that have not been strained. You can also strain yogurt yourself (see Page 317). If you find the nonfat too tangy, try low-fat which is less tart. *Stonyfield Low-Fat Plain Yogurt* has a slightly less saturated fat than most brands of low-fat yogurt.

❖ **Yogurt Best choice:** Buy plain fat-free or low-fat, yogurt with no sugars, sweeteners, artificial sweeteners or chemicals added! Mix in one of the following if desired.
  - Fruit, such as
    - wild blueberries
    - mashed banana
    - crushed pineapple with coconut extract
    - mashed strawberries
  - A small amount of raw honey, *Wax Orchards' Fruit Sweet,* maple syrup, or brown rice syrup along with chopped nuts.
  - A packet of *True Lemon* or *True Lime* with stevia.
  - Extracts such as vanilla, orange, maple, coconut or almond.
  - Add dry, natural cocoa powder plus one of the sweeteners listed below.
  - Sweetener if desired
    - *Stevia a* no-calorie sweet herb. See page 174 for brands using stevia extracts.
    - Sugar alcohol, such as xylitol. *Zsweet,* or *Organic Zero* made by *Wholesome Sweeteners, that* contains the sugar alcohol erythritol. A teaspoon and a half equals the sweetness of a teaspoon of sugar.
    - Luo han guo (fruit extract), such as *SweetFiber.*

Chocolate / Chocolate Chips

If you want the health benefits of chocolate choose, dark chocolate – not just any "chocolate." Avoid those with partially hydrogenated fats. Watch portion size. You only need 1-ounce chocolate to get health benefits. If you eat more the calories add up quickly.

The type of fat in chocolate is equal parts oleic, stearic and palmitic. Oleic is the heart healthy, monounsaturated fat, also found in olive oil. The other two, stearic and palmitic, are saturated fats. Although stearic is a saturated fat, it does not raise LDL cholesterol. One third of the fat in chocolate is in the form of stearic. That leaves only about one-third of the total fat or half of the saturated fat in chocolate as the type that raises cholesterol.

Dark chocolate has more of the healthy flavanols. The amount depends on how it is processed. The best source of cocoa flavanols is found in pure natural cocoa powder, like the type you use for baking, which is not dutched. If it has been dutched, you will see "cocoa treated with alkali" in the ingredients. This reduces flavanols. Instant hot chocolate is often treated with alkali.

Look for products that state the percentage of cocoa on the label, or the milligrams of antioxidants. Higher is better. Choose brands with 70% or more cocoa, such as *Dagoba, Omanhene 80%, Green and Black's, Scharffen Berger Bittersweet*. More cocoa means less sugars.

The *Mars* company uses the *Cocoapro* logo on some of its products, such as *Dove Dark*. This logo indicates that the cocoa beans have been handled to preserve the polyphenols with potential health benefits.

When checking ingredients, the first ingredient should be chocolate, cocoa beans or chocolate liquor, not sugars. See the example below:

❖ **Good choice:** Chocolate (unsweetened chocolate, sugar, cocoa butter) has less sugar since chocolate is listed before sugar.
❖ **Less desirable:** Chocolate (sugar, chocolate, cocoa butter…)

Although mini morsels are not always available in dark chocolate, the small size allows you to cut the amount in a recipe by half, and the small size allows them to give the illusion of more.

Cocoa nibs are simply roasted cocoa beans separated from their husks and broken into small bits, with a slightly bitter, intense flavor. They can be used in baking or as a snack. They can be found coated in cocoa powder with spices or chocolate covered.

White chocolate and carob have none of the benefits, since they do not contain any cocoa or chocolate liquor.

Chocolate Sauce

1 tablespoon unsweetened, natural cocoa
1 tablespoon *Fruit Sweet* (concentrated fruit juice blend)
1-2 teaspoons water
1/4 teaspoon vanilla

Blend all ingredients together, adding more water to thin if needed.

SERVING SUGGESTIONS
❖ Drizzle over fresh berries or other fruit.
❖ Drizzle over nonfat yogurt, topped with chopped nuts.

Fruit Sweet. Made by Wax Orchards from fruit juice concentrates. Tastes 1-1/2 times sweeter than sugar and twice as sweet as honey, yet contains 1/3 fewer calories than sugar.

TO CONVERT YOUR OWN RECIPES
❖ Substitute 2/3 cup *Fruit Sweet* per cup of sugar in the recipe. Reduce other liquids by 1/3 the amount of sweetener used. The conversion table below is a guideline for substitutions.

Sugar	*Fruit Sweet*	Reduce Liquid By
1 cup	2/3 cup	3-1/2 tablespoons
3/4 cup	1/2 cup	2-1/2 tablespoons plus 1/2 teaspoon
1/2 cup	1/3 cup	2 tablespoons
1/4 cup	2-1/2 tablespoons	1 tablespoon plus 1 teaspoon

Servings: 2

NUTRITION PER SERVING

Serving size   1 tablespoon
Calories   27
Protein   0.5 g
Carbohydrate*   6 g
(*5 g added sugars)
Fiber   1 g
Soluble fiber   0 g
Fat   0.4 g
Saturated fat   0.2 g
Cholesterol   0 mg
Sodium   0.5 mg
Potassium   41 mg
Calcium   3 mg
Omega-3   none

Peach Whip

16 ounces frozen, unsweetened peaches, **do not thaw**
1 (5- to 6-ounce) container *Fage 0%* Greek yogurt, or fat-free vanilla or peach yogurt
2 tablespoons sugar
1 packet stevia herbal sweetener
1 teaspoon vanilla extract
1 tablespoon triple sec or *Cointreau* liqueur (or orange juice)
1/4 teaspoon almond extract

1. Combine all ingredients in a food processor, let stand about 10 to 15 minutes, then blend until smooth and creamy. Do not allow peaches to completely thaw.
2. Serve immediately in four stemmed glasses. This is best eaten immediately after making.

HELPFUL HINT
This is best made in a food processor, since a blender is not able to break up the frozen peaches fast enough, and it will be melted and runny instead of a creamy consistency.

Servings: 4

NUTRITION PER SERVING

Serving size   1/2 cup
Calories   88
Protein   4 g
Carbohydrate*   21 g
(*6 g added sugar)
Fiber   2.2 g
Soluble fiber   1 g
Fat   0 g
Saturated fat   0 g
Cholesterol   0 mg
Sodium   13 mg
Potassium   88 mg
Calcium   56 mg
Omega-3   none

Bonus:
Vitamin C   (19% DV)
Iron   (16% DV)

Berry Sorbet

3/4	cup frozen mixed berries, do not thaw
3	tablespoons pomegranate or blueberry juice

1. Place berries in a small bowl food processor, and let stand about 15 to 20 minutes. Do not allow berries to completely thaw.
2. Add juice and process until consistency of soft-serve ice cream.
3. Serve, as this is best eaten immediately after making.

HELPFUL HINTS

This is best made in a food processor. If not served immediately, mixture will melt and become running instead of having a creamy consistency.

May use 1/4 cup each of blueberries, blackberries and raspberries.

Freeze extra juice for later use if desired. Increase quantities for the number of servings desired. Use a large food processor for larger quantities.

Servings: 1

NUTRITION PER SERVING

Serving size	3/4 cup
Calories	87
Protein	1 g
Carbohydrate*	21 g
(*no added sugars)	
Fiber	4.5 g
Soluble fiber	1 g
Fat	0.6 g
Saturated fat	0 g
Cholesterol	0 mg
Sodium	6 mg
Potassium	74 mg
Calcium	26 mg
Omega-3	7 mg

Bonus:	
Vitamin C	(19% DV)
Copper	(3% DV)
Magnesium	(3% DV)
Vitamin K	(14 mcg)

Silken Chocolate Ginger Dream

A rich, sweet and spicy treat. You don't need much of this to get your chocolate fix.

1   (12.3-ounce) box *Organic Silken Mori-Nu Tofu,* room temperature
2   teaspoons sugar or other desired sweetener
2   packets stevia herbal sweetener
2   tablespoons natural cocoa powder (not dutched)
1   teaspoon vanilla extract
1   teaspoon freshly grated or minced ginger
1/3 cup dark chocolate chips (*Ghirardelli 60% Cacao*) or grain-sweetened
     chocolate chips

1.   Open tofu and pour off the small amount of water. Place in a food processor. Add all the ingredients except chocolate and blend until shiny, smooth and creamy.
2.   Melt chocolate chips by microwaving. Stir after a minute. If not completely melted, heat 20 seconds more and stir again. May also melt chocolate on stove top with a double boiler.
3.   Add melted chocolate to processor and blend. Place 1/4 cup into small paper cups.
4.   Extra portions can be frozen. Thaw overnight in refrigerator.

SERVING SUGGESTIONS
❖   Place in whole-wheat phyllo cups (purchase from health food store or make).
❖   Place in edible, dark chocolate shot glasses.
❖   Crumble whole-wheat graham crackers or *Newman's Tops and Bottoms* to sprinkle over top.
❖   Place a dollop on a bowl of berries and top with a spritz of *Soyatoo Whipped Soy Topping.*

Organic Mori-Nu Silken Tofu may be sold in refrigerated sections of the grocery store. It does not require refrigeration until opened. It is important that tofu is at room temperature for this recipe. If it is cold when the chocolate is added, it will form tiny lumps instead of being smooth.

Servings: 5

NUTRITION PER SERVING

Serving size	1/4 cup
Calories	130
Protein	5 g
Carbohydrate*	14 g
(*1.7 g added sugar plus 5.6 g in chocolate)	
Fiber	1.6 g
Soluble fiber	0.3 g
Fat	7 g
Saturated fat	3 g
Cholesterol	0 mg
Sodium	26 mg
Potassium	137 mg
Calcium	27 mg
Omega-3 ALA	186 mg
Bonus:	
Copper	(7% DV)
Iron	(6% DV)
Magnesium	(5% DV)

Cheesecake

HELPFUL HINTS
- To freeze, cut into serving pieces, set on cookie sheet and freeze. When frozen, wrap and store until needed.

- To thaw, allow to stand overnight in refrigerator.

- Baking in a water bath is what keeps the cheesecake creamy.

Crust:
1/3	cup almonds
1	cup whole-wheat graham cracker crumbs (1/2 box *Healthy Valley Oat Bran*, crushed)
1	tablespoon butter
1	teaspoon walnut oil
1	egg yolk

Filling:
2	cups (1 pound) 1% cottage cheese (no-salt-added preferred)
6	ounces (3/4 cup) nonfat plain yogurt or Greek yogurt
8	ounces reduced-fat cream cheese
8	ounces fat-free cream cheese
1/2	cup sugar
5	packets (1 gram) stevia (*Sweet Leaf*) or 48 drops liquid stevia
2	tablespoons arrowroot (cornstarch may be used)
3	tablespoons fresh lemon juice
1/2	teaspoon grated lemon zest (yellow part only, as white is bitter)
1	teaspoon lemon extract
1	teaspoon vanilla extract
1	egg (omega-3 enriched)
1	egg white

1. Preheat oven to 325°F. The cheesecake must be baked in a water bath. This is a key to the cheesecake being creamy. To do this use a shallow roasting pan that the springform pan will fit inside without touching the outside edges. Line the outside of a 10-inch springform pan with two layers of heavy duty foil to prevent water from seeping in.
2. Make crust by placing all the ingredients in food processor and blending until no chunks of graham cracker remain and all ingredients are blended. Press mixture into the bottom of the foil-lined springform pan. Bake for 10 minutes. Remove and let cool while preparing filling.
3. Heat water for use in roasting pan to boiling.
4. To make filling, scoop cottage cheese and yogurt into a food processor and process. Stop and scrape bowl after about 30 seconds. Continue to process until no lumps remain.
   - Add cream cheese and process until smooth.
   - Add sugar, stevia, arrowroot, lemon, zest, lemon extract and vanilla. Blend again.
   - Add egg and egg white, and pulse until just blended.
5. Pour into baked crust. Set inside the roasting pan. Pour boiling water into roasting pan until it reaches 1/2-inch deep. Carefully set inside oven. Bake for 45 minutes. Turn off oven and leave slightly ajar by placing a potholder to leave the door open about an inch. Leave in oven for 1 hour. Then remove pan from water bath and allow to cool another hour on the countertop. Run a knife around the edge of the pan. Place in refrigerator uncovered and cool 3 hours.
6. Once thoroughly cooled, cover for storage. Open springform pan, removing outside ring. For a cheesecake with a softer texture, let stand 30 minutes at room temperature prior to serving. Keep leftover cheesecake in refrigerator up to 3 days or freeze. If the bottom crust becomes too wet when stored, cut into wedges and place on paper toweling before storing in refrigerator. The excess moisture will be absorbed, making the cheesecake more firm.

NOTE: If using 9-inch springform, bake 60 minutes.

Servings: 16

NUTRITION PER SERVING

Serving size	1 piece
Calories	130
Protein	9 g
Carbohydrate*	15 g
(*6 g added sugars)	
Fiber	1.1 g
Soluble fiber	0 g
Fat	4 g
Saturated fat	2.3 g
Cholesterol	25 mg
Sodium	170 mg
Potassium	97 mg
Calcium	105 mg
Omega-3 ALA	14 mg

Whole-Wheat Honey Banana Bread

Bowl One:
- 1   cup whole-wheat pastry flour or white whole-wheat flour
- 1/2   cup all-purpose flour
- 3/4   teaspoon baking soda

Optional:
- 1/3   cup toasted, chopped walnuts or pecans or 3 tablespoon whole flaxseeds, pulsed a few times in coffee mill to crack

Bowl Two:
- 1/4   cup canola oil
- 1/3   cup honey
- 1   cup mashed banana
- 1   teaspoon vanilla extract
- 1   egg (omega-3 enriched)

1. Preheat oven to 350°F.
2. Combine dry ingredients together in Bowl One. Set aside.
3. In Bowl Two stir all the ingredients together.
4. Dump contents of Bowl One into the wet ingredients in Bowl Two and stir by hand until just blended. Spoon into oiled 9 X 5-inch loaf pan.
5. Bake for 50 to 60 minutes or until toothpick inserted into the center comes out clean.

HELPFUL TIPS

When bananas get too ripe, peel, mash and freeze in 1-cup portions until ready to bake.

Whole-wheat pastry flour may be used instead of 1/2 cup all-purpose flour if desired.

Traditional whole-wheat flour will produce a much more dense loaf than the whole-wheat pastry flour or white whole-wheat flour.

Servings: 12

NUTRITION PER SERVING

Serving size	1 slice (3/4 inch thick)
Calories	145
Protein	2.6 g
Carbohydrate*	2 g
(*8 g added sugars)	
Fiber	2 g
Soluble fiber	0.3 g
Fat	5 g
Saturated fat	0.5 g
Cholesterol	18 mg
Sodium	85 mg
Potassium	123 mg
Calcium	8 mg
Omega-3 ALA	450 mg

Carrot Walnut Bar

HELPFUL HINT
Toasting walnuts and using an unrefined walnut oil will give a wonderful nutty flavor to the cake.

Bowl One

1/4	cup walnuts, toasted, chopped
1	cup whole-wheat pastry flour
3/4	cup all-purpose flour
3	tablespoons whole flaxseed, ground (about 1/4 cup when ground)
1	teaspoon baking soda
1	teaspoon cinnamon

Bowl Two

3	carrots, peeled and grated on a box grater (use small holes not the star shaped ones) or use a microplane to grate (1-1/2 cups loosely packed)
3	tablespoons walnut oil (or canola)
3/4	cup honey
1/4	cup carrot juice, pineapple juice or water
1/3	cup crushed pineapple, with liquid
1	teaspoon vanilla extract

1. Preheat oven to 350°F. Spray 9 X 9-inch pan with cooking spray.
2. Toast walnuts in dry pan over medium heat, then chop.
3. Combine dry ingredients in Bowl One.
4. Peel and grate carrots. Add to Bowl Two along with other wet ingredients. Stir.
5. Add dry ingredients from Bowl One to Bowl Two and stir until just blended.
6. Spoon into prepared pan.
7. Bake for 30 minutes or until center springs back when pressed with finger.
8. Cool. Cut into 16 pieces.
9. Wrap and freeze extra pieces.

Servings: 16

NUTRITION PER SERVING

Serving size	1 piece
	(2 1/4" X 2 1/4")
Calories	150
Protein	3 g
Carbohydrate*	26 g
(*13 g added sugars)	
Fiber	2 g
Soluble fiber	0.3 g
Fat	5 g
Saturated fat	0.5 g
Cholesterol	15 mg
Sodium	90 mg
Potassium	108 mg
Calcium	15 mg
Omega-3 ALA	750 mg

HELPFUL TIPS

Freeze extra pineapple if desired for later use. May serve bars with a dollop of plain, nonfat yogurt, drained (see Page 317), or Greek yogurt, sweetened with a little stevia if desired.

Measure oil into measure cup before measuring honey. The oil will coat the cup and the honey will slip out easily.

Chocolate Beany Cake

1	(15-ounce) can black beans, no-salt-added preferred, drained and rinsed (or black soy beans)
1/4	cup canola oil
1-1/4	cups water
2	eggs (omega-3 enriched)
1	package *Bob's Red Mill Whole-Grain Chocolate Cake Mix*

1. Preheat oven to 350°F. Spray 9 x 13-inch pan.
2. Combine black beans, oil and water in food processor and blend. Add eggs and pulse. Add cake mix and pulse until just blended.
3. Scrape batter into prepared pan and bake 25 minutes or until cake springs back when lightly touched with finger or toothpick inserted in center comes out clean.

Chocolate Beet Cake

Add 2 cups raw, peeled and grated beets to 1 package *Bob's Red Mill Whole-Grain Chocolate Cake Mix*. Follow package directions.

Servings: 24

NUTRITION PER SERVING

Serving size	1 piece (2-1/4" x 2")
Calories	118
Protein	4.5 g
Carbohydrate*	17 g
(*8 g added sugars from cake mix)	
Fiber	2.5 g
Soluble fiber	0.3 g
Fat	4 g
Saturated fat	0.5 g
Cholesterol	15 mg
Sodium	124 mg
Potassium	42 mg
Calcium	19 mg
Omega-3 ALA	230 mg

Fudgy Chocolate Pumpkin Cake

Pumpkin adds the nutrition of beta-carotene. You won't taste the pumpkin, but it adds moistness.

Servings: 24

1	package *Bob's Red Mill Whole-Grain Chocolate Cake Mix*
1	teaspoon pumpkin pie spice
1	(15-ounce) can pure pumpkin or 1 1/2 cups cooked mashed butternut squash
1	egg (omega-3 enriched)
1/4	cup canola oil
3/4	cup water
2	tablespoons mini chocolate chips

1. Preheat oven to 350°F. Spray 9 x 13-inch pan with nonstick spray.
2. Place cake mix, spice, pumpkin, egg, oil and water in bowl. Stir with spoon until smooth. It will be very thick.
3. Spread in prepared pan. Top with mini chocolate chips. If you plan to frost the cake, omit the chocolate chips.
4. Bake 30 to 35 minutes or until toothpick inserted near center comes out clean. Allow to cool. Cut into 24 pieces.
5. To bake as 30 mini muffins, bake for 12 to 15 minutes.

Frosting:

1/4	cup raw cashews
3	tablespoons water
1/4	package (or 3 ounces) of silken tofu (*Mori-Nu*)
2	tablespoons maple syrup
1/2	teaspoon vanilla
1/2	cup *Ghiradelli 60% Cacao Baking Chocolate Chips*

1. In food processor, blend cashews until finely chopped.
2. Add water, tofu, maple syrup and vanilla. Blend until well blended, scrape sides and blend again.
3. Melt chocolate chips and add to mixture, blending until combined. Chill about 30 minutes, then spread on cake.
4. Makes 1 cup frosting. May freeze extra, thaw in refrigerator overnight before using.

Oatmeal Chocolate Chip Cookie

A cookie is still a cookie no matter how healthy you try to make it. Make these and freeze them so that you can eat them in moderation. Make cookies small by using a tablespoon sized scoop. Adapted from recipe provided by Jennifer Reusch, R.D.

Bowl One:

3/4	cup old-fashioned rolled barley or rolled oats
1/2	cup whole-wheat pastry flour
1/2	cup all-purpose flour
1/4	cup of ground or milled flaxseed
1/2	teaspoon baking soda
1/8	teaspoon baking powder
1/2	cup mini chocolate chips
1/4	cup currants, craisins or dried cherries, chopped

Optional:

1/2	cup toasted walnuts or pecan, chopped

. . . .

Bowl Two:

2	tablespoons extra-virgin olive oil, walnut oil or canola oil
1/4	cup butter
3/4	cup brown sugar or *Sucanat*
1	teaspoon vanilla
1/2	teaspoon coconut extract
1	egg (omega-3 enriched)

1. Preheat oven to 400°F.
2. Measure all the dry ingredients into Bowl One. Set aside.
3. In Bowl Two combine all the wet ingredients, stirring to blend. If using *Sucanat* it does not dissolve as readily, so letting it stand overnight refrigerated will result in it dissolving.
4. Using a spoon, stir dry bowl ingredients into wet mixture until all is blended.
5. Using a tablespoon-sized scoop, drop onto prepared cookie sheets.
6. Bake for 10 minutes.
7. Remove from pans and cool on wire rack. When cooled, store in freezer.

HELPFUL TIPS

To bake two sheets, rotate between two shelves for even browning.
Start with one pan on lower shelf, and after 5 minutes, move it to the higher shelf and add a new pan to the lower shelf.
After baking 5 minutes longer, remove the first pan and rotate second pan up, adding a third pan to lower shelf and repeating until all are baked.

HELPFUL HINT
- If pans are sprayed with a cooking spray cookies will be flatter.

- *Sucanat* is a blend of evaporated cane juice and molasses.

- For a gluten free *version substitute Pamela's Baking & Pancake Mix* for the whole wheat and all purpose flour and omit the baking powder and baking soda. Use gluten free rolled oats

Servings: 42 (3-1/2 dozen)

NUTRITION PER SERVING

Serving size	1 cookie
Calories	79
Protein	1 g
Carbohydrate*	11 g
(*5 g added sugar)	
Fiber	1 g
Soluble fiber	0.1 g
Fat	3.5 g
Saturated fat	0.6 g
Cholesterol	5 mg
Sodium	19 mg
Potassium	47 mg
Calcium	10 mg
Omega-3 ALA	250 mg

Pumpkin Oatmeal Harvest Cookies

HELPFUL HINT
Date sugar is an unprocessed sweetener made from dehydrated dates. Look for it at a natural foods store. It is sweeter, so use 1/3 less than regular sugar when substituting.

Bowl One:

1	cup old-fashioned rolled oats or rolled barley
1	cup whole-wheat pastry flour
1/4	teaspoon baking soda
1	teaspoon pumpkin pie spice
1/3	cup craisins
1/2	cup chopped walnuts

Bowl Two:

1	cup canned pumpkin or mashed butternut squash
1/3	cup walnut oil or canola oil
1/2	cup date sugar, *Sucanat* or brown sugar
1	teaspoon vanilla
2	eggs (omega-3 enriched)

1. Preheat oven to 350°F.
2. Spray cookie sheet with nonstick cooking spray on the areas where you will drop cookies to save on clean up.
3. Measure all the dry ingredients into Bowl One. Set aside.
4. In Bowl Two combine all the wet ingredients, stirring to blend.
5. Using a spoon, stir dry bowl ingredients into wet mixture until all is blended.
6. Using a tablespoon-sized scoop, drop onto prepared cookie sheets. Press the top to flatten with a fork or the bottom of a juice glass.
7. Bake for 12 minutes.
8. Cool cookies on wire rack. When cooled, store in freezer.

Servings: 60 (5 dozen)

NUTRITION PER SERVING

Serving size	1 cookie
Calories	57
Protein	1 g
Carbohydrate*	6.6 g
(*0.4 g added sugar)	
Fiber	1 g
Soluble fiber	0.2 g
Fat	3 g
Saturated fat	0.3 g
Cholesterol	6 mg
Sodium	10 mg
Potassium	25 mg
Calcium	6 mg
Omega-3 ALA	350 mg

Bonus:
Vitamin A	(9% DV)

HELPFUL TIPS
To bake two sheets, rotate between two shelves for even browning.
Start with one pan on lower shelf, and after 6 minutes, move it to the higher shelf and add a new pan to the lower shelf.
After baking 6 minutes longer, remove the first pan and rotate second pan up, adding a third pan to lower shelf and repeating until all are baked.

RECIPE INDEX

A

Almond Butter
Granola Bar   426
Grilled Nut Butter   338
Nutty Rotini   335
Steel Cut Oats   312

Almonds
Apple & Spelt Berry Salad   376
Barley Nut Pilaf   328
Graham Cracker Breading   412
Spinach & Basil Pasta   389
Stuffed Pork Tenderloin   405
Wild Rice Spinach Salad   374

Apples
Breakfast Quinoa   314
Steel Cut Oats (option 2)   312
Muesli   315
Nutty Fruity Salmon Spread   338
Apple & Spelt Berry Salad with Raspberry
Vinaigrette   376

Apricots
Wild Rice Spinach Salad   368
Wild Rice Stuff Squash   368
Apricot bites   425

Arugula
Garden Salad   369
Pickled beets, snack   423
Warm Lentil Salad   379
Asian Chicken   402
Asian Noodles   336

Asparagus
Creamy Vegetable Soup   347
How to roast   354
How to prepare   291

Avocados
Green Salad w/ Salmon   377
Green Soybean Guacamole   429
Roasted beets, snack   423
Salsa variation   432
Veggie Pita Pocket   337
Avocado Fruit Smoothie   306

B

Baked Lemon Tempeh   298
Baked Oven French Toast   318
Baked Pasta & Cheese Florentine   393
Baked Vegetable Medley with
flaxseed topping   361

Bananas
Banana Blueberry Smoothie   305
Orange Banana Smoothie   304
Whole-Wheat Honey
Banana Bread   441

Barley
Barley Nut Pilaf   328
Cooking Guide   325
Cooking in a rice cooker   314
Multi Grain Mix   327
Quick Multi-Grain   328
Muesli (rolled flakes)   315

Barramundi
Quick meal Lemon Fish   301
Variation Mexicali Fish   411
Basic Grilled Fish   416
Basic preparation of Tofu   395
Basic Vinaigrette   371

Basil
Garden Herbed Dip   430
Garden Salad   369
Green, Orange Super Salad   373
Italian Pasta Salad   381
Parmesan Breading   412
Pecan Stuff Salmon   419
Pesto   390
Root & Bean Soup   348
Spinach & Basil Pesto   389
Sun Dried Tomato Basil Sauce   415
White Bean Tofu Shells   394
Basmati Rice Pilaf   332

Beans/Legumes
Beef and Beans Burger   406
Black Bean Salad   378
Black Bean Soup   350
Chicken Beany Burger   408
Italian Pasta Salad   381
Minestrone Soup   349
Root & Bean Soup   348
Vegetarian Chili   383
White Bean Spread   429
White Bean Tofu Stuff Shell   394

Beef
Beef And Beans Burger   406
Beef and Salsa, crockpot   301
Italian Beef & Chicken Patties   407
Safe cooking temperatures   291
Sandwich Spread   341
Soy and Beef Burger   406

Bell peppers see Peppers
Berry Sorbet   438
Berry Chicken   402

Beverages
Hot Chocolate   303
Hot Chocolate Teeccino   303
Choco-Berry Smoothie   304
Orange Banana Smoothie   304
Banana Blueberry Smoothie   305
Tropical Smoothie   305
Heart Smoothie   306
Avocado Fruit Smoothie   306
Black Bean Salad   378
Black Bean Soup   350
Black Beans and Brown Rice   299

Blueberries
Banana Blueberry Smoothie   305
Blueberry Walnut Bran Muffin   322
Choco-Berry Smoothie   304
Quick Dessert Idea   433
Bok Choy, preparation   291

Breads
Butternut Squash Bread with
Fruit and Nuts   324
Butternut Squash Rolls   320
Whole-Wheat Bread   323
Whole-Wheat Honey Banana Bread   451
Bread crumbs, make your own   284
Breakfast Burrito to Go   308
Breakfast ideas, quick   298

Broccoli
Broccoli Bean Dip   430
Broccoli Cauliflower Salad   380
Broccoli Corn Soup, Quick and Easy   349
Broccoli Couscous   333
Broccoli Pesto Penne   392
Broccoli Salmon Pizza   346

Brown rice, see rice
Brown rice syrup   375, 426

Brussels sprouts
How to prepare   291
Crumb Topped Oven-Roasted
Vegetables   356
Butternut Orange Sauce over Spaghetti
Squash   367

Burgers
Beef and Beans   406
Chicken Beany Burgers   408
Easy Salmon Burgers   407
Italian Beef & Chicken Patties   407
Salmon Beef Burgers   406
Soy and Beef Burger   406
Turkey Sausage   310
Turkey Beef Burgers   406
Tuscan Turkey Burgers   408

Butternut Squash
Butternut Squash Bread with Fruit and
Nuts   324
Butternut Squash Rolls   320
Butternut Orange Sauce   367
Creamy Butternut Sauce   367
Creamy Vegetable soup   347
Crumb Topped, Vegetables   356
Green & Gold Vegetable   362
Pumpkin Dip, variation   431
Pumpkin Oatmeal Cookies   446
How to prepare   292
Quick meals, creamy soup   300

C

Cake
Chcocolate Beany Cake   443
Chocolate Beet Cake   443
Fudgy Chocolate Pumpkin   444

Carrots
Asian Noodles   336
Barley Nut Pilaf   328
Black Bean Soup   350
Basmati Rice Pilaf   332
Confetti Vegetables with Dill   358
Creamy Lemon Salmon over
Multi Grains   420
Easy Italian Vegetables   359
Ginger Roasted Carrots   357
Green and Gold Vegetable
Bake   362
Italian Beef and Chicken Patties   407
Kale Salad   375
Lentil Taco Filling   384
Nutty Fruity Salmon   338
Oat Groat Pilaf   329
Rainbow Veggie Rice   331
Root & Bean Soup   348
Summer Vegetable Medley   360
Vegetarian Chili   383
Whole-Wheat Veggie Wrap   343
Carrot Walnut Bar   442

Cashews
Asian Noodles   336
Frosting   444

Cauliflower
Confetti Veggies with Dill   358
Broccoli Cauliflower Salad   380
Cheese toast   317
Cheesecake   440

Cherries, nutrition info 434
Chicken
   Asian Chicken 402
   Berry Chicken 402
   Beany Burgers 408
   Broccoli Stir-Fry 403
   Pesto Pasta 399
   Rice Primavera 400
   Rolls, Chicken 401
   Tuscan Chicken 401
   Vegetarian (Quorn) 399
Chickpeas (garbanzo)
   Hummus 428
   Root & Bean Soup 348
   Green salad with salmon 377
   Vegetarian Chili 383
Chili, vegetarian 383
Cracked 7-grain cereal 323
Chocolate
   Chocolate/chocolate chips 436
   Choco-Berry Smoothie 304
   Chocolate Beany Cake 443
   Chocolate Beet Cake 443
   Hot Chocolate 303
   Chocolate Pumpkin,
     fudgy cake 444
   Chocolate Sauce 437
   Heart Fuel Nutty Snack Mix 427
   Occasional snack 425
   Silken Chocolate Ginger Dream 439
Cocoa Powder, natural 303
   Hot Chocolate 303
   Silken Chocolate Dream 439
   Yogurt w/ cocoa 435
Confetti Veggies with Dill 358
Cookies
   Oatmeal Chocolate Chip 445
   Pumpkin Oatmeal Harvest 446
Cottage Cheese Spread 339
Couscous
   Cooking Guide 325
   Broccoli Couscous 333
Creamy Butternut Squash Sauce 367
Creamy Lemon Salmon over
   Multi Grains 420
Creamy Nut Butter 337
Creamy Parmesan Dressing 372
Creamy Vegetable Soup 347
Crispy Baked Fish 413
Crispy Tempeh Croutons 370
Crumb-Topped, Oven-Roasted
   Vegetables 356

D

Dark Green/Deep Orange Super
   Salad, Vinaigrette 373
DESSERT 433-446
   Quick dessert ideas 433
   Yogurt for dessert 435
Deviled Egg Substitute 339
Dip
   Garden Herbed Dip 430
   Green Soybean Guacamole 429
   Hummus 428
   Pumpkin Dip 431
   Rosemary-Roasted Red Pepper
     & Bean Dip 430
   Salsamole 422
   Simple Fresh Salsa 432
   Spinach Dip 431
   White Bean Spread 429
Double Baked Potatoes 300

Dressing
   Basic Vinaigrette 371
   Creamy Dressing 371
   Creamy Parmesan 372
   Honey French 372
   Maple-Vinaigrette 372
   Potato Salad 382
   Ranch Dressing 371

E

Easy Italian Vegetables 359
Easy Salmon Burgers 407
Eggplant
   Roasted Vegetables 354
   Summer Vegetable Medley 360
Eggs, scrambled 307
Egg, muffin veggie 309
Emerald Mashed Sweet Potatoes 365

F

Feta spread 340
Fettuccini with Tofu Alfredo 394
Fire-Roasted Tomatoes Lentils
   and Pasta 398
Fish, see also Salmon
   Basic Method for Baked
     "Oven-fried" Fish 412
   Crispy Baked Fish 413
   Grilled 353
   How to tell when done 409
   Poached 414
   Safe temperature 291
   Sauces for Poached Fish 415
   Stew 421
   Tartar Sauce 422
Flavorful Vegetable Stew 387
Flaxseeds
   Baked Pasta and Cheese
     Florentine 393
   Baked Vegetable Medley with
     Flaxseed Topping 361
   Banana Blueberry Smoothie 304
   Blueberry Walnut Bran Muffin 322
   Carrot Walnut Bar 442
   Cheese Toast 317
   Choco-Berry Smoothie 304
   Crumb Topped Oven Roasted
     Vegetables 356
   Flounder Mexicali 411
   Granola Bars 426
   Oatmeal Chocolate Chip
     Cookie 445
   Oven Fried Parmesan Chicken
     Nuggets 404
   Whole-Wheat Bread 323
Flounder Mexicali 411
French toast 318
Frosting, cake 444
Fruit Sweet
   Steel cut oats (option 1) 312
   Yogurt 435
   Chocolate Sauce 437
Fruity Cinnamon Rolled Oats
   with Oat Groats 313

G

Garden Herbed Dip 430
Garden Salad 369
Garlic, Roasted 355
Garlic Rosemary Sweet Potatoes 365
Garlic Spinach Sauté 364
Ginger Roasted Carrots 357

Ginger-Soy Grilled Salmon 417
Ginger Soy Marinated Tofu
   and Rice 396
Gluten Free
   see variation 445
Graham Cracker
   Breading, fish 412
   Cheesecake 445
Grain sweetened chocolate chips 439
Grains see rice, oats, couscous
   Cooking Guide 325
   Creamy Lemon Salmon 420
   Multi-Grain-A-Roni, quick 328
   Multi-grain Mix 327
   Quinoa Pilaf with Red & Yellow
     Peppers 379
   Toasted Grain Granola 316
   Tomato Rosemary Polenta Bake 386
Greens see also Salads
   Basic Cooking Method for Sautéed
     Greens 363
Granola
   Granola bars 426
   Toasted Grain Granola 316
Greek yogurt 288, 297, 425, 435,
   437, 440, 442
Green & Gold Vegetable Bake 362
Green Salad with Salmon
   and Vinaigrette Dressing 377
Green Soybean Guacamole 429
Grilled Nut Butter 338
Grilled salmon with Honey Mustard
   Dijon Sauce 416
Ground Beef Burger Variations 406

H

Harissa paste 387
Heart Fuel Nutty Snack Mix 427
Heart Smoothie 306
Honey French Dressing 372
Honey Rum Sweet Potatoes 366
Hot Chocolate Teeccino 303
Hulled barley, see barley
Hummus 428

I

Italian Beef and Chicken Patties 407
Italian Pasta Salad 381
Ingredients 283-8

J

Jicama what to look for 373

K

Kalamata Olives
   Feta Spread 340
   Italian Pasta Salad 381
   Hummus variation 428
Kale, see also spinach (may use kale instead)
   Basic Cooking Method for Sautéed
     Greens 363
   Baked Vegetable Medley w Flaxseed
     Topping 361
   Confetti Veggies with Dill 358
   Emerald Mashed Sweet Potatoes 365
   Garden Salad 369
   Green & Gold Vegetable Bake 362
   Kale Salad 375
   Tomato Rosemary Polenta Bake 386
Kamut
   Cooking Guide 325
Kidney beans, see beans
Kiwifruit, ideas 351, 433-4

L

Leafy greens, see salads
Lemon-Baked Tempeh   397
Lentil
   Fire Roasted Tomatoes Lentils and
      Pasta   398
   Lentil Taco Filling   384
   Pasta sauce (add red lentils)   388
   Warm Lentil Salad   379
Lundberg wild rice blend   374, 396

M

Mango
   Grilled   433
   Salsamole   422
Meatless Substitutes for chicken   399
Meals, Quick   299-301
Meatless Meals, see also Tofu, Tempeh
   Baked Pasta and Cheese
      Florentine   393
   Broccoli Pesto Penne 392
   Chicken Pesto Pasta with meatless
      option   399
   Fire Roasted Tomatoes Lentils
      and Pasta   398
   Flavorful Vegetable Stew   387
   Lentil Taco Filling   384
   Pasta sauce w/lentils   388
   Quick Minestrone Soup   349
   Spaghetti Squash Casserole   385
   Tomato Rosemary Polenta Bake   386
   Vegetarian Chili   383
   Veggie Egg Muffin   309
   Veggie Stuffed Pita Pocket
Menu Plan 7-DAY   294-7
Microwaved Old-Fashioned Rolled
      Oatmeal   311
Millet Cooking Guide   325
Minestrone Soup, Quick   349
Mori-Nu silken tofu
   Creamy Lemon Salmon   420
   Creamy Vegetable Soup   347
   Creamy Parmesan Dressing   372
   Fettuccini with Tofu Alfredo   394
   Frosting   444
   Garden Herbed Dip   430
   Honey Dijon Dipping Sauce   404
   Scrambled Tofu Egg   308
   Silken Chocolate Ginger Dream   439
   Tofu Egg Salad   342
   White Bean & Tofu Stuff Shells   384
Morning Star Farms Grillers Recipe
      Crumbles, see TVP
Muesli   315
Muffins   321-2
Multi-Grain-A-Roni, quick   328
Multi-grain Mix   327
Mushroom Melts, Portabella   342
Mustard
   Lower sodium brands   285
   Potato Salad   382
   Walnut Crusted Salmon   410

N

Nut Butter
   Asian Chicken   402
   Granola Bars   426
   Nut Butter Sandwich   337-8
   Nutty Rotini   335
   Steel Cut Oats, variation   312
   Yogurt Cheese, flavored   317

Nuts, see also almond, walnut,
cashew, pecan
   Broccoli Couscous   333
   Butternut Squash Bread   324
   Heart Fuel Nutty Snack   427
   Honey Rum Sweet Potato   366
   How to toast nuts   285
   Nutty Fruity Salmon   338
   Pesto   390
   Roasted Vegetable & Orzo   334
   Nutrition   427, see book 119

O

Oat Bran
   Breading for chicken   404
   Cheese Toast   317
   Chicken Burgers   408
   Cottage Cheese Spread   339
   Granola Bars   426
   Muesli   315
   Pumpkin Maple Muffins   321
   Topping for vegetables   361
   Turkey Sausage   310
Oat Groats
   Breakfast cereal   313
   Cooked in vegetable steamer   314
   Fruity Cinnamon Rolled Oats   313
   Know your oats   311
   Multi-Grain Mix   327
Oat Groat Pilaf   329
Oat Groats, whole   313
Oatmeal Chocolate Chip Cookie   445
Oats, Rolled Cold
   Muesli   315
   Toasted Grain Granola   316
Oats, Hot
Baked Steel-cut Oats   312
Betty's Baked Oatmeal   315
Microwaved Old Fashioned   311
   Steel Cut Oats   312
   Fruity Cinnamon Rolled   313
Oil
   Liquid fish oil, in salad dressing   371
Oil, toasted sesame
   Asian Noodles   336
   Pan Grill Marinated Tempeh   397
   Asian Chicken   402
   Ginger-Soy Grilled Salmon   417
Oil, Olive, extra-virgin, see book 62
Orange Banana Smoothie   304
Orzo, roasted vegetable   334
Oven-Baked French Toast   318
Oven-Fried Fish   412
Oven-Fried Parmesan Chicken
      Nuggets   404

P

Pan-Grilled Marinated Tempeh Slices   397
Parmesan Cheese
   Ingredient 285, 390
Parmesan Pesto Pizza   346
Parsnip
   Green and Gold Vegetable Bake   362
   Root & Bean Soup   348
Pasta
   Asian Noodles   336
   Baked Pasta and Cheese Florentine   393
   Broccoli Pesto Penne   392
   Chicken Pesto Pasta   399
   Fettuccini with Tofu Alfredo   394
   Fire Roasted Tomatoes Lentils and
      Pasta   398
   Italian Pasta Salad   381

Nutty Rotini   335
   Quick Minestrone Soup   349
   Roasted Vegetable & Orzo   334
   Spinach and Basil Pasta   389
   White Bean and Tofu Shells   394
Pasta sauce   388
Pastry flour, substitute whole-wheat 319
Peach Whip   437
Peanut butter, see nut butter
Pecan-Stuffed Salmon Filet   419
Penzeys Spices   286
Peppers, Bell
   Asian Noodles   336
   Baked Vegetable Medley   361
   Black Bean Salad   378
   Chicken Pesto Pasta   399
   Confetti Veggies w/ Dill   358
   Flavorful Vegetable Stew   387
   Ginger Soy Marinated Tofu   396
   Green & Gold Vegetable   362
   Green Salad w/ Salmon   377
   Lentil Taco Filling   384
   Rainbow Veggie Rice   331
   Salmon Wheat Berry Salad   375
   Seafood Stew   421
   Tomato Rosemary Polenta   386
   Whole-Wheat Veggie Wrap   343
Pesticides   351, 434
Pesto   390
Pesto Salmon Pita Pizza   346
Pilaf, Multi-Grain   331
Pine Nut, see Nuts
Pineapple
   Tropical Smoothie   305
   Carrot Walnut Bar   442
   Quick Dessert, grilled   433
Pita, Pizza   346
Pizza Crust   344
Pleasoning mini-mini salt   286
Poached Fish   414
Polenta   386
Pomegranate   434
Pork Tenderloin   405
Portabella Mushroom Melts   342
Potato Salad   382
Poultry See Chicken
Protein powder, whey
   Ingredients   287
   Choco-Berry Smoothie   304
   Avocado Fruit Smoothie   306
   Granola Bars   426
Pumpkin Dip   431
Pumpkin Maple-Pecan Oat Bran
      Muffin   321
Pumpkin Oatmeal Harvest Cookies   446

Q

Quinoa, breakfast   314
Quinoa Pilaf with Red & Yellow Peppers   330
Quorn chick'n tenders   399

R

Rainbow Veggie Rice   331
Ranch Dressing   371
Red bell pepper, see peppers
Rice, see also grain
   Basmati Pilaf   332
   Chicken Rice Primavera   400
   Ginger Soy Marinated Tofu
     and Rice   396
   How to cook   327
   Rainbow Veggie Rice   331
   Quick meals   299
   Wild Rice Spinach Salad   374
Roasted Beets   355Roasted Bell Peppers
355
     and Basil Sauce   391
Roasted Garlic   355
Roasted Vegetable & Orzo   334
Roasted Vegetables   354
Rolled oats see oats
Romaine, see Salad
Root & Bean Soup   348
Rosemary-Roasted Red Pepper
    and Bean Dip   430
Rotini, Nutty   335
Rye, how to cook   326

S

Safe Cooking Temperatures   291
Sage Green Beans with Walnuts   357
Salad
   Apple & Spelt Berry Salad   376
   Black Bean Salad   378
   Broccoli Cauliflower   380
   Dark Green/Deep Orange Super
     Salad   373
   Garden Salad   369
   Green Salad with Salmon   377
   Italian Pasta   381
   Kale Salad   375
   Potato Salad   382
   Salmon Wheat Berry Salad   375
   Tempeh Salad   379
   Warm Lentil Salad   379
   Wild Rice Spinach Salad   374
   Zucchini Julienne with Lemon and
     Chives   380
Salad Dressing   371-2
Salmon, canned
   Creamy Lemon Salmon over Multi
     Grain   420
   Easy Salmon Burgers   407
   Nutty Fruity Salmon   338
   Pesto Salmon Pizza   346
   Salmon Spread   341
   Salmon Wheat Berry Salad   375
Salmon, fresh/frozen
   Green Salad with Salmon   377
   Grilled Salmon with Honey Mustard
     Dijon   416
   Ginger Soy Grilled Salmon   417
   Salmon Beef Burgers   406
   Simply Seasoned Grilled
     Salmon   418
   Pecan Stuffed Salmon Filet
Salsa, Simple Fresh   432
Salsamole   422
Sandwich
   Cottage Cheese Spread   229
   Deviled Egg Substitute   339
   Grilled Nut Butter   338
   Ideas   337

Nutty Fruity Salmon   338
Sandwich Spread   341
Salmon Spread   341
Tofu Egg Salad   342
Whole-Wheat Veggie Wrap   343
Sauce
   Asian Chicken (peanut)   434
   Asian Noodles   336
   Berry Chicken   402
   Broccoli Pesto   392
   Butternut Orange   367
   Creamy Butternut   367
   Ginger-Soy   417
   Honey Mustard Dijon   416
   Quick Pizza   388
   Tartar Sauce   422
Sauce Dipping
   Ginger Mustard   404
   Honey Dijon   404
Sauce, Poached Fish
   Cucumber   415
   Lemon Herb   415
   Sun-Dried Tomato Basil   415
Sausage, Turkey   310
Sausage, soy   309
Sautéed Greens, basic cook
    method   363
Scrambled Tofu Egg   308
Seafood Stew   421
Seasoned Mayonnaise   340
Silken Chocolate Ginger Dream   439
Silken tofu see Mori-Nu silken tofu
Simple Fresh Salsa   432
Simply Seasoned Grilled Salmon   418
Smoothies, see beverages
Snack ideas   423-4, see also dessert
    ideas   433
Sorbet, Berry   438
Soups
   Black Bean Soup   350
   Creamy Vegetable Soup   347
   Root & Bean Soup   348
   Quick Minestrone Soup   249
   Quick & Easy Broccoli Corn
     Soup   349
Soy and Beef Burgers   406
Spaghetti Squash Casserole   385
Spelt berry   376
Spinach, see also Kale
   Baked Pasta and Cheese
     Florentine   393
   Chicken Pesto Pasta   399
   Chicken Rolls   401
   Garlic Spinach Saute 364
   Nutty Rotini   335
   Quick Minestrone Soup   349
   Rainbow Veggie Rice   331
   Spaghetti Squash Casserole   385
   Spinach and Basil Pasta   389
   Spinach Dip   431
   Spinach Parmesan   364
   Stuffed Pork Tenderloin   405
   Tuscan Turkey Burgers   408
   Veggie Egg Muffin   309
   Whole-Wheat Veggie Wrap   343
   Wild Rice Spinach Salad   374
Spaghetti Squash   385
Squash, see also Zucchini and Butternut
  Squash Yellow
   Chicken Broccoli Stir-Fry   403
   Roasted   354
   Garden Salad   369

Steel Cut Oats   312
Stevia   174
   Carrot Walnut Bar   442
   Cheesecake   440
   Yogurt sweetened   435
Stir-Fry, Chicken Broccoli   403
Stuffed Pork Tenderloin   405
Summer Vegetable Medley   360
Sun-Dried Tomatoes Basil Sauce   415
Sun-dried, soak/re-hydrate   287
Sweet Leaf, see stevia
Sweet Potato, see also butternut squash
  may substitute
   Honey Rum   366
   Sweet Potato Fries   366

T

Taco, Lentil   384
Tahini   428
Tamari/soy sauce   286
Tartar Sauce   422
Teeccino   303
Tempeh
   Crispy Crouton   370
   Lemon-Baked   397
   Marinated Pan Grill   397
   Tempeh Salad   379
Tenderloin, Pork   405
Thousand Island Spread   340
Toasted rolled grains, granola   316
Tofu Egg Salad   342
Tofu, Regular (not silken) see also
  Mori-Nu silken tofu
   Basic preparation   395
   Tofu, ginger soy marinated   396
   Tofu with Fire-Roasted Tomatoes   395
Tomatoes
   Black Bean Salad   378
   Italian Pasta Salad   381
   Lentils and Pasta   398
   Quick Minestrone Soup   349
   Salmon Wheat Berry Salad   375
   Salsamole   422
   Seafood Stew   421
   Summer Vegetable Medley   360
   Sun-Dried Tomatoes Basil Sauce   415
   Tofu w/Fire-Roast Tomato   395
   Tuscan Chicken   401
Tomato Rosemary Polenta Bake   386
Tortilla, brands to buy   287
Tortilla, Veggie Wrap   343
Tropical Smoothie   305
Trout, Grilled   416
Tuna, see salmon canned, may
  substitute tuna
Tuna, troll caught info 287
Turkey Beef Burgers   406
Turkey Sausage   310
Tuscan Chicken   401
Tuscan Turkey Burgers   408
TVP textured vegetable soy protein
   Ground meat, meatless   285
   Pasta sauce   388
   Soy and Beef Burgers   406
   Vegetarian Chili   383
   Veggie Egg Muffin 309

V

Vegetable Preparation   291
Vegetable recipe section   351
Vegetables, roasted, how to   354
Vegetables, tips to eat more   351
Vegetarian Main Dishes, see tofu,
   tempeh, meatless
Vegetarian Chili   383
Veggie Egg Muffin   309
Veggie Stuffed Pita Pocket   337
Vinaigrette, see dressing

W

Walnuts
   Carrot Walnut Bar   442
   Honey Rum Sweet Potato   366
   Sage Green Beans   357
   Walnut Crusted Salmon   410
Warm Lentil Salad   379
Water-bath for cheesecake   440
Wax Orchards, see Fruit Sweet
Wheat Berries
   Cooking   326
   Grind into flour   319
   Multi-grain mix   327
   Salmon salad   375
   Whole-Wheat Bread   323
Whey protein, see protein powder
White Bean Spread   429
White Bean & Tofu Stuffed Shells   394
Whole Grains, Cooking guide   325
Whole-wheat bread   323
Whole-wheat Graham Cracker Breading   412
Whole-Wheat Veggie Wrap   343
Wild Rice-Spinach Salad   374
Wild Rice Stuffed Squash   368

Y

Yogurt cheese   317

Z

Zesting peel, microplane   290
Zucchini
   Baked Vegetable Medley   361
   Flavorful Vegetable Stew   387
   Julienne,w/ lemon & chive   380
   Roasted Vegetables   354
   Summer Vegetable Medley   360
   Vegetarian Chili   383

INDEX

A

activity 4, 253
  effect on health 252
  optimal fitness, weight loss 259
advanced glycation end-products
  (AGE) 70
advanced testing 31-6
agave 170
Ahi 96-8, 111
ALA 93-5, 105, 113-4, 117, 120, 158
  in foods 117
alcohol 45, 172, 191, 201, 205
  coumadin 205
  triglycerides 45
  what is a drink 201
allicin 230
almonds 12, 53, 55, 87, 119-20,
  126, 225
  nutrition 120
  number per ounce 119
alpha linolenic acid, see ALA
amaranth, gluten free 145
anchovy 98, 109
angus, certified 68, 71-2
antibiotic free poultry 75
antioxidants 9, 62, 120, 138,
  199-201, 220, 223
  pecan 120
apo
  apo B 32, 131
  apo E 5, 32, 34
arteries 23, 39
artificial sweeteners 173
aspirin 35, 238
  flushing niacin 238
  hs-CRP 36
assessment, self 7, 41
  metabolic syndrome 41
Atlantic salmon 99, 111
average calories per day 266

B

barley 132, 137, see also recipe index
  rolled 54, 129, 149
  soluble fiber 132
  waxy hulless 138
bean flour 155
beans, see also legumes 130, 151-2,
  156
  Beano 130
  ways to add 152
beef 67, 73, 75, 77
  grass fed 75-6
  ground 67
  hormone free 77
beef. protein per ounce 162
beef, saturated fat 67
beef,de-fat, how to 73
berkley heart lab 32
beta carotene 211-3
  food source 211
  multi-vitamin 212
  vegetables rich in 353
  smoker 213
beta-glucan, barley
  oats 137
  prowashonupana 138
beverage, water 174
beverages 197, 246
bison 70

blood
  cholesterol 21
  lipid profile test 25
  pressure 189
    caffeine 199
    DASH 194
    effect of protein and fat 58
    fish oil 93, 192
    lifestyle changes to lower 190
    physical activity 252
    potassium 192
    sea salt 183
    sodium 19, 181
    soy nuts 191
    systolic, diastolic 30
    vitamin D 217
  test, vitamin D 217
BMI chart 263
body fat 266
bone health
  sodium 183
  vitamin K 204
bottled water 197
bran, wheat germ 145
Brazil nuts 136, 209, 220-1, 226
breads
  eating out 246
  low glycemic 168
  three steps for choosing 145
butter
  almond, cashew, seed 123
  tips use less 87
  vs margarine 85

C

c-reactive protein 36
CAD, see coronary artery disease
caffeine 199, 200
cage free 79
calcium 220-1
  foods, table 221
calcium score 39
calorie intake for weight loss 266
calories 14, 20, 259, 266, 276-7
  in 2,000 steps 253
  burned to maintain weight 14, 256
  of exercise daily 255
  fat burning mode 259
  to raise HDL 259
cancer
  grill meats 70
  red meat 69
cancers, vitamin D 215
canned salmon 99
canola oil 7, 36, 46, 58-64, 86, 93, 113,
  117-8, 126, 200, 218
carbohydrates 19, 47, 163-4, 178
  better choices, poor choices 164
  refined 43, 46
carrots, glycemic load 166
cheese 67, 247
  serving size 272
chia seeds 117, 120
Chicken breast, nutrition 79
chicken, broasted 80
chickens, hormone free 76
cholecalciferol, Vitamin D 216
cholesterol 3, 21, 89
  alcohol 201
  blood test, lipid profile 25

convert mg/dl to mmol/l 24
  eggs 89
  HDL 22
  LDL see also LDL 22, 26-28
  shrimp 89
  testing 5
    advanced testing 31-36
  what your numbers should be 30
cinnamon 46, 229
CLA (conjugated linoleic acid) 76
cocoa 50, 197, 201
coconut oil 68
cod liver oil 104, 107
coenzyme Q10 230
coffee 197, 199
  benefits 199
  like beverage Teecino 200
  paper filters 199
  whiteners
cold pressed oil 63
CoQ10 230
corn syrup 170
coronary artery disease (CAD)
  23, 31, 94
coumadin see also warfarin,
  vitamin K 203
crackers, 3 steps for choosing 145
CRP 36
crystalline fructose 169
CT scan 40
  calcium score 39

D

dairy 273
DASH diet 55, 194
deli meats, saturated fat 68
desserts, eating out 249
DHA
  see EPA
  ALA, EPA 94
  marine algae 101
diabetes 177
diabetic sample menu 180
diastolic 190
diet, portfolio 55
dietary fiber 127
dietary supplements 227
dining out 241
  avoid trans fat 242
  sodium 249
  tips 244
    appetizers 246
    beverages 246
    breakfast 245
    entrees 247
    fast food 245
    salads 248
    sandwiches 247
    sodium reduce 249
    soups 246
dinner plate diagram 276
DNA test 36
doctor, lipidologist 32
drain fat ground meat 72
drink alcohol 201
drug
  niacin 236
  warfarin/coumadin 203
drugs raise LDL, triglycerides 27
dry beans/legumes 151

E

E2/E2 36
EBCT 39
eating out, see dining out
EGCG 200-1
Eggland egg 64, 90, 117
egg whites 90
   protein 162
eggs 89
electron beam 39
enriched grain, nutrients missing 144
EPA 103-4
erythritol 173
exercise see also physical activity 251
   Borg Scale 258
   raise HDL 259
   record activities 261
   strength training 260
   weight loss 259
EWG, environmental working group 95
expeller pressed oil 63
extra virgin olive oil 36, 53, 62-4, 83, 86,
   230, 244

F

fat allowance 8,16, 61, 86-7
fat diagram 57
fatty acids in oils and fats 59
fat, choosing 61
fat effect on health 60
fat, interesterified 86
fat, omega-3 93
fat, saturated 67
fat, tips for eating healthy balance 64
fat, trans 83
fiber see also soluble fiber
   daily allowance 17
   four month plan 129
   sample menu 56, 130
   statin drugs 131
fish, see also salmon 65, 92, 93
   allergic 101
   barramundi 101
   farmed salmon 99
   fried 99
   how much to eat 97
   mercury, high 95
   mercury, low 96
   oil 103
      supplements 103
   ounces per week for EPA DHA 98
   sablefish 100
   selenium 220
   smoked 99
   supplements 103
   table, omega-3 content of various fish
      109-112
   trout 101
fish oil labels 104
   brands, EPA/DHA 104
   prescription 108
   vs cod liver oil 107
flavanoids 200-1
flax, flaxseed see also ALA
   65, 94, 113-6, 125
   baking 115
   food source table 117
   nutrition 56, 125
   oil 59, 61, 105, 113-4
      vs fish oil 114
   prostate cancer 114
   storage, how to handle 115

tips 116
   whole vs ground 115
   yellow, solin 115
flour 164
   barley 138
   bean 155
   choosing foods made from 145
   white whole wheat 319
   whole wheat pastry 319,
flush, niacin
   decrease 237
   no flush niacin 237
folate 90, 120, 151, 212, 214
food
   labels, fiber 128
   sources Vitamins
      C foods 215
      D foods 216
      E foods 218
   sources minerals
      calcium 221
      magnesium 193
      potassium 193
      selenium 220
food journals, weight loss 267
foods
   fast 245
   high GI 165, 167
   organic 146
four simple ways 3
framingham 10-year risk 37-8
free range 79
fructose 168-9
fruit juice 175
fruit sweet 172
fruits 272
   potassium 193
   serving, what is 272
frying foods 63

G

game meats 77
garlic 230
gas 154
   beano 130
   ways to decrease 154
GI glycemic index 165
GL glycemic load 165
gluten free whole grain 145
grades of beef 71
grain mill 149, 155, 319
grains 143-4
   gluten free 145
   whole 143
grapefruit 50
   and statin drugs 50
grapeseed oil, poly-unsaturated 60
grass fed beef
   100% 75
   vs organic 75
gravy 73
green tea 200, 205
grilling 70
ground meat saturated fat 73
ground beef, de-fat 73
guggulipids 232

H

hardness, water 185
HATS trial 235
hazelnuts 119, 124, 126, 136, 209, 211,
   218, 225
HCA, grilling 70

HDL see also cholesterol)
   alcohol 47
   how to increase 47
   lowered by 47
   niacin 48
   non HDL 27
health claim
   nuts 119
   olive oil 62
   phytosterols 228
   soluble fiber 137
   soy foods 157
heart
   attack 23
   disease risk factors 30
   healthy plate 49
   rate 256, 258
      Borg Scale 258
      fat burning 259
      maximum 257
      medication effect 258
      reserve 258
      target 257
   scan 39
heat, high cooking oil 63
herbs, stevia 174
high blood pressure 189
high fructose corn syrup, HFCS 168
HNE 6
homocysteine 35
hormone free beef 77
hormones in poultry 76
honey 172
hs-CRP 36
hulled barley 138
hypertension stages 30

I

IDL 29
iliac crest 41
indole-3-carbinole 353
inflammation 4, 35-6, 61, 70, 83
INR (international normalized ratio) 203-6
insulin 177
   vitamin D 217
insulin resistance 42
intact grains 146
INTERHEART study 55
intensity (low vs high in exercise) 259
interesterification 87
iodine 183, 225
IP6 phytate 158
iron 212, 220
   molasses 172
   in multi vitamin 212
isoflavones supplements 158-9

J

jams no sugar 175
JNC-7 190
juices 175, 274
   and coumadin 204
   and grapefruit 50

L

labels
   and antibiotics 76
   and fish oil 104
   and soluble fiber 127
   and no trans fat 84
   and whole grain 143
lamb, red meat 69
l-carnitine 34

LDL 22, 26
    drugs that raise 27
    effect of different fats 60
    fish oil 105
    fructose 169
    goal 26-7, 38
    particle numbers 33
        and soy 158
    risk factors 30
    soluble fiber 12
    tea 200
legumes 151, 155, 157, 165
    ways to add 152
    ways to decrease gas 154
lentils 152, 154
    chana dal 168
lifestyle
    assessment 7
    and blood pressure 190
    and diet 267
    effect on lipids 12
    and metabolic 43
light tuna, canned 96
linoleic 57
lipidologist 32
lipids 21
Lipo-Profile test, NMR 32
lipid profile 25
lipoprotein a, see Lp(a)
lipoprotein lipase 23
lipoproteins 5, 21
liver
    cod 107
    makes cholesterol 89
loin, meat cut 72
Lovaza prescription fish oil 106
low fat diet
    and triglycerides 22
Lp(a) 5, 32, 34, 83
    and trans fat 83
Lyon diet heart study 55

M
macadamia 119, 125
magnesium 192
    food sources 193
marbling, meat 71, 75, 247
margarine 85
    and interesterification 86
    and stanol 228
maximum heart rate see heart rate
meal planning plate method 275
meat 69
    game saturated fat 78
    labels (lean and extra lean) 71
    organic vs grass 75
    saturated fat in various cuts 73-4
Mediterranean diet 55
menu eating out 242
mercury fish 95-6
mercury (fish oil) 105
metabolic syndrome 41, 44, 163, 165, 169
    self assessment 41
    how to treat 44
Metamucil 131
Metamucil (psyllium) 129
millet 145-6
minerals 211, 220, 225
monacolins, red yeast 233
monounsaturated fats 63, 84, 194
montina, grain 145-6
multi-vitamin 211
myoglobin in meat 69

N
niacin 34, 36, 47-8, 223, 235-40
    and flushing 236
    no-flush 237
    Slo-Niacin 235-6
    tps to reduce flushing 238
Niaspan, niacin 236
nitric oxide 120
NMR Lipo-Profile 32
non HDL 27, 28
northern pike, mercury 97
Nurses' Healthy study 84, 253
nut butters 122-3, 126, 272-3
nutritional needs, eight steps 13
nuts 119
    and health claim 119
    butters 122
    number in one ounce 119
    nutrition table 125
    raw 121
    roasted 121

O
oat bran 127-9, 137-9
oats 137-9
oils 59
    choosing cooking 62
    cold pressed 63
    coconut 58-61, 68, 117
    expeller pressed 63
    extra light 62
    extra virgin 62
    fatty acids 59
    heating 63
olive oil 62-66
    margarine 86
o-mega-Zen3 101
omega-3 93
omega-3
    ALA 113
    EPA DHA in fish 92
    flax 105
    in salmon 100
    supplements 103
omega-6 61
OmniHeart study 58, 194
optimal fitness level 259
organic 76, 146

P
PABA 223
PAH, grilling 70
palm
    kernel oil 60, 87
    oil in peanut butter 122
palmitate 213
paper filters, coffee 199
partially hydrogenated oils 16, 54, 60, 68,
    84-7, 122, 200, 228
particle size LDL 32
pastures, beef 75
PCBs 95, 105
peanut butter 123, 126
peanuts 120, 125
pearled barley 137-8
pecans 120, 125
pedometer 253
    how to add steps 254
personal trainer 261
pesticides in vegetable 351
physical activity 251-2
    calories expended 256
    fat burning mode 259

self assessment 252, 255
    moderate activities 255
phthalate, plastic 198
phytochemicals 120, 144, 199, 212
phytosterols plant sterols 227-8
phytosterolemia 228
plant stanol 12, 227
pistachios 119-20, 125
plate, heart healthy 49
    1500-1700 calorie 276
plant sterols 227-9, 234
plaque 5, 22-3, 39
plastic codes 198
policosanol 232
polymeal study 55
polyphenols 200-1
Pomona 175
pork 69, 72
portfolio diet 55-56
portion, serving 271
potassium 192-3
    food sources 193
    free seasoning 185
    salt 185
poultry 67, 76, 79, 80
    broasted 80
    saturated fat in various types 81
protein 162, 272
    food sources 162
    how much you need 18
psyllium 12, 127, 131, 137, 140
PureVia 174

Q
quiz answers 279-81
quinoa see recipe section

R
rancid 108, 114, 126
ratio
    cholesterol 29
    waist to hip 265
raw, nuts 121
RDA 226
Rebiana 174
red meat and cancer 69
red yeast extract 232-4
reserve, heart rate 258
resistant starch, beans 153
restaurant foods 241
retinol 213, 223
reynolds risk score 37
rhabdomyolysis 231
rice bran oil 59, 61, 117, 218
rice, red yeast 233
risk
    10 year 37-8
    factors 27
rooibos tea 201
rotisserie chicken 80,82,183

S
sablefish 100, 110
salicylates 36
salmon 110, 216
    canned 99
    farmed 99
    farmed vs wild 99
    selenuium 220
    vitamin D 216

salt, see also sodium
  cooking to reduce sodium   186
  iodized   183
  sea   183
  sensitivity   181
  softened water   198
  substitutes   185
  tips for less sodium   185
salt (sodium)   181
sample menu, see appendix C
sardines   96, 110
saturated fat   12-3, 21, 47, 56, 60, 64,
    67-8, 74, 87
  daily allowance chart   16
  lauric   68
  in lean meat   71
scan, heart   39
scan, CTA   40
sea salt   183
seafood see fish
second-hand smoke   4
sedentary   13-5, 253, 259
seeds   113, 117, 119-20, 125, 218
self-assessments, see appendix C
selenium   220
serving, what is   272
serving size practice   274
shrimp   89
simvastatin   131
size, serving   271, 274
sleep   4, 36, 43-4
slo-niacin   236
small particles LDL   32
smoke   4, 40, 63
smoked fish   99
snack see page 423
sodium   181-2, 188
  and bone health   183
  cooking to reduce   186
  daily allowance   19
  in teaspoon salt   182
  in water   185
  tips for less   184
  where we get   188
soluble fiber   17, 20, 33, 36, 55-6, 127-41,
    151, 153, 161, 169, 227
  finding on label   128
  four month plan   129
  goal   17
  sample menu   130
  statin drugs   131
  table, content in foods   132-136
soups   246
  eating out   184
  making in two steps   73
  sodium   182
sorghum   145-7
soy
  foods   117, 157
    breast cancer   159
    fermented   158
    nuts   191
    protein health claim   157
    ways to increase whole soy foods   160
spinach, lutein   213
sports drinks   198
stanols see plant sterols
starch/grain   272-3
statin drugs
  and Coenzyme Q 10   230
  and small particles   33
  and soluble fiber   131

steps
  8 for nutritional needs   13
  to heart rate   257
stevia   174
strength training   260
  personal trainer   261
stretching   255, 260
sucralose, splenda   173, 175
sugar alcohol   172
sugar, artificial substitutes   173
sugar, herbal   174
sugars   19, 171
  teaspoons of hidden in foods   171
  tips to use less   175
supplements   211, 229, 232
  not FDA approved   229
sweeteners   168, 171-4
systolic   189-90
  blood pressure   30, 189

T

tables page 223   203, 211, 215, 223-4, 281,
   see also appendix B for list of tables
tahini   123
tea   197, 200-1
  green and coumadin   205
  red, rooibos   201
teecino   200
teff   145-6
tempeh   136, 158, 272
tenderloin   70, 72, 74
testing   5
  assess overall risk   5
  genetic   36
  vitamin D   217
tocotrienols   137-8, 217, 224
tofu   159
trainer, how to choose personal   261
no trans fat   84
trans fats   16, 61, 83, 85
  nurses' health study   84
  ruminant   83
  safe amount   84
triglycerides   30, 45
  and alcohol   201
  and fish oil   103
  and HFCS   169
  lower, how to   45
    vitamin D   43
troll caught tuna   65, 97
trout   101
True lemon and lime   197
Truvia   174
tuna   111
  ahi, yellowfin   96
  albacore   46, 65, 92, 96-7, 100, 111, 279
  low mercury   65
types of fat diagram   57
type 2 diabetes   177

U

ubiquinone   230
UL vitamin and minerals   223-226
USP   212

V

VAP test   32
vegetable serving   272
  tips to eat more   351-3 see also recipe
index   351
venison   67
vegetable, cruciferous list   353

vinegar
  and glycemic index   167
  test vitamins dissolve   212
vitamin
  see tables page 223
  B vitamins   214
  C food sources   215
  D3   215-6
    blood test   217
  E   217
    food source vitamin E, table   218
  K-content of foods   207-209
  K, amount per meal   204
Vitamin mineral supplements   183, 211
  how to take   213
  what to look for   212
VLDL   23, 29

W

waist circumference (WC)   28, 265
waist measurement   42
walking   253
  steps per mile   253
walnuts   113, 117, 119-20, 125, 136
warfarin, see also vitamin K   203
  amount vitamin K per meal   204
  fish oil   205
  juices   204
  tips for taking
water   197-8
  softener   185, 198
  bottled   197
watermelon   135, 165, 208, 215
Web sites, see appendix A
weight   14, 18, 20, 27, 33, 143-4, 150,
    177- 8, 183, 259, 263-4, 266-7, 277
  BMI   263
  calories to maintain   266
  food journal   267
  lifestyle changes to cut calories   269
  serving size 1500-1700 calorie   276
  why you may not lose   270
wheat   144, 146-7, 164-5, 272
  germ   145
whole grain   143
  gluten free   145
  tips for adding   148
  whole intact grains   146
  whole grain ground into flour   147
  whole grains, not whole   147
wholesome sweeteners (Zero)   173
whole wheat flour   319
wild salmon   99
wine, red   50-1, 201
women
  AHA guidelines   27
  HDL   30
  LDL-P   31
  LP(a)   34
  pattern B   33
  triglycerides   29
  visceral fat   43

Y

yeast, red   232-3

Further Reading and Resources

1. _____ "Dietary Reference Intakes for Energy, Carbohydrate, Fiber, Fat, Fatty Acids, Cholesterol, Protein, and Amino Acids." *National Academy Press.* www.nap.edu/openbook.php?isbn=0309085373.

2. _____ "ATP III Guidelines At-A-Glance Quick Desk Reference." www.nhlbi.nih.gov/guidelines/cholesterol/atglance.pdf.

3. Wu X., et al. "Lipophilic and Hydrophilic Antioxidant Capacities of Common Foods in the United States." *Journal of Agricultural and Food Chemistry* 52 (2004): 4026-4037.

4. Gaziano, J. M., et al. "A Prospective Study of Consumption of Carotenoids in Fruits and Vegetables and Decreased Cardiovascular Mortality in the Elderly." *Annals of Epidemiology* 5 (1995): 255-260.

5. Bansal, S., et al. "Fasting Compared With Nonfasting Triglycerides and Risk of Cardiovascular Events in Women." *Journal of the American Medical Association* 298 (2007): 309-316.

6. Jenkins, David J. A., et al. "Effects of a Dietary Portfolio of Cholesterol-Lowering Foods vs Lovastatin on Serum Lipids and C-Reactive Protein." *Journal of the American Medical Association* 290 (2003): 502-510.

7. Ostlund, Richard E., Jr., et al. "Inhibition of Cholesterol Absorption by Phytosterol-Replete Wheat Germ Compared with Phytosterol-Depleted Wheat Germ." *American Journal Clinical Nutrition* 77 (2003): 1385-1389.

8. Nigris, F. "Pomegranate Juice May Clear Clogged Arteries." *Proceedings of the National Academy of Sciences* 102 (2005): 4896-4901.

9. Grundy, Scott M., et al. "Primary Prevention of Coronary Heart Disease: Guidance from Framingham. A Statement for Healthcare Professionals from the AHA Task Force on Risk Reduction." *Circulation* 97 (1998): 1876-1887.

10. Gardner, C. D., et al. "Association of Small Low-Density Lipoprotein Particles with the Incidence of Coronary Artery Disease in Men and Women." *Journal of the American Medical Association* 276 (1996): 875-881.

11. Cromwell, W. C., et al. "LDL Particle Number and Risk of Future Cardiovascular Disease in the Framingham Offspring Study - Implications for LDL Management." *Journal of Clinical Lipidology* 1 (2007): 583-592.

12. Bostom, A. G., et al. "A Prospective Investigation of Elevated Lipoprotein(a) Detected by Electrophoresis and Cardiovascular Disease in Women. The Framingham Heart Study." *Circulation* 90 (1994): 1688–1695.

13. Davakis, E., et al. "Whole Flaxseed Consumption Lowers Serum LDL-Cholesterol and Lipoprotein(a) Concentrations in Postmenopausal Women." *Nutrition Research* 18 (1998): 1203-1214.

14. Davies, Michael J., et al. "Black Tea Consumption Reduces Total and LDL Cholesterol in Mildly Hypercholesterolemic Adults." *Journal of Nutrition* 133 (2003): 3298S-3302S.

15. Jenkins, David J. A., et al. "Effect of a Diet High in Vegetables, Fruit, and Nuts on Serum Lipids." *Metabolism* 46 (1997): 530-537.

16. Jenkins, David J. A., et al. "Dose Response of Almonds on Coronary Heart Disease Risk Factors: Blood Lipids, Oxidized Low-Density Lipoproteins, Lipoprotein(a), Homocysteine, and Pulmonary Nitric Oxide: A Randomized, Controlled, Crossover Trial." *Circulation* 106 (2002): 1327.

17. Derosa, G., et al. "The effect of L-carnitine on Plasma Lipoprotein(a) Levels in Hypercholesterolemic Patients with Type 2 Diabetes Mellitus." *Clinical Therapeutics* 25 (2003): 1429-1439.

18. Bravata, Dawn M., et al. "Association Between Impaired Insulin Sensitivity and Stroke." *Neuroepidemiology* 25 (2005): 69-74.

19. _____ "The Effect of Metformin and Intensive Lifestyle Intervention on the Metabolic Syndrome: The Diabetes Prevention Program Randomized Trial." *Annals of Internal Medicine* 142 (2005): 611-619.

20. Duncan, G. E., et al. "Exercise Training, without Weight Loss, Increases Insulin Sensitivity and Postheparin Plasma Lipase Activity in Previously Sedentary Adults." *Diabetes Care* 26 (2003): 57-62.

21. Slentz, C. A., et al. "Effects of the Amount of Exercise on Body Weight, Body Composition, and Measures of Central Obesity: STR-RIDE-a Randomized Controlled Study." *Archives of Internal Medicine* 164 (2004): 31-39.

22. Brown, V. W. "Effects of Lifestyle Interventions on High-Density Lipoprotein Cholesterol Levels." *Journal of Clinical Lipidology* 1 (2007): 7-19.

23. Vollmer, W. M., et al. "Effects of Diet and Sodium Intake on Blood Pressure: Subgroup Analysis of the DASH-Sodium Trial." *New England Journal of Medicine* 344 (2001): 3-10.

24. de Lorgeril, M., et al. "Mediterranean Diet, Traditional Risk Factors, and the Rate of Cardiovascular Complications after Myocardial Infarction: Final Report of the Lyon Diet Heart Study." *Circulation* 99 (1999): 779–785.

25. Jenkins, David J. A., et al. "Effects of a Dietary Portfolio of Cholesterol-Lowering Foods vs Lovastatin on Serum Lipids and C-Reactive Protein." *Journal of the American Medical Association* 290 (2003): 502-510.

26. Jenkins David J. A., et al. "Direct Comparison of a Dietary Portfolio of Cholesterol-Lowering Foods with a Statin in Hypercholesterolemic Participants." *American Journal Clinical Nutrition* 81 (2005): 380-387.

27. Djoussé, L., et al. "Fruit and Vegetable Consumption and LDL Cholesterol: the National Heart, Lung, and Blood Institute Family Heart Study." *American Journal of Clinical Nutrition* 79 (2004): 213-217.

28. Franco, Oscar H., et al. "The Polymeal: a More Natural, Safer, And Probably Tastier (than the Polypill) Strategy to Reduce Cardiovascular Disease by more than 75%." *British Medical Journal* 329 (2004): 1447-1450.

29. Yusuf, S., et al. "Effect of Potentially Modifiable Risk Factors Associated with Myocardial Infarction in 52 Countries (the INTER-HEART study): Case-Control Study." *The Lancet* 364 (2004): 937-952.

30. Jula, Antti, et al. "Effects of Diet and Simvastatin on Serum Lipids, Insulin, and Antioxidants in Hypercholesterolemic Men. A Randomized Controlled Trial." *Journal of the American Medical Association* 287 (2002): 598-605.

31. _____ "A Randomized Controlled Trial of a Moderate-Fat, Low-Energy Diet Compared with a Low Fat, Low-Energy Diet for Weight Loss in Overweight Adults." *International Journal of Obesity Related Metabolic Disorders* 25 (2001): 1503-1511.

32. Kris-Etherton, Penny M., et al. "AHA Science Advisory. Lyon Diet Heart Study: Benefits of a Mediterranean-style, National Cholesterol Education Program/American Heart Association Step I Dietary Pattern on Cardiovascular Disease." *Circulation* 103 (2001): 1823-1825.

33. Howard, B. V., et al. "Low-Fat Dietary Pattern and Risk of Cardiovascular Disease: the Women's Health Initiative Randomized Controlled Dietary Modification Trial." *Journal of the American Medical Association* 295 (2006): 655–666.

34. McKeown, Nicola M., et al. "Whole-Grain Intake is Favorably Associated with Metabolic Risk Factors for Type 2 Diabetes and Cardiovascular Disease in the Framingham Offspring Study." *American Journal Clinical Nutrition* 76 (2002): 390-398.

35. Appel, Lawrence J., et al. "Effects of Protein, Monounsaturated Fat, and Carbohydrate Intake on Blood Pressure and Serum Lipids Results of the OmniHeart Randomized Trial." *Journal of the American Medical Association* 294 (2005): 2455-2464.

36. Hu, Frank B. "Plant-Based Foods and Prevention of Cardiovascular Disease: An Overview." *American Journal Clinical Nutrition* 78 (2003): 544S-551S.

37. Ascherio, Alberto, et al. "Dietary Fat and Risk of Coronary Heart Disease in Men: Cohort Follow Up Study in the United States" *British Medical Journal* 313 (1996): 84-90.

38. Klipstein-Grobusch, K., et al. "Dietary Iron and Risk of Myocardial Infarction in the Rotterdam Study." *American Journal Epidemiology* 149 (1999): 421-428.

39. Ascherio, A., et al. "Dietary Iron Intake and Risk of Coronary Disease Among Men." *Circulation* 89 (1994): 969-974.

40. Mozaffarian, D., et al. "Trans Fatty Acids and Cardiovascular Disease." *New England Journal of Medicine* 354 (2006): 1601-1613.

41. Miller, G. J., et al. "Lipids in Wild Ruminant Animals and Steers." *Journal of Food Quality* 9 (1986): 331-343.

42. Willett, W. C., et al. "Intake of Trans Fatty Acids and Risk of Coronary Heart Disease Among Women." *Lancet* 341 (1993): 581-585.

43. Mensink, R., et al. "Effect of Dietary Trans Fatty Acids on High Density and Low Density Lipoprotein Cholesterol Levels in Healthy Subjects." *New England Journal of Medicine* 323 (1990): 439-445.

44. Sundram, K., et al. "Stearic Acid-rich Interesterified Tat and Trans-rich Fat Raise the LDL/HDL Ratio and Plasma Glucose Relative to Palm Olein in Humans." *Nutrition and Metabolism* 4 (2007): 3.

45. De Oliveira e Silva, Elizabeth R., et al. "Effects of Shrimp Consumption on Plasma Lipoproteins." *American Journal Clinical Nutrition* 64 (1996): 712-717.

46. Hu, Frank B., et al. "A Prospective Study of Egg Consumption and Risk of Cardiovascular Disease in Men and Women." *Journal of American Medical Association* 281 (1999): 1387-1394.

47. Fernandez, M. L. "Dietary Cholesterol Provided by Eggs and Plasma Lipoproteins in Healthy Populations." *Current Opinion in Clinical Nutrition and Metabolic Care* 9 (2006): 8-12.

48. Seierstad, S. L., et al. "Dietary Intake of Differently Fed Salmon; the Influence on Markers of Human Atherosclerosis." *European Journal of Clinical Investigation* 35 (2005): 52-59.

49. Bell, J. G., et al. "Altered fatty Acid Compositions in Atlantic Salmon (Salmo Salar) Fed Diets Containing Linseed and Rapeseed Oils can be Partially Restored by a Subsequent Fish Oil Finishing Diet." *Journal of Nutrition* 133 (2003): 2793-2801.

50. Kris-Etherton, Penny M., et al. "Fish Consumption, Fish Oil, Omega-3 Fatty Acids, and Cardiovascular Disease." *Circulation* 106 (2002): 2747.

51. Mortensen A., et al. "Comparison of the Effects of Fish Oil and Olive Oil on Blood Lipids and Aortic Atherosclerosis in Watanabe Heritable Hyperlipidaemic Rabbits." *British Journal of Nutrition* 80 (1998): 565-573.

52. Melanson, S. F. "Mercury Levels in Fish Oil Capsules." *Archives of Pathology and Laboratory Medicine* 129 (2005): 74-77.

53. Metcalf, R. G., et al. "Effects of Fish-Oil Supplementation on Myocardial Fatty Acids in Humans." *American Journal Clinical Nutrition* 85 (2007): 1222-1228.

54. Harris, W. S. "Fish Oils and Plasma Lipid and Lipoprotein Metabolism in Humans: A Critical Review." *Journal of Lipid Research* 30 (1989): 785-807.

55. Marcovina, Santica M., et al. "The Lugalawa Study. Fish Intake, Independent of Apo(a) Size, Accounts for Lower Plasma Lipoprotein(a) Levels in Bantu Fishermen of Tanzania." *Arteriosclerosis, Thrombosis, and Vascular Biology* 19 (1999): 1250-1256.

56. Gruppo Italiano per lo Studio della Sopravvivenza nell'Infsrto Miocardico. "Dietary Supplementation with n-3 Polyunsaturated Fatty Acids and Vitamin E after Myocardial Infarction: Results of the GISSI-Prevenzione Trial." *Lancet* 354 (1999): 447–455.

57. Burr, M. L., et al. "Effects of Changes in Fat, Fish, and Fibre Intakes on Death and Reinfarction: Diet And Reinfarction Trial (DART)." *Lancet* 2 (1989): 757-761.

58. Morris, M. C., et al. "Does Fish Oil Lower Blood Pressure? A Meta-Analysis of Controlled Trials." *Circulation* 88 (1993): 523–533.

59. Wang, C., et al. "n-3 Fatty Acids from Fish or Fish-oil Supplements, but not Alpha-Linolenic Acid, Benefit Cardiovascular Disease Outcomes in Primary- and Secondary-Prevention Studies: a Systematic Review." *American Journal Clinical Nutrition* 84 (2006): 5-17.

60. Zhao G., et al. "Dietary alpha-linolenic Acid Reduces Inflammatory and Lipid Cardiovascular Risk Factors in Hypercholesterolemic Men and Women. *Journal of Nutrition* 134 (2004): 2991-2997.

61. Jiang, Rui, et al. "Nut and Seed Consumption and Inflammatory Markers in the Multi-Ethnic Study of Atherosclerosis." *American Journal of Epidemiology* 163 (2006): 222-231.

62. Kris-Etherton, P. M., et al. "Nuts and their Bioactive Constituents: Effects on Serum Lipids and Other Factors That Affect Disease Risk." *American Journal Clinical Nutrition* 70 (1999): 504S-511S.

63. Sabaté, Joan. "Nut Consumption and Body Weight." *American Journal Clinical Nutrition* 78 (2003): 647S-650S.

64. Jenkins, David J. A., et al. "Viscous Fibers, Health Claims, and Strategies to Reduce Cardiovascular Disease Risk." *American Journal Clinical Nutrition* 71 (2000): 401-402.

65. Olson, Beth H., et al. "Psyllium-Enriched Cereals Lower Blood Total Cholesterol and LDL Cholesterol, but Not HDL Cholesterol, in Hypercholesterolemic Adults: Results of a Meta-Analysis." *The Journal of Nutrition* 127 (1997): 1973-1980.

66. Moreyra, Abel E., et al. "Effect of Combining Psyllium Fiber with Simvastatin in Lowering Cholesterol." *Archives of Internal Medicine* 165 (2005): 1161-1166.

67. Behall, K. M., et al. "Diets Containing Barley Significantly Reduce Lipids in Mildly Hypercholesterolemic Men and Women." *American Journal Clinical Nutrition* 80 (2004): 1185-1193.

68. Anderson, J. W., et al. "Hypocholesterolemic Effects of Oat-Bran or Bean Intake for Hypercholesterolemic Men." *American Journal Clinical Nutrition* 40 (1984): 1146-1155.

69. Kirby, R. W., et al. "Oat-Bran Intake Selectively Lowers Serum Low-Density Lipoprotein Cholesterol Concentrations of Hypercholesterolemic Men." *Journal of Clinical Nutrition* 34 (1981): 824-829..

70. Winham, Donna M., et al. "Pinto Bean Consumption Reduces Biomarkers for Heart Disease Risk." *Journal of the American College of Nutrition* 26 (2007): 243-249.

70. Cassidy, A., et al. "Factors Affecting the Bioavailability of Soy Isoflavones in Humans after Ingestion of Physiologically Relevant Levels from Different Soy Foods." *Journal of Nutrition* 136 (2006): 45-51.

71. Anderson, J. W., et al. "Meta-Analysis of the Effects of Soy Protein Intake on Serum Lipids." *New England Journal of Medicine* 333 (1995): 276–282.

72. Sacks, F. M., et al. "Soy Protein, Isoflavones, and Cardiovascular Health. An American Heart Association Science Advisory for Professionals from the Nutrition Committee." *Circulation* 113 (2006): 1034-1044.

73. Frost, G., et al. "The Relevance of the Glycaemic Index to our Understanding of Dietary Carbohydrates" *Diabetic Medicine* 17 (2000): 336–345.

74. Liu, S., et al. "A Prospective Study of Dietary Glycemic Load, Carbohydrate Intake, and Risk of Coronary Heart Disease in US Women." *American Journal Clinical Nutrition* 71 (2000): 1455–1461.

75. Ceriello, A., et al. "Meal-Induced Oxidative Stress and Low-Density Lipoprotein Oxidation in Diabetes: The Possible Role of Hyperglycemia." *Metabolism* 48 (1999): 1503–1508.

76. Cavin, J. "Pathophysiologic Mechanisms of Postprandial Hyperglycemia." *American Journal of Cardiology* 88 (2001): 4–8.

77. Basciano, H., et al. "Fructose, Insulin Resistance, and Metabolic Dyslipidemia." *Nutrition and Metabolism* 2 (2005): 1-14.

78. Swanson , J. E., et al. "Metabolic Effects of Dietary Fructose in Healthy Subjects." *American Journal Clinical Nutrition* 55 (1992): 851-856.

79. Reiser, S., et al. "Blood Lipids and their Distribution in Lipoproteins in Hyperinsulinemic Men Consuming Three Different Levels of Sucrose." *Journal of Nutrition* 111 (1981): 1045-1057.

80. Hollenbeck, C. B. "Dietary Fructose Effects on Lipoprotein Metabolism and Risk for Coronary Artery Disease." *American Journal Clinical Nutrition* 58 (1993): 800S–809S.

81. Reiser S. "Effects of Dietary Sugars in Metabolic Risk Factors Associated with Heart Disease." *Nutrition and Health* 3 (1985): 203–216.

82. Havel, P. J. "Dietary Fructose: Implications for Dysregulation of Energy Homeostasis and Lipid/Carbohydrate Metabolism." *Nutrition Review* 63 (2005):133-157.

83. Wylie-Rosett, J., et al. "Carbohydrates and Increases in Obesity: Does the Type of Carbohydrate Make a Difference?" *Obesity Research* 12 (2004):124S-129S.

84. Bray, George A. "Consumption of High-Fructose Corn Syrup in Beverages May Play a Role in the Epidemic of Obesity." *American Journal Clinical Nutrition* 79 (2004): 537-543.

85. Bantle J. P., et al. "Effects of Dietary Fructose on Plasma Lipids in Healthy Subjects." *American Journal Clinical Nutrition* 72 (2000): 1128–1134.

86. http://www.ers.usda.gov/Data/foodconsumption/FoodAvailSpreadsheets.htm#sweeteners

87. Fleck, F. "WHO Resists Food Industry Pressure on its Diet Plan." *British Medical Journal* 328 (2004): 973.

88. Davidson, T., et al. "A Pavlovian Approach to the Problem of Obesity." *International Journal of Obesity* 28 (2004): 933-935.

89. Sacks, F. M., et al. "Effects on Blood Pressure of Reduced Dietary Sodium and the Dietary Approaches to Stop Hypertension (DASH) Diet." *New England Journal of Medicine* 344 (2001): 3-10.

90. _____ "Dietary Reference Intakes: Water, Potassium, Sodium, Chloride, and Sulfate." National Academies Press, 2004

91. Havas, S., et al. "The Urgent Need to Reduce Sodium Consumption." *Journal of the American Medical Association* 298 (2007): 1439-1441.

92. Welty, F. K., et al. "Effect of Soy Nuts on Blood Pressure and Lipid Levels in Hypertensive, Prehypertensive, and Normotensive Postmenopausal Women" *Archives of Internal Medicine* 167 (2007): 1060-1067.

93. Blais, C. A., et al. "Effect of Dietary Sodium Restriction on Taste Responses to Sodium Chloride: A Longitudinal Study." *American Journal Clinical Nutrition* 44 (1986): 232-243.

94. Whelton, P. K., et al. "Magnesium and Blood Pressure: Review of the Epidemiologic and Clinical Trial Experience." *American Journal of Cardiology* 63 (1989): 26G-30G.

95. Patki, P. S., et al. "Efficacy of Potassium and Magnesium in Essential Hypertension: A Double Blind, Placebo Controlled, Crossover Study." *British Medical Journal* 301 (1990): 521–523.

96. Rissanen, T., et al. "Fish Oil-Derived Fatty Acids, Docosahexaenoic Acid and Docosapentaenoic Acid, and the Risk of Acute Coronary Events: The Kuopio Ischaemic Heart Disease Risk Factor Study." *Circulation* 102 (2000): 2677-2679.

97. Mori, T. A., et al. "Docosahexaenoic Acid but not Eicosapentaenoic Acid Lowers Ambulatory Blood Pressure and Heart Rate in Humans." *Hypertension* 34 (1999): 253-260.

98. Van Dusseldorp, M., et al. "Cholesterol-Raising Factor from Boiled Coffee Does Not Pass a Paper Filter." *Arteriosclerosis and Thrombosis* 11 (1991): 586-593.

99. Mukamal, K. J., et al. "Alcohol consumption and Risk for Coronary Heart Disease in Men with Healthy Lifestyles." *Archives of Internal Medicine* 166 (2006): 2145-2150.

100. Szmitko, P. E., et al. "Red Wine and Your Heart." *Circulation* 106 (2002): 1465-1469.

101. Greenblatt, D. J. "Cranberry Juice and Warfarin: Is There An Interaction?" *Anticoagulation Forum Newsletter* 10 (2006): 3.

102. Fairfield, K. M., et al. "Vitamins for Chronic Disease Prevention In Adults: Scientific Review." *Journal of the American Medical Association* 287 (2002): 3116-3126.

103. Dwyer, J., et al. Estimation of Usual Intakes: What We Eat in America." *The Journal of Nutrition* 133 (2003): 609S-623S.

104. Richer, S., et al. "Double-Masked, Placebo-Controlled, Randomized Trial of Lutein and Antioxidant Supplementation in the Intervention of Atrophic Age-Related Macular Degeneration: The Veterans LAST Study (Lutein Antioxidant Supplement Trial)." *Optometry* 4 (2004): 216-230.

105. _____ "Dietary Reference Intakes for Thiamin, Riboflavin, Niacin, Vitamin B6, Folate, Vitamin B12, Pantothenic Acid, Biotin, and Choline" National Academy Press. http://books.nap.edu/openbook.php?isbn=0309065542.

106. Vieth, R., et al. "Vitamin D in Congestive Heart Failure." *American Journal Clinical Nutrition* 83 (2006): 731-732.

107. Wang, T., et al. "Vitamin D Deficiency and Risk of Cardiovascular Disease." *Circulation* 117 (2008): 503-511.

108. Carter, N. B. "Plant Stanol Ester: Review of Cholesterol Lowering Efficacy and Implications for Coronary Heart Disease Risk Reduction." *Preventive Cardiology* 3 (2000): 121-130.

109. Miettinen, T. A., et al. "Plant Sterols in Serum and in Atherosclerotic Plaques of Patients Undergoing Carotid Endarterectomy." *The Journal of American College of Cardiology* 45 (2005): 1794-1801.

110. Weingartner, Oliver, et al. "Vascular Effects of Diet Supplementation with Plant Sterols." *Journal of the American College of Cardiology* 51 (2008): 1553-1561.

111. Khan, A., et al. "Cinnamon Improves Glucose and Lipids of People With Type 2 Diabetes." *Diabetes Care* 26 (2003): 3215-3218.

112. Gardner, C. D., et al. "Effect of Raw Garlic vs Commercial Garlic Supplements on Plasma Lipid Concentrations in Adults with Moderate Hypercholesterolemia." *Archives of Internal Medicine* 167 (2007): 346-353.

113. Singh, R. B., et al. "Effect of Coenzyme Q10 on Risk of Atherosclerosis in Patients with Recent Myocardial Infarction." *Molecular and Cellular Biochemistry* 246 (2003): 75-82.

114. Berman, M., et al. "Coenzyme Q10 in Patients with End-Stage Heart Failure Awaiting Cardiac Transplantation: A Randomized, Placebo-Controlled Study." *Clinical Cardiology* 27 (2004): 295-299.

115. Mortensen, S. A., et al. "Dose-Related Decrease of Serum Coenzyme Q10 during Treatment with HMG-CoA-reductase Inhibitors." *Molecular Aspects of Medicine* 18 (1997): S137-S144.

116. Ghirlanda, G., et al. "Evidence of Plasma CoQ10-Lowering Effect by HMG-CoA Reductase Inhibitors: A Double-Blind, Placebo-Controlled Study." *Journal of Clinical Pharmacology* 33 (1993): 226-229.

117. Strey, C. H., et al. "Endothelium-ameliorating Effects of Statin Therapy and Coenzyme Q10 Reductions in Chronic Heart Failure." *Atherosclerosis* 179 (2005): 201-206.

118. Singh, R. B., et al. "Effect on Absorption and Oxidative Stress of Different Oral Coenzyme Q10 Dosages and Intake Strategy in Healthy Men." *Biofactors* 25 (2006): 219-224.

119. Lonn, E., et al. "Effects of Long-term Vitamin E Supplementation on Cardiovascular Events and Cancer: A Randomized Controlled Trial The HOPE and HOPE-TOO Trial Investigators." *Journal of the American Medical Association* 293 (2005): 1338-1347.

120. Szapary, P. O., et al. "Guggulipid for the Treatment of Hypercholesterolemia: A Randomized Controlled Trial." *Journal of the American Medical Association* 290 (2003): 765-772.

121. Heiner, K., et al. "Effect of Policosanol on Lipid Levels Among Patients with Hypercholesterolemia or Combined Hyperlipidemia: A Randomized Controlled Trial." *Journal of the American Medical Association* 295 (2006): 2262-2269.

122. Heber, D., et al. "An Analysis of Nine Proprietary Chinese Red Yeast Rice Dietary Supplements Implications of Variability in Chemical Profile and Contents." *The Journal of Alternative and Complementary Medicine* 7 (2001): 133-139.

123. Zhao, Xue-Qiao, et al. "Safety and Tolerability of Simvastatin Plus Niacin in Patients with Coronary Artery Disease and Low High-Density Lipoprotein Cholesterol (The HDL Atherosclerosis Treatment Study)." *The American Journal of Cardiology* 93 (2004): 307-312.

124. Birjmohun, R. S., et al. "Efficacy and Safety of High-Density Lipoprotein Cholesterol-increasing Compounds: A Meta-Analysis of Randomized Controlled Trials" *Journal of the American College of Cardiology* 45 (2005): 185-197.

125. Meyers, C. D., et al. "Varying Cost and Free Nicotinic Acid Content in Over-the-Counter Niacin Preparations for Dyslipidemia." *Annals of Internal Medicine* 139 (2003): 996-1002.

126. Knopp, R. H., et al. "Equivalent Efficacy of a Time-Release Form of Niacin (Niaspan) given once-a-night versus Plain Niacin in the Management of Hyperlipidemia" *Metabolism* 47 (1998): 1097-1104.

127. Cheung, M. C., et al. "Antioxidant Supplements Block the Response of HDL to Simvastatin-Niacin Therapy in Patients with Coronary Artery Disease and Low HDL." *Arteriosclerosis, Thrombosis and Vascular Biology* 21 (2001): 1320.

128. Pate, R. R., et al. "Physical Activity and Public Health. A recommendation from the Centers for Disease Control and Prevention and the American College of Sports Medicine." *Journal of the American Medical Association* 273 (1995): 402-407.

129. Physical Activity and Health: A report of the Surgeon General. U.S. Department of Health and Human Services, Centers for Disease Control and Prevention. (1999) http://www.cdc.gov/nccdphp/sgr/sgr.htm.

130. Podewils, L. J., et al. "Physical Activity, APO E Genotype, and Dementia Risk: Findings from the Cardiovascular Health Cognition Study." *American Journal of Epidemiology* 161 (2005): 639-651.

131. Fletcher, G. F., et al. "Exercise Standards for Testing and Training: A Statement for Healthcare Professionals from the American Heart Association" *Circulation* 104 (2001): 1694-1740.

132. Whaley, M. *ACSM Guidelines for Exercise Testing and Prescription, 7th Edition*, Lippincott Williams and Wilkins. Philadelphia, 2006.

133. La Forge, R. "Cardiorespiratory Fitness." *ACE Personal Trainer Manual*. 3rd Edition, 2003.

134. Bassett, D.R., et al. "Physical activity in an Old Order Amish community." *Medicine and Science in Sports and Exercise* 36 (2004): 79–85.

135. Colditz, G. A., et al. "Weight, Weight Gain, Activity, and Major Illnesses: The Nurses' Health Study" *International Journal Sports Medicine* 18 (1997): S162-S170.

136. Ogden, C. L., et al. "Prevalence of Overweight and Obesity in the United States 1999-2004." *Journal of the American Medical Association* 295 (2006): 1549-1555.

137. _____ "Dietary Reference Intakes for Energy, Carbohydrate, Fiber, Fat, Fatty Acids, Cholesterol, Protein, and Amino Acids." National Academies Press http://books.nap.edu/openbook.php?record_id=10490&page=936.

138. James, W. P. T., et al. *Human Energy Requirements: A Manual for Planners and Nutritionists.* Oxford Medical Publications, 1990.

139. Kragelund, C. "A Farewell to Body-Mass Index." *Lancet* 366 (2005): 1589-1591.

140. Jansen, Ian, et al. "Waist circumference and health risk." *American Journal Clinical Nutrition* 79 (2004): 379-384.

141. Dalton, M., et al. "Waist Circumference, Waist-Hip Ratio and Body Mass Index and their Correlation with Cardiovascular Disease Risk Factors in Australian Adults." *Journal of Internal Medicine* 254 (2003): 555-563.

142. McArdle, William D., et al. "Essentials of Exercise Physiology." Lippincott. 2005.

143. Dansinger, Michael L., et al. "Comparison of the Atkins, Ornish, Weight Watchers, and Zone Diets for Weight Loss and Heart Disease Risk Reduction." *Journal of the American Medical Association* 293 (2005): 43-53.

144. Kragelund, C., et al. "Impact of Obesity on Long-term Prognosis Following Acute Myocardial Infarct." *International Journal of Cardiology* 98 (2005): 123-131.

145. Frankenfield, D. C., et al. "Validation of Several Established Equations for Resting Metabolic Rate in Obese and Non-Obese People." *Journal of the American Dietetic Association* 103 (2003): 1152-1159.

146. Gunther, C. W., et al. "Dairy Products Do Not Lead to Alteration in Body Weight or Fat Mass in Young Women in a 1-Year Intervention." *American Journal Clinical Nutrition* 81 (2005): 751–756.

147. Wing, R. R., et al. "Long Term Weight Loss Maintenance." *American Journal of Clinical Nutrition* 82 (2005): 222S-225S.

148. Tudor-Locke, C., et al. *The Art and Science of Step Counting.* Trafford Publishing, Victoria Canada. 2003.

149. Yusuf, S., et al. "Obesity and the Risk of Myocardial Infarction in 27,000 Participants from 52 Countries: A Case–Control Study." *Lancet* 366 (2005): 1640-1649.

150. French, M. A., et al. "Cholesterolaemic Effect of Palmitic Acid in Relation to other Dietary Fatty Acids." *Asia Pacific Journal Clinical Nutrition* 11 (2002): S401–S407.

151. Schulman, S. P., et al. "L-Arginine therapy in acute myocardial infarction. The Vascular Interaction with Age in Myocardial Infarction (Vintage MI) Randomized Clinical Trial." *Journal of The American Medical Association* 295 (2006): 58-64.

152. Doutreleau, S., et al. "Chronic L-Arginine Supplementation Enhances Endurance Exercise Tolerance in Heart Failure Patients." *International Journal of Sports Medicine* 27 (2006): 567-572.

153. Gaddi, A., et al. "Controlled Evaluation of pantethine, a Natural Hypolipidemic Compound, in Patients with Different Forms of Hyperlipoproteinemia." *Atherosclerosis* 50 (1984): 73-83.

Appendix A: Web Sites

www.bhlinc.com - Berkeley HeartLab proprietary LDL and HDL tests

www.liposcience.com - NMR LipoProfile test, direct measure of LDL particles

www.thevaptest.com -Test that directly measures LDL and other components

www.trackyourplaque.com - Program designed around heart scan calcium score

www.alderspring.com – Grass-fed organic beef

www.texasgrassfedbeef.com – Grass-fed beef

www.eatwellguide.org - Source for sustainably raised meat, poultry

www.wildgame.com – Game-raised, free-range animals

www.nal.usda.gov/fnic/foodcomp/search - Nutrition database

www.vitalchoice.com - Wild Alaskan salmon and great newsletter with recipes

www.gotmercury.org - Mercury calculator to help make healthy seafood choices

www.marylouseafoods.com/marketplace - Troll caught, low-mercury albacore tuna

www.papageorge.com - Troll caught low mercury albacore tuna

www.nutru.com, www.water4net, www.devanutrition.com – Algae-based omega-3

www.consumerlab.com - Independently tests and evaluates nutritional supplements

www.flaxcouncil.ca, www.flaxrd.com - Source for flax recipes and ideas

www.nuthealth.org - International tree nut council

www.futtersnutbutters.com - Nut butters from many different nuts and seeds

www.kingarthurflour.com – Waxy, hulless variety of barley Prowashonupana, high in soluble fiber

www.montina.com - Indian rice grass

www.glutenfreemall.com – Gluten-free grains

www.bobsredmill.com, www.naturespath.com, www.hodgsonmill.com, - Source for whole-grain foods

www.penzeys.com – Source for many no salt added spices and seasonings

www.beanogas.com - Beano to reduce gas from foods

www.beanflour.com - Bean flour

www.cancerrd.com - good source of information on soy and breast cancer, includes a question-and-answer section, as well as recipes

www.glycemicindex.com, www.mendosa.com - Glycemic index and load

www.sweetsavvy.com - Natural sweeteners including recipes with various sweeteners

www.permaculture.com - Pomona, for making jams without any sweetener

www.healthyheartmarket.com -Low sodium food items

www.pleasoning.com, www.dcdistributors.com – Low-sodium, no potassium seasonings

www.sweetleaf.com - Stevia herbal sweetener

www.alsosalt.com - Salt substitute with potassium but less bitter aftertaste

www.nhlbi.nih.gov/health/public/hbp/dash -DASH diet

www.truelemon.com - Dry lemon and lime powder to add to water

www.teeccino.com - Caffeine free herbal beverage that tastes like coffee

www.strongwomen.com - Strength training program suitable for doing at home

www.accumeasurefitness.com - Body fat calipers

www.mypyramidtracker.gov, www.fitday.com – Web-based food journal

www.healthyweight4life.net - Plan for weight loss, 16-week

Appendix B: Tables

Table 3.1	The Effect Diet And Lifestyle Have On LDL, HDL And Triglycerides	12
Table 4.1	Calories To Maintain Current Weight	14
Table 4.2	Calories If Weight Loss Desired	15
Table 4.3	Saturated Fat Gram Allowance	16
Table 4.4	Adequate Intake For Fiber	17
Table 4.5	Protein - How Much You Need	18
Table 6.1	What Your Numbers Should Be	30
Table 7.1	Find Your 10-Year Risk With Framingham Heart Disease Risk Assessment	37
Table 13.1	Fatty Acids In Various Oils And Fats	59
Table 13.2	The Type Of Fat And The Effect It Has On Your Heart	60
Table 13.3	Choosing Fats	61
Table 15.1	Ground Meat	73
Table 15.2	Beef Choice Cuts	74
Table 15.3	Pork Cuts	74
Table 15.4	Lamb	74
Table 15.5	Veal	74
Table 16.1	Game Meat	78
Table 17.1	Broasted Chicken	80
Table 17.2	Poultry	81
Table 19.1	Amount Of Omega-3 (EPA + DHA) In 3.5 Oz Of Fish	92
Table 20.1	Daily Amounts Of Omega-3 For Healthy Adults	95
Table 20.2	Approximate Ounces Of Fish Per Week To Provide 1,000 mg EPA/DHA	98
Table 21.1	AHA's Recommendations For Omega-3 Fatty Acid Intake (EPA + DHA)	103
Table 21.2	Amount Of EPA/DHA Per Capsule Of Some Brands Of Fish Oil	104
Table 21.3	Seafood Nutrition	109-112
Table 22.1	Omega 3 – ALA (Alpha Linoleic Acid) In Foods	117
Table 23.1	Number Of Nuts And Seeds In 1 Ounce	119
Table 23.2	Nuts And Seeds Nutrition	125
Table 24.1	Soluble Fiber	132-136
Table 28.1	Where Do You Find Protein?	162
Table 32.1	Effect Of Lifestyle Changes On Blood Pressure	191
Table 32.2	Foods Rich In Potassium	193
Table 32.3	Foods Rich In Magnesium	193
Table 34.1	Vitamin K Content Of Foods	207-209
Table 35.1	Food Sources Of Vitamin C	215
Table 35.2	Food Sources Of Vitamin D	216
Table 35.3	Natural Food Sources Of Vitamin E	218-219
Table 35.4	Food Sources Of Selenium	200
Table 35.5	Calcium In Foods	221
Table 35.6	Vitamins (function, upper-level for adults, RDA or AI, food sources)	223-224
Table 35.7	Minerals (function, upper-level for adults, RDA or AI, food sources)	225-226
Table 39.1	Maximum Heart Rate By Age	257
Table 40.1	Adult BMI	264

Appendix C: Tips, Self-Assessments, Sample Menu

Tips

Tips To Make Your Plate Healthier 53

Tips For Eating A Healthy Balance Of Fats 64

Tips For Using Less Solid Fats Such As Butter Or Margarine......................87

Tips To Reduce Mercury And Pollutants When Choosing Fish 96

Tips To Include Flax In Your Daily Diet 116

Tips For Adding Whole Grain To Your Diet...49

Tips To Use Less Sweetener 175

Tips For Less Sodium..184-185

Tips For Taking Warfarin (*Coumadin*) 206

Tips To Reduce Flushing From Niacin 238

Tips For Eating Heart Healthy When Eating Out 244

More Helpful Sections

How To Convert Cholesterol And Glucose Units 24

Ways To Use Nut Butters 123

Four-Month Plan To Start Adding Soluble Fiber To Your Diet 129

Three Steps For Choosing Foods Made From Flour 145

Gluten-Free Whole Grains 145

Whole, Intact Grains 146

Simple Ways To Add Beans And Lentils 152

Ways To Increase Whole Soy Foods In Your Diet 160

Better Carbohydrate Choices 164

How To Use Glycemic Index (GI) And Glycemic Load (GL) 167

Lifestyle Changes That May Lower Your Blood Pressure...........................190

Bottom Line To Control Blood Pressure 195

Dining To Reduce Sodium 249

Simple Lifestyle Changes To Cut Calories..269

What Is A Serving?..272

Self-Assessments

How Smart 4 Your Heart Is Your Lifestyle?...7

Self Assessment For Metabolic Syndrome 41

Self-Assessment of Physical Activity Part 1 252

Self-Assessment of Physical Activity Part 2 255

Sample Menu

Portfolio Diet Sample Meal Plan (1,500 Calories) 56

Sample Menu With 20 Grams Soluble Fiber 130

Sample Heart Healthy Diabetic Menu 180

7-Day Menu Plan (No Wheat or Refined Grains) 294

7-Day Menu Plan (With Whole Grains) 296

MEASURE EQUIVALENTS

3 teaspoons = 1 tablespoon
4 tablespoons = 1/4 cup
16 tablespoons = 1 cup

1/3 cup = 5 tablespoons +1 teaspoon
1/2 cup = 8 tablespoons
3/4 cup = 12 tablespoons

1 cup = 8 fluid ounces
3/4 cup = 6 fluid ounces
1/2 cup = 4 fluid ounces
2 tablespoons = 1 fluid ounce

1 pint = 2 cups
1 quart = 2 pints
1 quart = 4 cups
1 gallon = 4 quarts
1 gallon = 16 cups

1 teaspoon = 5 milliliters
1 tablespoon = 15 milliliters
1 cup = 240 milliliters

1 quart = 1 liter
1 ounce = 28 grams
1 pound = 454 grams

Fluid ounces multiply by 29.57 to get grams
Ounces, dry multiply by 28.35 to get grams
Pounds multiply by 453.6 to get grams
Quarts multiply by 0.946 to get liters

NOTES

NOTES

Smart 4 Your Heart